Dilemmas in ERCP

Daniel K. Mullady
Editor

Dilemmas in ERCP

A Clinical Casebook

Springer

Editor
Daniel K. Mullady
Division of Gastroenterology
Washington University in St.
Louis School of Medicine
St. Louis, MO
USA

Additional material to this book can be downloaded from https://link.springer.com/book/10.1007/978-3-030-12741-1.

ISBN 978-3-030-12740-4 ISBN 978-3-030-12741-1 (eBook)
https://doi.org/10.1007/978-3-030-12741-1

This Springer imprint is published by the registered company Springer Nature Switzerland AG
The registered company address is: Gewerbestrasse 11, 6330 Cham, Switzerland

Preface

Welcome to *Dilemmas in ERCP: A Clinical Casebook.* Given its invasiveness, multitude of possible interventions, and potential complications, it is not uncommon to face a dilemma (i.e., a problem involving a difficult choice) when performing ERCP.

The subjects covered in this book are challenging scenarios in ERCP. When encountering these during ERCP, one is not always faced with a dilemma per se. However, through the presentation of clinical situations through case-based format, the authors have highlighted difficult management decisions encountered when performing ERCP. In sharing their personal cases, the authors demonstrate how to approach dilemmas and optimize efficacy and safety through a thoughtful, experience-based, and evidence-based approach. The cases serve as a basis for concise discussion followed by summary "take-home" bullet points and list of references. This book is meant to be high yield and clinically relevant to the practice of modern, therapeutic ERCP. I hope that this is an interesting read and helpful to your clinical practice.

The authors include former advanced endoscopy fellows at Washington University in St. Louis who I have had the privilege of helping to train, current colleagues within the Interventional Endoscopy Section at Washington University in St. Louis, and colleagues from peer institutions who I have had the opportunity to work with during training, on committees, or on research projects. I am immensely grateful to all of them for contributing their time and expertise to this book. They are an extremely accomplished and excellent group of physicians, and I am humbled to call them colleagues.

St. Louis, MO, USA Daniel K. Mullady

Contents

Contributors

A. Aziz Aadam Assistant Professor of Medicine, Division of Gastroenterology, Northwestern Memorial Hospital, Chicago, IL, USA

Leen H. Al-Sayyed Transplant Hepatologist, Saint Luke's Hospital of Kansas City, Kansas City, MO, USA

Osama Altayar Gastroenterology Fellow, Division of Gastroenterology, Washington University School of Medicine, St. Louis, MO, USA

Motaz H. Ashkar Gastroenterology Fellow, Division of Gastroenterology, Washington University in St. Louis, School of Medicine, St. Louis, MO, USA

Jason G. Bill Advanced Endoscopy Fellow, Division of Gastroenterology, Washington University School of Medicine in St. Louis, St. Louis, MO, USA

Christopher G. Chapman Assistant Professor of Medicine, University of Chicago Medicine, Center for Endoscopic Research and Therapeutics (CERT), Chicago, IL, USA

Antonio R. Cheesman Gastroenterology Fellow, Division of Gastroenterology, Icahn School of Medicine at Mount Sinai, New York, NY, USA

Natalie Cosgrove Assistant Professor of Medicine, Division of Gastroenterology, Washington University in St. Louis, School of Medicine, St. Louis, MO, USA

Koushik Das Assistant Professor of Medicine, Division of Gastroenterology, Washington University School of Medicine, St. Louis, MO, USA

Christopher J. DiMaio Associate Professor of Medicine, Division of Gastroenterology, Icahn School of Medicine at Mount Sinai, New York, NY, USA

Jeffrey J. Easler Assistant Professor of Medicine, Division of Gastroenterology and Hepatology, Indiana University School of Medicine, Indianapolis, IN, USA

Cassandra Fritz Instructor of Medicine, Internal Medicine, Washington University School of Medicine/Barnes Jewish Hospital, Saint Louis, MO, USA

Christopher Fritzen Gastroenterology, Hepatology and Nutrition, Children's Healthcare of Atlanta, Emory University School of Medicine, Atlanta, GA, USA

Larissa Fujii-Lau Gastroenterology, University of Hawaii, Queens Medical Center, Honolulu, HI, USA

Srinivas Gaddam Assistant Professor of Medicine, Division of Digestive and Liver Diseases, Cedars-Sinai Medical Center, Los Angeles, CA, USA

Neil Gupta Associate Professor of Medicine, Department of Gastroenterology, Loyola University Medical Center, Maywood, IL, USA

Stephen Hasak Gastroenterology Fellow, Division of Gastroenterology, Washington University in St. Louis School of Medicine, St. Louis, MO, USA

Sreeni Jonnalagadda Gastroenterology, Saint Luke's Hospital of Kansas City, Kansas City, MO, USA

Jaclyn Kagihara University of Hawaii, Queens Medical Center, Honolulu, HI, USA

Rajesh N. Keswani Associate Professor of Medicine, Division of Gastroenterology, Northwestern Memorial Hospital, Chicago, IL, USA

Jennifer M. Kolb Gastroenterology Fellow, Division of Gastroenterology and Hepatology, University of Colorado Anschutz Medical Center, Aurora, CO, USA

Vladimir M. Kushnir Associate Professor of Medicine, Division of Gastroenterology, Washington University School of Medicine in St. Louis, St. Louis, MO, USA

Richard S. Kwon Associate Professor of Medicine, Division of Gastroenterology, University of Michigan, Ann Arbor, MI, USA

Gabriel D. Lang Assistant Professor of Medicine, Division of Gastroenterology, Washington University in Saint Louis, Saint Louis, MO, USA

Ernesto M. Llano Gastroenterology Fellow, University of Chicago Medicine, Center for Endoscopic Research and Therapeutics (CERT), Chicago, IL, USA

Rizwan Mahmood Gastroenterology Fellow, Department of Gastroenterology, Loyola University Medical Center, Maywood, IL, USA

Michael B. McCabe Gastroenterology Fellow, Division of Gastroenterology and Hepatology, University of Virginia Health System, Charlottesville, VA, USA

Dhairya Mehta Gastroenterology Fellow, University Hospitals Cleveland Medical Center, Gastroenterology and Liver Disease, Cleveland, OH, USA

Fahad Faisal Mir Gastroenterology Fellow, Saint Luke's Hospital of Kansas City, Kansas City, MO, USA

Mayssan Muftah Internal Medicine Resident, Department of Medicine, Emory University School of Medicine, Atlanta, GA, USA

Daniel K. Mullady Professor of Medicine, Division of Gastroenterology, Washington University in St. Louis School of Medicine, St. Louis, MO, USA

Anand Singla Assistant Professor of Medicine, Division of Gastroenterology, University of Washington Medical Center, Seattle, WA, USA

Zachary L. Smith Assistant Professor of Medicine, Division of Gastroenterology and Liver Disease, University Hospitals Digestive Health Institute, Case Western Reserve University School of Medicine, Cleveland, OH, USA

Anna Tavakkoli Assistant Professor of Medicine, Division of Gastroenterology, University of Texas, Southwestern, Dallas, TX, USA

Andrew Y. Wang Associate Professor of Medicine, Division of Gastroenterology and Hepatology, University of Virginia Health System, Charlottesville, VA, USA

Sachin Wani Associate Professor of Medicine, Division of Gastroenterology and Hepatology, University of Colorado Anschutz Medical Center, Aurora, CO, USA

Field F. Willingham Associate Professor of Medicine, Division of Digestive Diseases, Emory University School of Medicine, Atlanta, GA, USA

Department of Gastroenterology, Children's Healthcare of Atlanta, Emory University School of Medicine, Atlanta, GA, USA

Chapter 1 Cholangiogram Interpretation

Stephen Hasak and Daniel K. Mullady

Case Presentation

A 73-year-old female with no significant prior medical history presented with 7 days of progressive abdominal pain, dark urine, nausea, and jaundice. Initial laboratory evaluation revealed a total bilirubin of 9 mg/dl, alkaline phosphatase of 472 U/L, aspartate transaminase of 116 U/L, alanine transaminase of 224 U/L, and white blood cell count of 16.1 K/mm^3. She underwent imaging with magnetic resonance imaging/magnetic resonance cholangiopancreatography (MRI/MRCP) which revealed a 1.5-cm hepatic hilar lesion consistent with at least Bismuth IIIa versus IV cholangiocarcinoma with right and left ductal dilation. The tumor appeared to abut the

S. Hasak · D. K. Mullady (✉)
Division of Gastroenterology, Washington University in St. Louis School of Medicine, St. Louis, MO, USA
e-mail: mulladyd@wustl.edu

D. K. Mullady (ed.), *Dilemmas in ERCP*,
https://doi.org/10.1007/978-3-030-12741-1_1

right hepatic artery, main portal vein, right portal vein, and takeoff of the left portal vein. She underwent ERCP at her local hospital with placement of a plastic biliary stent in the right intrahepatic duct. Brushings for cytology noted atypical glandular epithelial cells consistent with adenocarcinoma.

She was then transferred for surgical evaluation. Despite stent placement her bilirubin increased to 11.9 mg/dl. Her case was discussed in multidisciplinary hepatobiliary conference, and it was decided that extended right hepatectomy may be feasible. For hypertrophy of the left lobe, she was referred for repeat ERCP for removal of the right-sided stent and stenting of left-sided biliary tree, which was still significantly dilated.

Following removal of the previously placed right-sided stent, ERCP was performed with opacification of the main bile duct, hepatic duct bifurcation, right main hepatic duct, and right intrahepatic branches. The left ducts could not be opacified with gentle occlusion cholangiogram. After much effort, the left biliary tree was accessed with a 0.025″ angled wire through a sphincterotome. The left main hepatic duct was shown to contain a single severe stenosis, and a 10 Fr by 10 cm biliary stent with a full external pigtail and a full internal pigtail was placed into the left hepatic duct (Figs. 1.1 and 1.2). She was discharged with follow-up plans to see medical oncology for neoadjuvant chemotherapy and IR-guided portal vein embolization.

The dilemma in this case is localizing pathology to the left or right biliary systems and ideally having multidisciplinary input prior to attempting biliary decompression. Identification of the appropriate sided intrahepatic duct was critical. The patient initially had stenting of the right side, which was the incorrect side of the liver to stent since the patient required a right hepatectomy. Additionally, this intervention did not lead to improvement of bilirubin and led to the need for repeat short-interval ERCP to stent the appropriate side of the liver.

Introduction

ERCP has been performed by gastroenterologists and surgeons for nearly 50 years. Since its inception to the

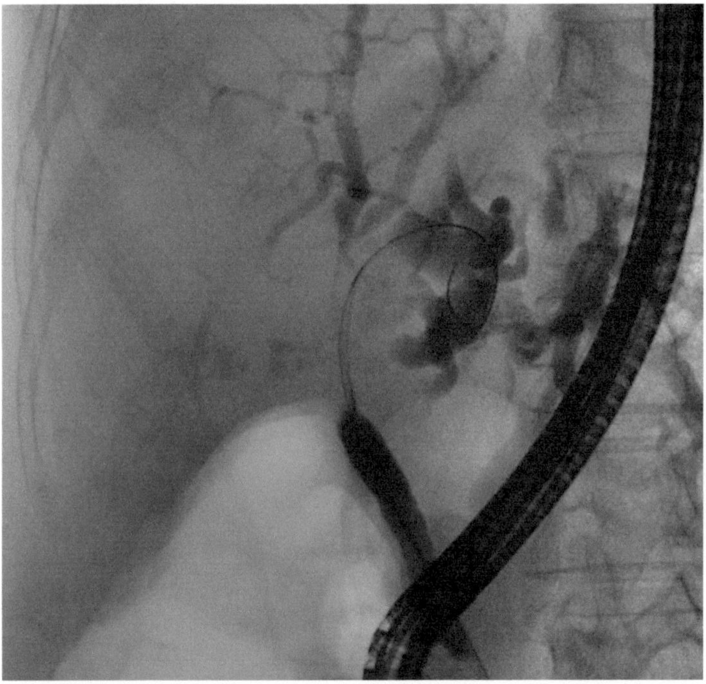

FIGURE 1.1 Opacification and wire access of the left biliary tree and extrahepatic bile duct with severe stricture of the common hepatic and left main ducts

present day, there has been a continuous shift in ERCP from an exclusively diagnostic test with the ability only to obtain fluoroscopic images of the pancreatic and biliary ducts to an almost therapeutic procedure with a wide variety of indications and therapeutic maneuvers. This shift has been due to two main factors: (1) improvements in cross-sectional imaging, particularly MRI/MRCP, and the emergence of endoscopic ultrasonography (EUS) which provide less invasive and more accurate images of the pancreatobiliary system and (2) improvements in through-the-scope technology which enable a wide variety of therapeutic maneuvers, many of which are discussed in other chapters in this book.

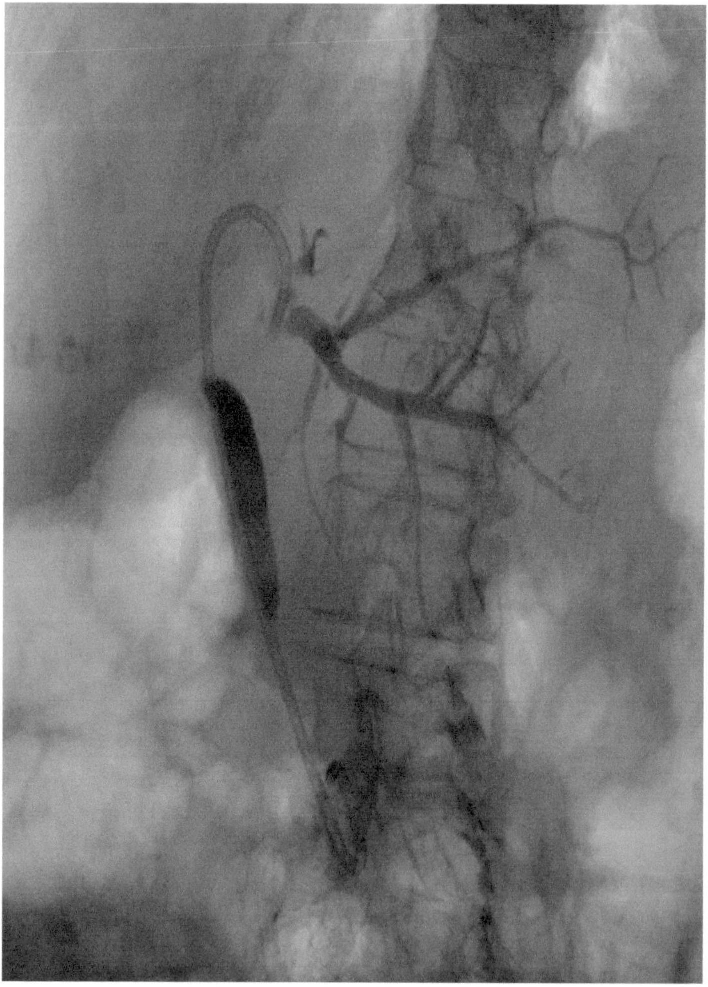

FIGURE 1.2 Cholangiogram showing double pigtail stent traversing the hilar stricture with proximal end in the left biliary tree

Obtaining good-quality cholangiography requires a thorough understanding of the biliary anatomy, knowing the limitations of cholangiography obtained endoscopically, and facility in use of fluoroscopy equipment to optimize imaging.

This is as imperative to procedural success as any other maneuver performed during ERCP [1, 2].

The above cases highlight some of the difficulties in obtaining high-quality cholangiograms and interpreting them correctly. This chapter will focus on the difficulties in obtaining and interpreting cholangiograms as well as strategies to improve image quality and interpretation.

Diagnosis/Assessment

Data are lacking regarding optimal performance and interpretation of cholangiography obtained via ERCP. Additionally, there is inherent limitation of recreating three-dimensional anatomy with two-dimensional technology. This section will focus on preprocedural, intra-procedural, and post-procedural considerations and techniques to optimize cholangiography and the subsequent interpretation (Table 1.1).

A thorough understanding of normal biliary anatomy is essential for all providers performing ERCP. Biliary anatomy is complex and variable, and providers need to be well-versed in interpreting normal and variant anatomy. It is useful to have a readily available images of normal and variant anatomy in the ERCP suite [1]. Errors can occur when the endoscopist fails to identify anatomical variants or interprets the anatomy inaccurately. Additionally, endoscopists should be well-versed in understanding the cholangiographic correlates of segmental liver anatomy [2].

Normal Anatomy

In the majority of patients, the right main hepatic duct is formed by the confluence of the right posterior and the right anterior ducts (Figs. 1.3 and 1.4) [3–6]. The right posterior duct usually passes posteriorly to the anterior duct, joining it at the left medial side to form the right hepatic duct (Fig. 1.4) [5, 6]. Segmental bile ducts from liver segments II–IV unite to form the left hepatic duct (Fig. 1.3) [7].

Table 1.1 Key considerations for optimizing cholangiogram performance and interpretation

Time relative to procedure	Consideration/ technique	Notes
Pre-procedure	Understanding normal anatomy and variants	Self-directed learning, training, experience
	Individual patient data review/ clinical situation	Record/imaging review, discussion with referring provider, multidisciplinary conference, is there a need for further imaging prior to ERCP?
Intra-procedure	Room/suite setup	Staff training, digital imaging, fluoroscopy equipment (rotatable C-arm, portable C-arm, fixed C-arm, flat table with overhead carriage), anesthesia
	Patient positioning	Semi-prone (left ducts fill before right), supine (right ducts fill before left), Trendelenburg, right lateral, patient movement to visualize specific anatomy
	Fluoroscopy arm movement	Easier to perform than patient repositioning, but does not change the effect of gravity on contrast pooling
	Cholangiogram performance	Scout radiograph prior to contrast injection, image resolution of various equipment and contrast agents, balloon occlusion or injection force to identify underfilled ducts

Table 1.1 (continued)

Time relative to procedure	Consideration/ technique	Notes
	Contrast density	Standard— strictures and pancreatic duct anatomy; dilute— small stones in large ducts
Post-procedure	Documentation	Thorough documentation of findings and therapies/ interventions necessary for continued care, radiology interpretation
	Radiology interpretation	Routinely done but helpful in selective cases with subtle findings

Common Variants

Variant biliary anatomy usually relates to differences in confluence of the left main, right anterior, and right posterior ducts. A common variant of the major ducts is the failure of fusion of the anterior and posterior right segmental ducts resulting in an absence of the right main hepatic duct, which occurs in 11% of patients [4]. In these patients, the right anterior, right posterior, and left hepatic ducts form a confluence at the common hepatic duct, sometimes referred to as a "trifurcation" (Fig. 1.5) [7, 8]. In 16% of patients, the right posterior duct drains directly into the left hepatic duct proximally to the confluence (Fig. 1.6) [7, 8]. In 6% of patients, the RPD drains into the common hepatic duct (Fig. 1.7) [8]. The right and left ducts usually join just outside the porta hepatis, but the union can be much lower so that a common duct is not formed. In these cases, the cystic duct can insert into the right hepatic duct. An accessory right posterior hepatic duct may insert at the cystic duct or common hepatic duct [7]. There is variation in the formation of the left hepatic duct from segmental bile ducts, with three primary patterns of

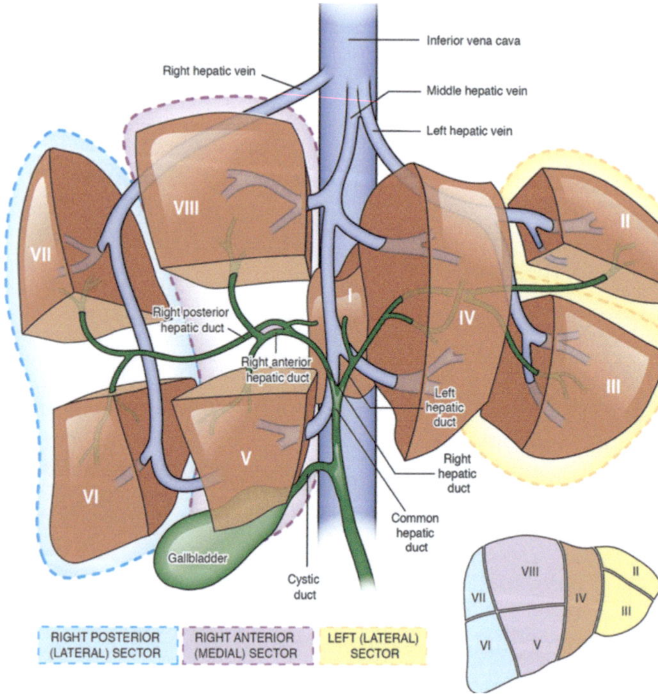

Figure 1.3 *Normal biliary anatomy and corresponding* hepatic segments and sectors as they relate to ERCP and biliary drainage

confluence [8]. Typically, the cystic duct joins the common bile duct about halfway from the hilum to the papilla, but the junction of the cystic duct is also variable [7]. This is important surgically because, if unrecognized during cholecystectomy, ligation of the cystic duct beyond the insertion of the cystic duct will result in bile duct injury. Failure to recognize variants can lead to difficult bile leaks following surgery and lead to delayed clinical improvement if not recognized during ERCP [9]. If there is a concern for a bile leak, initial imaging with MRCP may be useful to clarify anatomy because small, transected, and disconnected ducts will not opacify on ERCP [9]. If ERCP is performed prior to surgery, a good cholangiogram can highlight variant anatomy and help to minimize the risk of bile duct injury [10, 11].

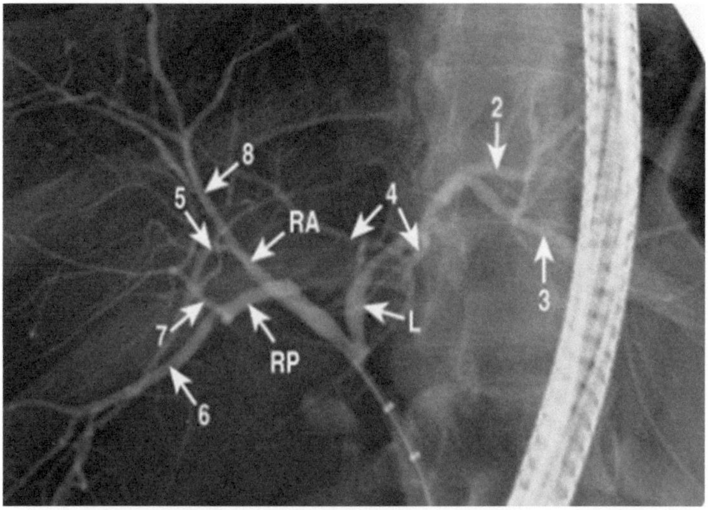

FIGURE 1.4 Normal duct anatomy—Type 1 right hepatic duct

Patient Anatomy/Review of Imaging/Records

In addition to understanding normal anatomy, understanding the individual patient's case prior to any procedure is important to maximize the chance of therapeutic success and minimize harm to the patient. In many cases, a complete understanding of a patient's biliary anatomy is not vital if an extrahepatic lesion such as a common bile duct stone or stricture can be identified and alleviated. However, in perihilar or intrahepatic disease processes, a better understanding on the individual patient's biliary ductal anatomy is vital. Such knowledge includes an understanding of any previous surgeries that could affect procedural approach and anatomy, such as bariatric surgery, liver transplantation, and prior liver resection, and review of any prior imaging. In cases where biliary anatomy is unclear, a pre-procedure MRCP may be helpful [1, 11–13].

An understanding of the expected goal(s) of the procedure is vital, and a thorough review of all imaging and clinical data should be performed prior to meeting the patient. If appropriate, an office visit should be scheduled to allow the

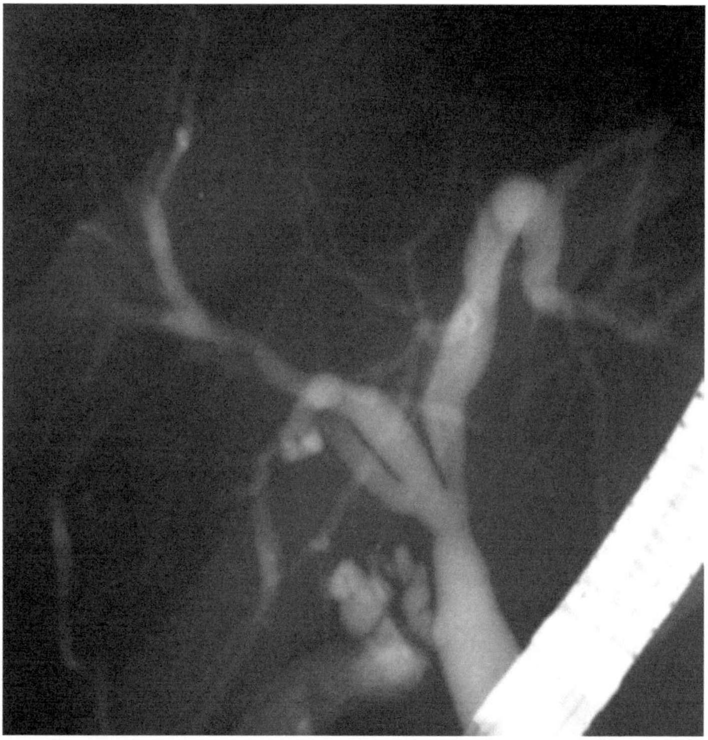

FIGURE 1.5 Trifurcation of the main biliary confluence—Type 2 right hepatic ducts

provider a more thorough review of the patient's imaging and other data and allow for a more in-depth discussion of risks, procedural goals, and alternatives.

Multidisciplinary Conference

Many centers have multidisciplinary conferences involving surgeons, diagnostic and interventional radiologists, endoscopists, and oncologists to discuss challenging cases, diagnostic dilemmas, or therapeutic options. This provides

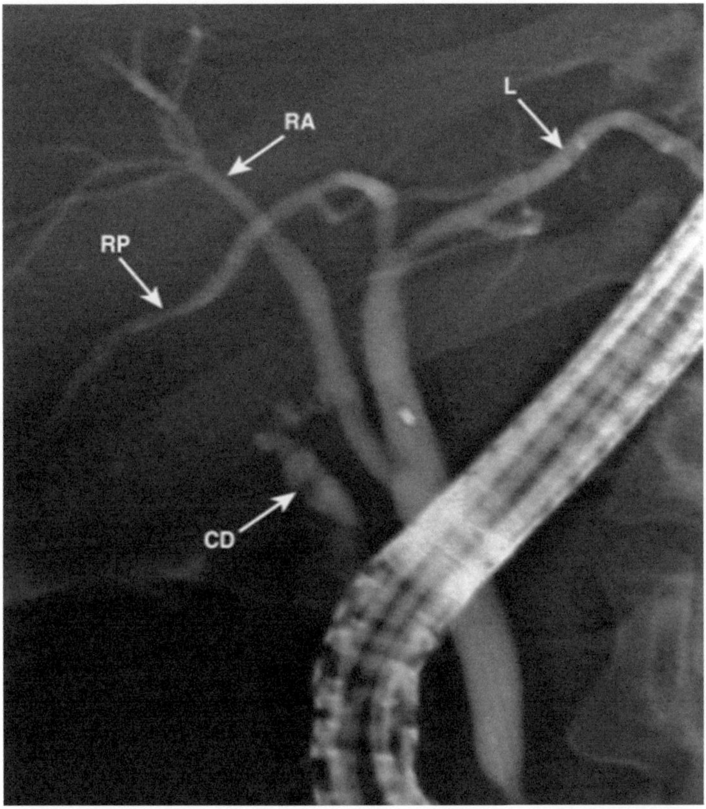

FIGURE 1.6 Right posterior duct draining into left hepatic proximal to the confluence—Type 3 hepatic duct

opportunities for better understanding of anatomy, treatment goals, and procedural limitations. Knowing the ultimate treatment plan, such as plans for subsequent surgery, is also necessary to ensure appropriate diagnostic images acquired for review, and appropriate therapy is performed. The benefits of collaboration have been borne out in multiple studies where a review of all data by providers from multiple specialties led to change in management in 25–30% of patients [14–16].

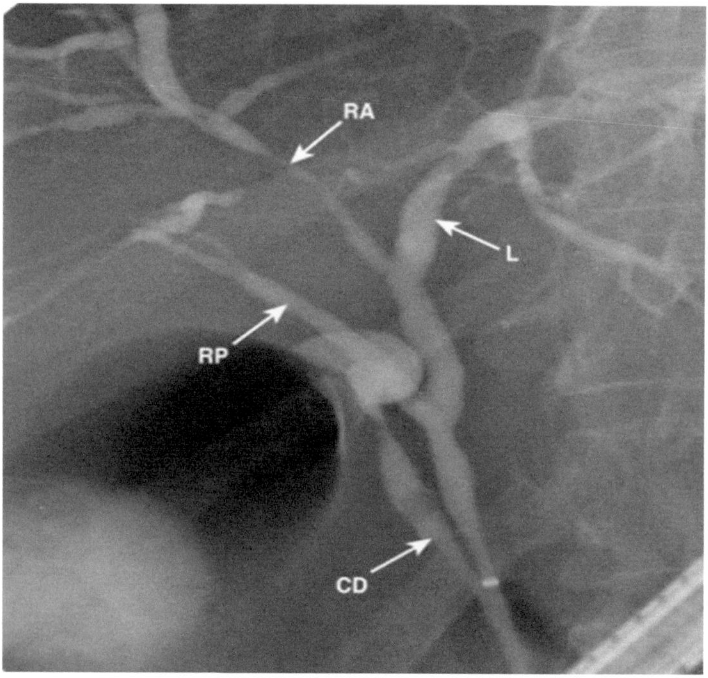

FIGURE 1.7 Right posterior duct drains into the common hepatic duct—Type 4 right hepatic ducts

Imaging Modalities

During pre-procedure planning, diagnostic ERCP has largely been replaced by CT and MRI/MRCP. These imaging modalities are widely available and noninvasive and provide highly accurate imaging of the biliary tree. CT and MRI have various protocols, which reconstruct anatomy in cross-sectional planes or other three-dimensional views, allowing users to visually grasp the complex anatomy of the bile ducts.

MRCP enables rapid, noninvasive evaluation of both the biliary tree and pancreatic duct without the use of intravenous contrast. MRCP provides better spatial and temporal resolution. CT, on the other hand, is more widely and rapidly available and more rapidly performed and may provide more reliable information on the number and location of stones due to artifacts [5]. However, it exposes patients to radiation and is less sensitive in detecting smaller, distal stones or periampullary lesions and benign or malignant strictures.

Being able to accurately determine the location of a stricture in reference to the hepatic bifurcation can sometimes be made much easier during ERCP if imaged previously on MRCP. Accurate determination of biliary pathology by using MRCP before ERCP can also allow for appropriate procedural planning [17]. This can be especially important for selecting areas for contrast injection and drainage of hilar lesions so as to minimize the risk of post-ERCP cholangitis. In addition, using MRCP to guide biliary stent placement patients with inoperable hilar obstruction has been demonstrated to reduce the overall cost of treatment [18].

Training/Education

At this point, there are no objective standards for ensuring competency in radiologic interpretation of cholangiograms. However, in order to maximize success in performing ERCP, it is critical for trainees to gain a thorough anatomical understanding during fellowship. To date, the focus of training and competency assessment has been on technical aspects of ERCP, such as cannulation and therapeutic maneuvers [19]. Various studies have proposed minimal procedure numbers as thresholds to achieving competence, with a systematic review in 2015 suggesting 160–400 ERCPs for competence [20]. In reality, trainees learn and acquire ERCP skills at different rates [21]. A recent training assessment includes questions about evaluation of trainee cholangiogram performance and interpretation [19]. There are still limits to this assessment method because there are no standard methods of performing and viewing cholangiograms. Therefore, trainee learning is largely dependent on the individual trainer. Most agree that a fourth year of advanced endoscopy training is required to achieve proficiency and certification in pancreaticobiliary endoscopy due to the increased scope and complexity of pancreaticobiliary endoscopy [20]. In this dedicated year of pancreaticobiliary, endoscopy trainees will get significant experience in cholangiogram interpretation through procedural volume, mentor-directed learning, and participation in multidisciplinary conferences to review pre-procedure imaging. However, future efforts should focus on developing standardized training in cholangiogram interpretation and competency assessment.

Intra-Procedural Considerations

There are a number of intra-procedural considerations and techniques to optimize performing and interpreting cholangiograms during ERCP.

Positioning

The patient's position should be agreed upon and understood by the anesthesia provider, the endoscopist, and the nurses and/or technical assistants. IV fluid lines, grounding wires, and ECG leads should be out of field of examination whenever possible. Historically, patients were placed prone, which created a favorable orientation for X-rays to pass through the patient between the fluoroscopy source and the detector. However, this is a difficult position for anesthesiologists to maintain a patent airway, so most often patients are placed in the semi-prone or modified prone position with the right chest elevated off the table using a shoulder roll or pillow [1, 2, 22]. The supine position is also used when performing ERCP but can be the most difficult position in which to access the descending duodenum, and secretions tend to pool over the ampulla. Additionally, the operator is usually required to stand facing away from the patient which can be a less than optimal ergonomic position. The supine position may be requested by the anesthesia provider for a morbidly obese patient because in the event of respiratory depression or a code [22]. Additionally, supine positioning provides better delineation of the hilar biliary anatomy [23]. When ERCP is performed in the supine position, endotracheal intubation is mandatory to decrease the risk of aspiration [23]. Left lateral decubitus position is not ideal for ERCP due to the unusual projection of the radiologic image obtained during fluoroscopy. The directions taken by the opacified bile and pancreatic ducts are unfamiliar in the left lateral projection [2]. However, if a large, J-shaped stomach makes it difficult to access and intubate the pylorus with the duodenoscope, transiently repositioning the patient to the left lateral position will often facilitate passage of the scope into the second portion of the duodenum [2].

It is important that the endoscopist understands how the biliary anatomy will appear with the patient in different positions. Because contrast is denser than bile, it flows to dependent portions of ducts. The left and caudate lobes will be in the dependent position in the semi-prone position, as they are located anteriorly [24]. Therefore, the left lobe will fill earlier preferentially compared to the right side (Fig. 1.8a) [7, 25]. In this case, a greater injection force may be required to adequately fill the right ducts and should not be mistaken for underlying pathology. Complete visualization of the right side is important as the right side often has variant anatomy and to detect subtle findings, such as primary sclerosing cholangitis. Adequate filling is assured with visualization and delineation of the tertiary segments. Conversely, filling of the right system without opacification of the left may indicate pathology of the left biliary tree [26].

If visualization of the right intrahepatic system is not obtained with injection and still needed, a catheter can be passed over a wire directly into the intrahepatic system. Balloon occlusion of the common bile duct can be performed for more rapid and effective filling of the intrahepatic ducts [7]. Repositioning the patient in the supine or right lateral decubitus positions allows preferential right-sided filling and can be considered if right-sided visualization is still not obtained despite the above maneuvers but is less than practical to do [26]. Right-sided filling can also be accomplished by tilting the table to head down (Trendelenburg) and tilting the patient rightward.

Other patient positioning can be considered in certain circumstances. Left lateral or fully prone positions will allow preferential filling of the left ductal systems. Trendelenburg positioning can aid in filling of the intrahepatic ducts bilaterally (Fig. 1.8b) [7]. In certain circumstances, lesions can be obscured by an oblique segment of the common hepatic duct, which forms a pronounced bend in some patients. The left oblique or left lateral position can allow better visualization. Likewise, rotation of the fluoroscopy C-arm can allow better evaluation of this segment [26].

There are a variety of lesions or artifacts that can be difficult to differentiate. The cystic duct can overlay the CBD. In this setting, rotation of the C-arm or patient is needed to separate superimposed ducts [2]. The pancreatic duct can overlay the CBD, which also requires changing angles to separate the ducts. In cases where stones mimic tumor, the endoscopist can change the angle of the C-arm or change the position of the patient [24]. Injection and withdrawal of contrast can help differentiate mobile stones from the tumor [1]. Occasionally, vascular impressions can mimic stones [27]. In such cases, it may be helpful to review pre-procedure imaging and compare with fluoroscopy.

Room Setup/Fluoroscopy Equipment

The planned setup of the endoscopic unit is also vital for performance of pancreaticobiliary endoscopy and optimizing imaging interpretation. Placement of fluoroscopy equipment and imaging monitors should be planned to make performance and viewing easy. All personnel should be trained in radiation safety and provided equipment to minimize exposure.

FIGURE 1.8 (**a**) Initial left lobe filling. This lobe fills preferentially because contrast medium is heavier than the bile and flows down into the dependent left lobe with the patient prone. This could be mistaken for complete biliary filling. (**b**) When the patient is tilted head down 20° and more volume is added, the right lobe can be viewed. Wire access and balloon occlusion of the right hepatic duct may facilitate right system cholangiogram as well

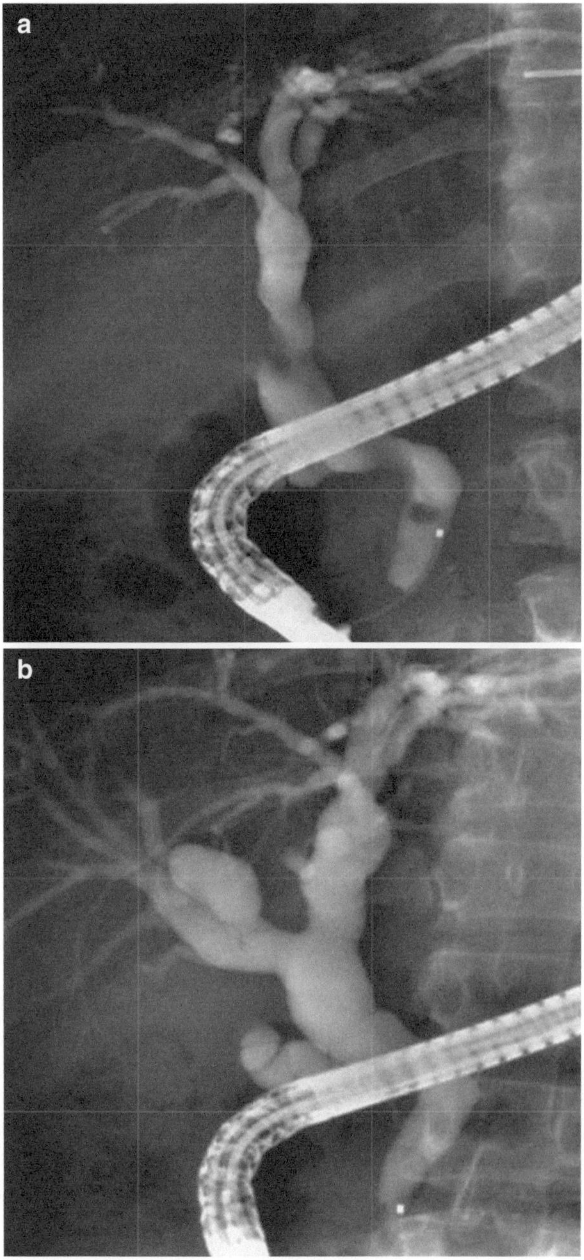
a
b

Exposure should be monitored and reported quarterly. A well-trained staff and dedicated anesthesia provider allow the endoscopist to focus on the procedure, including performance and interpretation of fluoroscopy.

Large centers typically perform ERCP in a dedicated fluoroscopy suite with digital imaging equipment. Optimal images are obtained with the aid of 180-degree rotatable C-arm, which provides for a wide variety of fluoroscopic projection angles. The ability to rotate the fluoroscopy is helpful in defining ductal strictures, separating ducts at the bifurcation, rotating the cystic duct off the bile duct, and assessing takeoff of ductal systems because pathology can be missed when performing a cholangiogram in only one body plane [7, 26]. It is important to remember that there is no standardized approach to viewing and delineating the ducts. In coronary angiography there are standardized views, such as right anterior oblique (RAO) and left anterior oblique (LAO) projections, in which there is an idea of how the coronary vessels should appear [28]. This standardization has not been created for ERCP. Therefore, it is important to understand the patient position and use the C-arm to adjust the projection and have an idea of where ducts should be. Easy manipulation of magnification and rapid image sequence acquisition are possible with the digital system. There are other fluoroscopy modalities used which have advantages and disadvantages. Portable C-arms are typically used when a case is performed outside of the fluoroscopy suite such as in the operating room or ICU. In these cases, the patients are typically too sick to travel to the fluoroscopy suite and have some other reasons why the procedure is performed in the nonstandard setting. Clearly, the benefit of the portable C-arm is that it can be moved and allows procedures to be performed on patients that need procedures but are otherwise too sick to travel away from critical care providers. These can also be used in setting where space is limited and allows rotation similar the rotatable C-arm. The image quality obtained from these is typically less than those obtained from fixed C-arm units [7]. Flat tables with fixed overhead carriages are used in some settings, including radiology suites. When these are used, patients may need to be rotated to clarify findings and separate ducts. In some instances, this might involve rotating the patient into the supine position to better visualize the bifurcation. These provide high-quality images but expose the patient and ERCP team to higher radiation doses [7].

Cholangiograms

Scout radiographs should be taken before the injection of contrast to provide a baseline image and delineate any abnormalities that could interfere with interpretation after contrast is injected. Baseline findings that should be identified and documented before ERCP include pneumobilia, presence of surgical clips or contrast from recent CT scan, rib calcifications, and pancreatic calcifications, particularly in the area of the distal bile duct [1]. Scout radiographs are best taken centered over the intended area of interest. There is no standardized approach with some scout films taken before introducing the duodenoscope and some scout films obtained with the duodenoscope in position but before cannulation.

Sequence of films is also important with the number of films determined by the diagnostic concern. The sphincter of Oddi should be filmed when it is relaxed and contrast filled to avoid misdiagnosis of pseudo-obstruction. Early contrast films can demonstrate small stones that can be obscured by high-density contrast. Various contrast agents are available and can be diluted as needed. High-osmolality contrast media is the standard agent for ERCP due to its lower cost compared to low-osmolality contrast media [29]. Dilute contrast may help visualize small gallstones within large ducts, but strictures and pancreatic duct anatomy are better visualized with full-strength contrast [29]. The disadvantage of diluting contrast is the need for increased volume, poorer image quality, and the introduction of air during syringe changes [29]. Films in various positions help understand the influence of gravity and contrast on the cholangiogram. Pathology in tortuous ducts may not been seen in one plane. Failure to recognize complete obstruction of left or right intrahepatic ducts is not uncommon. A sequence of films moving from prone to supine can separate the two lobes to avoid this error [25]. Likewise, early images of the bifurcation are also important, because extensive filling of dilated intrahepatics above a hilar lesion can then overlay and obscure the bifurcation [6].

Image resolution is also important for clear delineation of the biliary tree and is related to satisfactory opacification. Image density is related to concentration of contrast and peak kilovoltage (kVp). 85–95 kVp is average for average-sized patients [30]. Larger patients may require increased power (kilovolt-ampere (kVA)) [3]. Lower kVp increases exposure time with respiratory or cardiac motion affecting study quality [31].

The location of the duodenoscope can obscure pathology in some instances and can limit visualization of the entire distal common bile duct. To visualize this area, the duodenoscope should be advanced into the "long position," so that the entire cholangiogram can be visualized and fluoroscopic images can be obtained [2]. If the distal segment cannot be completely evaluated with the duodenoscope in the long position, withdrawing the duodenoscope into the stomach after contrast can be performed. It is also important to move the scope, patient, or C-arm such that the duodenoscope is not overlying/obscuring visualization of the CBD [1].

Post-procedural Considerations

Diagnostic Radiology Interpretation

Initially, radiologists were an integral part in ERCP because it was unfamiliar for the endoscopist. ERCPs were largely diagnostic, so involving radiologists with knowledge of imaging interpretation and use of fluoroscopy equipment made sense. At first, radiologists were even present, while ERCP was performed and provided real-time interpretation.

Radiologists are currently less involved due to decades of experience in performing and interpreting ERCP by endoscopists. Endoscopists have become quite comfortable interpreting fluoroscopic images with improvements in the quality of fluoroscopic imaging and with increased ERCP experience. Still, radiologists commonly provide post-procedure interpretation of static images provided by the endoscopists. However, their ability to reconstruct what was done during ERCP after the procedure is very limited, as they do not have access to the live, dynamic images. In fact, data suggests discrepancies between interpretations by endoscopists and radiologists are high. In one study, the radiology report did not report the findings of 50% of cases in which definite pathology was seen by the endoscopist [31]. Another study showed radiologist-endoscopist discordance rates in reading pancreatograms and cholangiograms of 38% and 47%, respectively [32].

In most settings where radiologic interpretation is routinely performed, it is important that the spot radiographs document in a stepwise manner the procedure being performed. If therapeutic procedures are performed, they should be clearly communicated to the radiologist interpreting the images. Good documentation of procedure processes, findings, and interventions is critical to optimizing radiologist interpretation.

Conclusion

An understanding of normal and common variant anatomy provides a foundation for accurate cholangiogram interpretation. Training in ERCP, typically during a fourth year of fellowship, allows sufficient time to gain a better grasp of biliary anatomy and how to optimize delineation of biliary anatomy via cholangiography in individual cases.

Cases should be approached systematically to optimize cholangiogram interpretation. Pre-procedure review of imaging, prior ERCP films, clinical symptoms, and goals of the procedure provides a road map for accurate "live" cholangiogram interpretation and guide appropriate interventions. Questions about imaging and desired outcomes can be discussed with referring providers and in multidisciplinary conferences. These conferences also provide continuing education opportunities for physicians outside of fellowship.

Comfort with equipment and staff is vital for the success of ERCP. Knowledge of the pros and cons of different fluoroscopy equipment is important. Patient positioning can be guided by comorbidities and anesthesia preference but ultimately should be chosen to optimize cholangiography in each patient which may vary by location of pathology. The fluoroscopy unit/C-arm can be rotated, and patients can be tilted or moved during the procedure to uncover obscured or poorly visualized anatomy or lesions.

Case Outcomes

In this case, pre-procedure review of imaging, prior ERCP films, and clinical course was vital. The goals of the ERCP were discussed in multidisciplinary conference, and it was determined that drainage of the left system was needed to reduce risk of cholangitis and to induce hypertrophy of the planned remaining liver after right trisectionectomy. The right side was dilated and was planned to be removed. All attempts were made to minimize opacification because there was no plan to drain the right side. Initially, the left ducts could not be opacified initially, so position and technique changes led to visualization of a left main duct stenosis.

At follow-up 2 months later, her CT was unchanged, and bilirubin improved to 5.7 mg/dl. Repeat ERCP for stent exchange was performed over a guidewire due to the severity of the hilar stricture. A subsequent MRI showed no significant changes. Her bilirubin normalized over time, and she was started on neoadjuvant gemcitabine/cisplatin. Repeat ERCP for stent exchange was performed 2 months following the previous procedure. On cholangiogram, the left and right main and left and right intrahepatic ducts were dilated. Balloon dilation of the hepatic duct bifurcation was performed (Fig. 1.9). Following this, a biliary stent was placed extending into the left biliary ducts, and one biliary stent was placed extending into the right anterior duct (Fig. 1.10). She tolerated four cycles of chemotherapy but then presented with malaise, fever, and leukocytosis, concerning for cholangitis. She was started on broad-spectrum antibiotics, and repeat ERCP was performed.

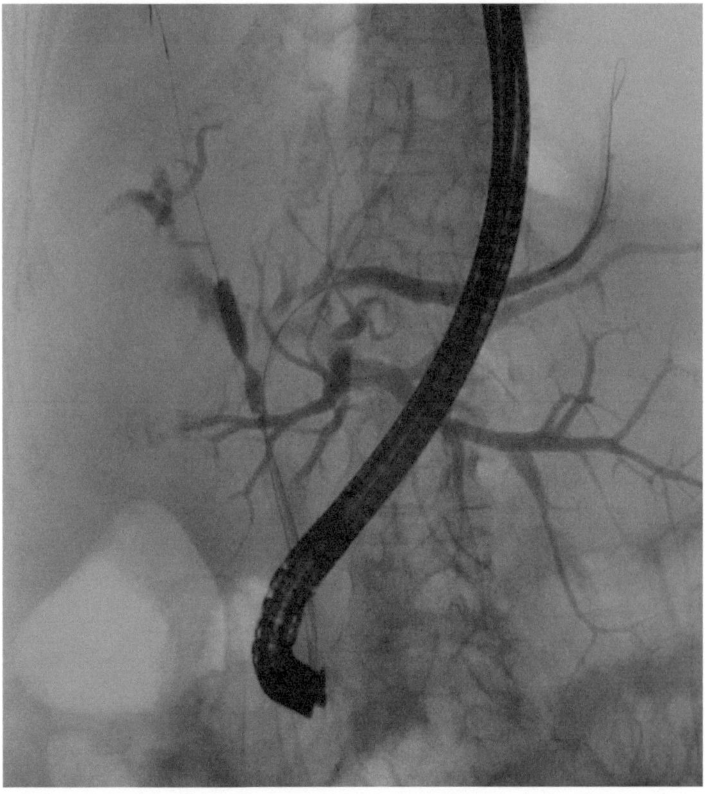

FIGURE 1.9 Follow-up ERCP for bilateral drainage after unilateral stenting of the left did not normalize bilirubin. The figure shows wire access to both left and right biliary trees with balloon dilation of a tight stricture of the right main duct

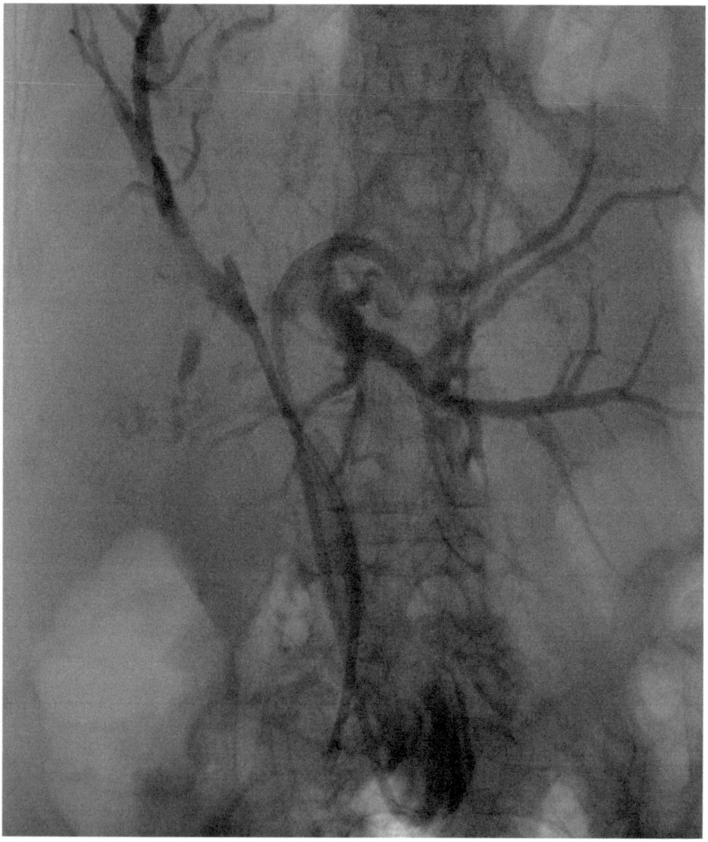

FIGURE 1.10 Cholangiogram showing stents within the right anterior and left biliary tree

The known hilar stenosis was dilated with a balloon to facilitate stent exchange. Contrast injection was limited due to concerns for cholangitis. The previously placed stents were exchanged. Her leukocytosis and jaundice improved. She subsequently underwent right portal vein embolization to induce hypertrophy of the left liver remnant in preparation for right hepatic trisectionectomy. Unfortunately, she developed disease progression with increase in the size of her known mass and new metastatic lesions in both hepatic lobes.

Pearls and Pitfalls

- It is critical for all practitioners performing ERCP to have a thorough understanding of the normal biliary anatomy and common hilar variants.
- Training in cholangiogram interpretation is largely dependent on the trainers, and competency develops at varying rates.
- While there is no standardized training program or means of assessment, skill in interpreting cholangiograms can be improved with dedicated training in interventional endoscopy, by discussing difficult cases with radiology and by attending multidisciplinary rounds with radiology and surgeons.
- For suspected hilar biliary obstruction, obtain good cross-sectional imaging, ideally with MRI/MRCP to provide a road map for subsequent ERCP.
- Prior to ERCP, obtain multidisciplinary input from surgeons and oncologists regarding tissue acquisition and surgical planning.
- When performing ERCP for perihilar obstruction, limit contrast injection to identification of stricture, and then gain wire access, with further injection performed proximal to the obstruction.
- Compare ERCP images with MRC images to optimize accuracy of determining laterality.
- Beware of misinterpreting right posterior ductal system for the left. This can be remedied by maximizing rotation of the C-arm and by comparing ERCP to MRCP images.
- A good understanding of how patients' position affects the appearance of anatomy on a cholangiogram can assist to clarify questions of specific anatomy. C-arm rotation is also critical for uncovering confusing anatomy.
- Understand how gravity will affect the course of injected contrast and how varying contrast densities can highlight different pathologies.

- Consult with radiologists in cases of complicated anatomy; good documentation will optimize their ability to assist in difficult cases and will provide a road map for repeat procedures.

References

1. Ballie J. ERCP from soup to nuts: evaluation, preparation, execution, and follow-up. ERCP and EUS: a case BAsed approach. New York: Springer Science; 2015. p. 57–76.
2. Baron TH, Kozarek RA, Carr-Locke DL. ERCP2. Philadelphia: Elsevier; 2013.
3. Zeman RK, Burrell MI. Biliary imaging techniques. In: Gallbladder and bile duct imaging: a clinical radiologic approach. New York: Churchill Livingstone; 1987. p. 47–104.
4. Sarawagi R, Sundar S, Raghuvanshi S, et al. Common and uncommon anatomical variants of intrahepatic bile ducts in magnetic resonance cholangiopancreatography and its clinical implication. Pol J Radiol. 2016;81:250–5.
5. Okada M, Fukada J, Toya K, et al. The value of drip infusion cholangiography using multidetector-row helical CT in patients with choledocholithiasis. Eur Radiol. 2005;15:2140–5.
6. Wang AY, Yachimski PS. Endoscopic management of pancreatobiliary neoplasms. Gastroenterology. 2018;154:1947–63.
7. Chandrasekhara V, Elmunzer BJ, Khashab M, Muthusamy VR. Clinical gastrointestinal endoscopy. Philadelphia: Elsevier Health Sciences; 2018.
8. Hyodo T, Kumano S, Okada M. CT and MR cholangiography: advantages and pitfalls in perioperative evaluation of biliary tree. Br J Radiol. 2012;85:887–96.
9. Kapoor V, Baron RL, Peterson M. Bile leaks after surgery. Am J Roentgenol. 2004;182:451–8.
10. Woods M, Traverso LW, Kozarek R, et al. Biliary tract complications of laparoscopic cholecystectomy are detected more frequently with routine intraoperative cholangiography. Surg Endosc. 1995;9:1076–80.
11. Costi R, Gnocchi A, Di Mario F, Sarli L. Diagnosis and management of choledocholithiasis in the golden age of

imaging, endoscopy and laparoscopy. World J Gastroenterol. 2014;20:13382–401.

12. Hekimoglu K, Ustundag Y, Dusak A, et al. MRCP vs. ERCP in the evaluation of biliary pathologies: review of current literature. J Dig Dis. 2008;9:162–9.
13. Soto J, Barish MA, Yucel E, et al. Magnetic resonance cholangiography: comparison with endoscopic retrograde cholangiopancreatography. Gastroenterology. 1996;110:589–97.
14. Brauer DG, Strand MS, Sanford D, et al. Utility of a multidisciplinary tumor board in the management of pancreatic and upper gastrointestinal diseases: an observational study. HPB (Oxford). 2016;19:133–9.
15. van Hagen P, Spaander MC, van der Gaast A, et al. Rotterdam Oesophageal Tumor Study Group. Impact of a multidisciplinary tumour board meeting for upper GI malignancies on clinical decision making: a prospective cohort study. Int J Clin Oncol. 2013;18:214–9.
16. Boniface MM, Wani SB, Schefter TE, et al. Multidisciplinary management for esophageal and gastric cancer. Cancer Manag Res. 2016;8:39–44.
17. Yeh T, Jan YY, Tseng J, et al. Malignant perihilar biliary obstruction: magnetic resonance cholangiopancreatographic findings. Am J Gastroenterol. 2000;95:432–40.
18. Harewood GC, Baron TH. Cost analysis of magnetic resonance cholangiography in the management of inoperable hilar biliary obstruction. Am J Gastroenterol. 2012;97:1152–8.
19. Wani S, Keswani R, Hall M, et al. A prospective multicenter study evaluating learning curves and competence in endoscopic ultrasound and endoscopic retrograde cholangiopancreatography among advanced endoscopy trainees: the rapid assessment of trainee endoscopy skills study. Clin Gastroenterol Hepatol. 2017;15:1758–67.
20. Shahidi N, Ou G, Telford J, Enns R. When trainees reach competency in performing ERCP: a systematic review. Gastrointest Endosc. 2015;81:1337–42.
21. Wani S, Hall M, Wang AY, et al. Variation in learning curves and competence for ERCP among advanced endoscopy trainees by using cumulative sum analysis. Gastrointest Endosc. 2016;83:711–9.
22. Aman M, Sinha AC. Challenges of performing out of operating room anesthesia on the morbidly obese. In: Out of the operating room anesthesia. Cham: Springer; 2016. p. 369–85.

23. Dumonceau JM, Garcia-Fernandez FJ, Verdun F, et al. Radiation protection in digestive endoscopy: European Society of Digestive Endoscopy (ESGE) Guideline. Endoscopy. 2012;44:408–24.
24. Ansel H, Silvis SE, Rohrmann C. Text and atlas of endoscopic retrograde cholangiopancreatography. New York: Igaku-Shoin; 1995.
25. Gardner T, Baron TH. Optimizing cholangiography when performing endoscopic retrograde cholangiopancreatography. Clin Gastroenterol Hepatol. 2008;6:734–40.
26. Turner M, Cho SR, Messmer J. Pitfalls in cholangiographic interpretation. Radiographics. 1987;7:1067–105.
27. Benson E, Page RE. A practical reappraisal of the anatomy of the extrahepatic bile ducts and arteries. Br J Surg. 1976;63:853–60.
28. Aquilina O, Grech V, Felice H, et al. Normal adult coronary angiography. Images Paediatr Cardiol. 2006;8:1–17.
29. Mishkin D, Carpenter S, Croffie J, al e. ASGE technology status evaluation report: radiographic contrast media used in ERCP. Gastrointest Endosc. 2005;62:480–4.
30. El-Hennawy H, El-Kahlout EA, Bedar E, et al. Laparoscopic intraoperative cholangiography interpretation by surgeons versus radiologists, a comparative study review of 200 cholangiographies. ISRN Minim Invasive Surg. 2012;2012:1–5.
31. Khanna N, May G, Bass S, et al. Postprocedural interpretation of endoscopic retrograde cholangiopancreatography by radiology. Can J Gastroenterol. 2008;22:55–60.
32. Kucera S, Isenberg G, Chak A, et al. Postprocedure radiologist's interpretation of ERCP x-ray films: a prospective outcomes study. Gastrointest Endosc. 2007;66:79–83.

Chapter 2
Sedation in ERCP

Fahad Faisal Mir, Leen H. Al-Sayyed, and Sreeni Jonnalagadda

Case Presentation

Our patient is a very pleasant 64-year-old Caucasian male with known history of pancreatic adenocarcinoma with metastatic disease to the liver who presented to the emergency room with increasing abdominal pain and abnormal liver chemistries. He does have chronic baseline abdominal pain but presented with worsening epigastric abdominal pain. The pain was reported as sharp and constant, radiating throughout his abdomen, with no aggravating or alleviating factors. He also had associated nausea and non-bloody non-bilious emesis.

He was diagnosed with pancreatic cancer 2 years before presentation and had plastic biliary stents placed which were replaced by a 10 mm × 6 cm uncovered biliary metal stent. Due to tissue ingrowth into the stent, it was replaced by a 10 mm × 4 cm fully covered biliary metal stent 6 months before this presentation. His bilirubin was normal 3 weeks before presentation, but on admission it was found to be 5.2 mg/dL, alanine aminotransferase was 90 IU/L, aspirate aminotransferase was 106 IU/L, and alkaline phosphatase was 237.

He underwent endoscopic retrograde cholangiopancreatography (ERCP) under monitored

F. F. Mir · L. H. Al-Sayyed · S. Jonnalagadda (✉)
Saint Luke's Hospital of Kansas City, Kansas City, MO, USA
e-mail: sjonnalagadda@saint-lukes.org

D. K. Mullady (ed.), *Dilemmas in ERCP*,
https://doi.org/10.1007/978-3-030-12741-1_2

anesthesia care (MAC). His Mallampati score was determined to be 2 and American Society of Anesthesiologists (ASA) score was 3. The patient was placed in prone position with capnographic and oxygenation monitoring. Propofol was used for anesthesia induction and maintenance. 900 cc of fluid was aspirated from the stomach with additional food residue remaining. A narrowing was identified in the post-bulbar duodenum. Given the large amount of food present in the stomach, the procedure was terminated without further intervention.

Pre-procedure Assessment

The American Society of Anesthesiologists (ASA) Practice Advisory defines pre-anesthesia evaluation as the process of clinical assessment that precedes the delivery of anesthesia care for surgery and for nonsurgical procedures [2]. This process can start a few weeks before an elective ERCP or emergently if indicated. The aim of pre-anesthesia evaluation is to assess the patient's ability to tolerate the anesthesia for the procedure. Adequate preparation improves procedure outcomes and patient satisfaction and decreases complications, cost, and mortality. The anticipated difficulty of airway interventions in case of an emergency often helps determine whether the procedure is best performed within a traditional endoscopy suite equipped with fluoroscopy or within a more controlled environment such as the operation theater where the tools required for advanced endotracheal intubation are readily available.

Patient Risk Factors

American Society of Anesthesiologists-Physical Status (ASA-PS)

The ASA-PS classification system evaluates the overall health status of the patient. The higher the ASA-PS class, the higher the risk of complications from anesthesia and prolonged hospital stay. Functional status of the patient can help identify the patient at risk and predict perioperative complications (Table 2.1). Each patient will need to have a focused history

TABLE 2.1 ASA-PS classification, modified from ASA guidelines

ASA PS Classification	Definition	Examples, including, but not limited to:
ASA I	A normal healthy patient	Healthy, non-smoking, no or minimal alcohol use
ASA II	A patient with mild systemic disease	Mild diseases only without substantive functional limitations. Examples include (but not limited to) current smoker, social alcohol drinker, pregnancy, obesity ($30 < BMI < 40$), well-controlled DM/HTN, and mild lung disease
ASA III	A patient with severe systemic disease	Substantive functional limitations; one or more moderate to severe diseases. Examples include (but not limited to) poorly controlled DM or HTN, COPD, morbid obesity ($BMI \geq 40$), active hepatitis, alcohol dependence or abuse, implanted pacemaker, moderate reduction of ejection fraction, ESRD undergoing regularly scheduled dialysis, premature infant PCA < 60 weeks, and history (>3 months) of MI, CVA, TIA, or CAD/stents.
ASA IV	A patient with severe systemic disease that is a constant threat to life	Examples include recent (<3 months) MI, CVA, TIA, or CAD/stents, ongoing cardiac ischemia or severe valve dysfunction, severe reduction of ejection fraction, sepsis, and DIC, ARD or ESRD not undergoing regularly scheduled dialysis
ASA V	A moribund patient who is not expected to survive without the operation	Examples include ruptured abdominal/thoracic aneurysm, massive trauma, intracranial bleed with mass effect, and ischemic bowel in the face of significant cardiac pathology or multiple organ/system dysfunction
ASA VI	A declared brain-dead patient whose organs are being removed for donor purposes	

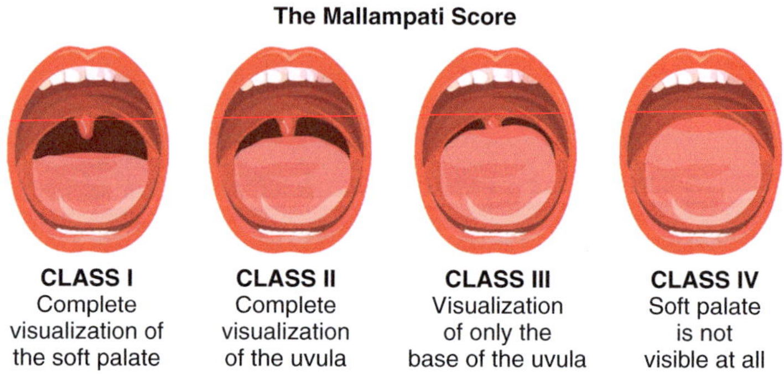

FIGURE 2.1 The modified Mallampati classification for difficult laryngoscopy and intubation. (Reproduced with permission from: Brown CA. Approach to the difficult airway in adults outside the operating room. In: UpToDate, Post TW (Ed), UpToDate, Waltham, MA. (Accessed on 1/25/2019) Copyright © 2019 UpToDate, Inc. For more information visit www.uptodate.com.) [5]

and physical examination that at a minimum should include an assessment of the airway and pulmonary and cardiac exam. Laboratory tests, imaging, and consultations with cardiology and pulmonary specialists are decided upon case by case. This will help to plan and anticipate the type of complications that may occur and thus prevent them [3].

Airway Evaluation

Safe airway management begins with pre-procedural evaluation of airway. This includes evaluating the head and neck for anatomical challenges, medical history, body habitus, neck circumference, and mouth opening, among other factors. Mallampati score (Fig. 2.1) is highly predictive of difficult airway intubation. The ASA Task force [4] has published specific prognostic factors that predict difficult airways, and these include congenital or acquired disease of the nose, tongue, teeth, temporomandibular joint, and cervical spine, previous narcosis with and without endotracheal intubation, obesity, snoring and obstructive sleep apnea, previous pro-

Table 2.2 Anthropometric parameters predictive of difficult airway. Modified from ASA guidelines for management of difficult airway [4]

Mobility of the neck and its shape
Mandibular hypoplasia or micrognathia
Mobility of the temporomandibular joint
Interdental distance
Conditions of teeth, denture fixed or mobile, protrusion of the incisors, dimension of the tongue in relation to the oral cavity
Chin-thyroid distance
Mallampati score
Mandibular protrusion test
Chin-sternum distance

longed intubation and/or difficult airway report, and history of tracheostomy. Other specific anthropometric parameters, predictive of difficult airway, are shown in (Table 2.2).

Obstructive Sleep Apnea (OSA)

Patients with OSA are at a greater risk for developing sedation-related complications during endoscopic procedures. Full polysomnography represents the gold standard for the diagnosis of OSA. However, it is an overnight study that is costly. There are several screening tools with high predictability for OSA. The STOP-BANG questionnaire (Table 2.3) represents a highly sensitive bedside tool that is particularly useful to screen for patients with severe OSA. A score of 3 or more correlates with a higher rate of postprocedural complications [6].

Patients with a higher body mass index (BMI) have an increased frequency of needing airway manipulation during advanced endoscopic procedures. A study has shown independent predictors of airway maneuvers needed for patients under deep sedation to include male sex, ASA class of 3 or higher, and increased BMI [7].

Table 2.3 STOP-BANG Questionnaire

STOP-BANG Questionnaire
1. Do you Snore loudly (louder than talking or loud enough to be heard through closed doors)? Yes/No
2. Do you often feel Tired, fatigued, or sleepy during daytime? Yes/No
3. Has anyone Observed you stop breathing during your sleep? Yes/No
4. Do you have or are you being treated for high blood Pressure? Yes/No
5. BMI 35 kg/m2? (BMI ________) Yes/No
6. Age 50 years or older? Yes/No
7. Neck circumference 40 cm? (neck circumference ________cm) Yes/No
8. Gender male? Yes/No

Note. A score of 3 or greater denotes a high risk for obstructive sleep apnea

Sedation Considerations Specific to ERCP

Sedation for ERCP can range from moderate to deep sedation or general anesthesia. Even in patients receiving propofol who are not intubated, in the author's experience, patients are unarousable with pain stimuli, and as such, their level of sedation straddles the divide between deep sedation and general anesthesia. In our hospital system, all ERCPs are performed under the care of a dedicated anesthesia provider. For most endoscopists who perform ERCP infrequently and average 30–90 minutes of procedure time, our anesthesia providers prefer to administer general anesthesia with endotracheal intubation. On the other hand, when an expert and experienced endoscopist is performing a procedure where the actual procedure time is usually expected to be 10–30 minutes, deep sedation with propofol alone or in a combination regimen is preferred, allowing for faster recovery and turn-around time in the ERCP suite.

Choice of Deep Sedation Versus General Anesthesia in ERCP

In one study, the depth of sedation was serially assessed during ERCP; 85% of patients met criteria for at least deep sedation during the procedure [8]. Therefore, patients receiving propofol for ERCP and endoscopic ultrasound (EUS), targeted for deep sedation, should be managed by a provider who is adequately trained in the administration of general anesthesia, airway management, and rescue maneuvers (Table 2.4).

Raymondos et al. [9] in a retrospective study assessed the indications for ERCP procedures under general anesthesia (GA) versus conscious sedation. Study results showed that patients with primary sclerosing cholangitis and liver transplants in whom painful dilations were planned received GA more frequently than conscious sedation, which in turn was utilized more in patients with neoplasms and cholelithiasis. ERCP under conscious sedation showed a higher failure and termination rate compared to ERCP under GA in these select patients. Inadequate sedation and patient discomfort were the main reasons for ERCP failure under conscious sedation. Repeating the procedure under GA improved success rate to 83%. It is noteworthy that the overall complication rate associated with therapeutic interventions during ERCP was significantly lower in patients who were under GA in this study. This is due to patient immobility and duodenal peristalsis which made the procedure technically easier [10]. The widespread use of propofol typically results in deeper sedation than use of opiates and benzodiazepines for conscious sedation and, as practiced currently, reduces the incidence of inadequate sedation and discomfort.

Patients at higher risk of aspiration due to gastroparesis, suspected gastric outlet obstruction, duodenal strictures or those who are expected to have a complex ERCP due to painful stricture dilation, pancreatic instrumentation, large-volume cystogastrostomy, and patients with increased intra-abdominal pressure or inadequate fasting time prior to

Table 2.4 Levels of sedation as defined by ASA [3]

	Minimal sedation anxiolysis	**Moderate sedation/ analgesia ("conscious sedation")**	**Deep sedation/analgesia**	**General anesthesia**
Responsiveness	Normal response to verbal stimulation	Purposeful response to verbal or tactile stimulation	Purposeful response following repeated or painful stimulation	Unarousable even with painful stimulus
Airway	Unaffected	No intervention required	Intervention may be required	Intervention often required
Spontaneous ventilation	Unaffected	Adequate	May be inadequate	Frequently inadequate
Cardiovascular function	Unaffected	Usually maintained	Usually maintained	May be impaired

ERCP are best done with GA with endotracheal intubation. A safe practice involves gastric decompression with a nasogastric tube overnight in patient with gastric outlet obstruction to reduce risk for aspiration during endotracheal intubation and extubation. During deep sedation or GA, pharyngeal reflexes are depressed, increasing the risk of aspiration of gastric contents. Therefore, endotracheal intubation will secure the airways and consequently minimize the risk of aspiration. General anesthesia with intubation should be considered when the ERCP is predicted to be complex and prolonged. Such cases will have a higher aspiration risk. ERCP complexity can be predicted using different scoring systems. The one published by the Quality Committee of the American Society of Gastrointestinal Endoscopy (ASGE) grades complexity from 1 to 4 [11]. Grade 1 and 2 procedures are considered technically less challenging and typically can be completed in a relatively short time compared to more complex (grades 3 and 4) ERCPs [11]. It can be a useful tool to ascertain the optimal type of anesthesia in each case.

Other related patient factors to be considered when choosing between deep sedation and GA include an underlying heart disease, chronic pulmonary obstructive disease (COPD), and obstructive sleep apnea, as the risk of aspiration is increased in these cases. General anesthesia with airway secured and ventilatory support may be a better choice in these patients. In select patients with anticipated short duration of procedure time and marginal cardiorespiratory status, occasionally our anesthesiologists prefer MAC to GA as extubation in some patients can prove problematic. While the benefits of GA in complex and painful cases outweigh the limitations supporting GA in these selective cases [2, 3], the ultimate choice of modality is best made by the anesthesiologist following consultation with the endoscopist, taking into account patient factors as well as endoscopist expertise and procedure complexity and duration.

Deep sedation without endotracheal intubation has been shown to be safe and effective in ERCP [12]. Unless patient characteristics dictate general anesthesia, most grade 1 and 2 and many grade 3 ERCPs can be safely performed using deep propofol sedation without endotracheal intubation [13]. On the other hand, for more complex procedures, the patient's safety and tolerance is a significant factor in determining procedural success, and general anesthesia with intubation may be preferable, especially if prolonged ERCP is expected. ERCP in healthy, nonobese patients who are expected to have a short procedure time is done under deep sedation with monitored anesthesia care (MAC). When compared to general anesthesia with intubation, in a study of 438 patients, the risk of adverse events was higher in the general anesthesia group (35.6%) compared to the MAC group (25.7%) but without significant difference in complications in either group [12]. MAC achieves many of the general anesthesia goals including sedation, anxiolysis, analgesia, and amnesia in addition to continued monitoring. In addition, it allows for faster recovery, improved patient tolerance of the procedure, and satisfaction afterward.

Patient-controlled sedation (PCS) is a delivery of sedative medications during unpleasant diagnostic and therapeutic procedures that are initiated and controlled by the patient [14]. PCS originated from patient-controlled analgesia (PCA). Patient-maintained sedation (PMS) is a modification of PCS that describes sedation which is initiated by an anesthesia provider and maintained by the patient at the level desired by the patient [15]. Using propofol alone or in combination with remifentanil or alfentanil, the success rate of PCS during ERCP is comparable to that during colonoscopy [16]. This protocol has been shown to be comparable to anesthesiologist-administered propofol. However, it has limitations and may not be an option for every patient, especially if she/he has a higher ASA-PS. It also cannot be utilized in emergency cases [15]. It can be promising in non-emergent ERCPs in the outpatient endoscopy units. Multicenter studies are still needed to validate PCS use in ERCP procedures.

Intra-procedural Considerations

Patient Monitoring During ERCP

When patients are sedated with propofol, electroencephalogram (EEG) monitoring enables more effective titration of propofol dosage for sedation and is associated with faster patient recovery [17]. Bispectral index (BIS) monitoring is an EEG-based method which quantifies the depth of anesthesia by analyzing the EEG and using a complex algorithm to generate an index score [18]. The EEG-guided method was originally evaluated for facilitation of sedation in ERCP [19]. It provides an objective measurement of the level of consciousness in sedated patients which helps titration of propofol for desired effect.

Monitoring of the patient is achieved by frequent automated assessment of blood pressure, continuous heart rate, capnography, electrocardiogram, and pulse oximetry monitoring. In critically ill patients or others with significant comorbidities, for instance, severe aortic stenosis, continuous arterial blood pressure monitoring may provide the most accurate and timely monitoring. Capnography monitors the respiratory activity and may act as an early warning system for hypoxemia. In a randomized controlled trial, microstream capnographic monitoring of respiratory activity was associated with significantly reduced hypoxemia, major hypoxemia, apnea, as well as reduced oxygen requirements in patients undergoing ERCP and EUS [20, 21]. Equally important is observing the patient's chest wall movement and regular evaluation of the level of sedation by stimulating the patient. Continuous monitoring will help to anticipate respiratory derangement which allows for early intervention in case of respiratory depression, hypoxemia, hypotension, or patient pain and discomfort.

Patient Positioning During ERCP

Patient positioning during ERCP varies based on endoscopist preference. The typical options are to perform the entire procedure in prone position or to start in the left lateral position and rotate the patient to prone position once the duodenum has been intubated. In the authors' experience and opinion, performing ERCP in prone position allows any oral secretions to track away from the oropharynx and reduces aspiration risk. On the other hand, occasionally, ERCP is performed in the supine position, particularly in the setting of altered anatomy or instability. In the supine position, there is a heightened concern for aspiration, particularly during longer procedures, and endotracheal intubation should be performed.

Oxygen Administration and Airway Management During ERCP

Close monitoring of the airway, respiration, and oxygenation is critical for safe sedation, and spontaneous ventilation should be preserved during deep sedation. Supplemental oxygen is routinely provided to all patients regardless of the level of sedation to prevent hypoxemia [22], more so if a patient is undergoing propofol sedation [23]. Oxygen concentration and saturation goal should be individualized according to patient's need and preexisting chronic lung disease.

There are multiple oxygen delivery systems for patients undergoing procedural sedation. Both low-flow, providing up to 15 L/min of oxygen, and high-flow systems are widely utilized. Oxygen can be delivered via standard nasal cannula, simple face mask, venturi mask, or non-rebreathing masks which deliver varying fractions of inspired oxygen (FiO2). The choice of which device is typically tailored to the clinical situation, patient and provider preference, reliability, and ease of use. For instance, in some patients with a history of sleep apnea or obesity, the use of a nasal trumpet along with nasal cannula can make a significant difference in the ability to maintain oxygen saturation. Inability to effectively heat and humidify gas can limit the utility of low-flow modalities in certain situations [24, 25].

Venturi mask – a high-flow system – can provide a flow rate of 60 L/min or greater and is superior at providing supplemental oxygen at precise concentrations. However, some patients may not tolerate these devices due to anxiety or a sensation of obstruction created by the mask [26]. Humidified heated high-flow nasal oxygen (HFNO) delivered through nasal cannula is designed to overcome some of these limitations. HFNO studies report increased patient comfort, less mucosal desiccation, improved clearance of pulmonary and airway secretions, a reduction in work of breathing, and enhanced oxygen delivery [27]. Moreover, a study has demonstrated decreased use of GA when HFNO is available in the endoscopy unit for patients undergoing ERCP and EUS [28]. Provision of HFNO and deep sedation was associated with decreased procedure and anesthesia-only times. It also improves access to the airway and gastrointestinal tract compared to oxygen delivery masks, and it is less bulky than nasal continuous positive airway pressure devices [28].

Data suggest that the Gastro-Laryngeal Tube (GLT) is an effective and secure device for airway management and for use during performance of ERCP (Fig. 2.2). The use of GLT for ERCP has been shown to decrease the rate of desaturations during ERCP (60% compared to 0%) when no airway device is used. The satisfaction score for the endoscopist was also significantly higher in the GLT group. This instrument has been shown to be safe and effective in maintaining airway and oxygen saturation [29, 30].

Another study evaluated the feasibility of using the laryngeal mask airway (LMA) instead of the endotracheal tube during ERCP. The LMA can be placed with the patient prone, obviating the need to change position. It also shortens the extubation time compared with endotracheal intubation [31]. Nevertheless, the use of LMA in the prone position requires more care because it can easily dislodge by manipulation during the procedure and it does not secure the patient's airway in case of aspiration of gastric fluids. There are a few commercial versions of modified laryngeal mask airway with a dedicated channel for the insertion of a duodenoscope. This is occasionally employed in high-risk patients as a means to avoid endotracheal intubation. A study sought

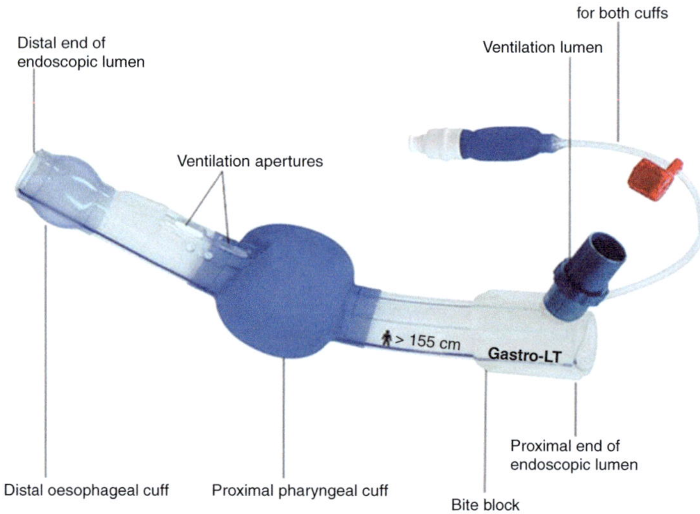

FIGURE 2.2 Gastro-Laryngeal Tube & its use in endoscopic retrograde cholangiopancreatography. (Published with permission from **VBM-Medical Inc.**)

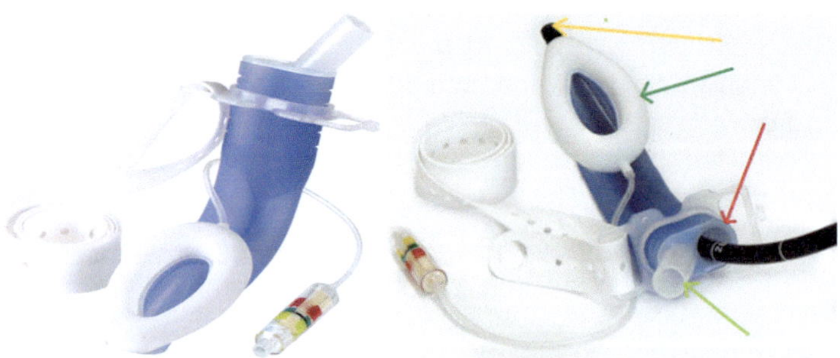

FIGURE 2.3 The gastrolaryngeal mask (GLM) with 2 separate channels, one for endoscope access and the other for gastric and airway access. It also allows for End tidal CO_2 monitoring [33]

to determine LMA® Gastro™ Airway (Fig. 2.3) efficacy for clinical use in upper gastrointestinal endoscopy and yielded a high rate of endoscopy success, along with an excellent airway insertion rate [32, 33].

Medications Used in Sedation in ERCP

When ERCP is performed under deep sedation without endotracheal intubation, propofol has emerged to be the drug of choice for sedation. Intravenous sedation with propofol for ERCP is more effective than sedation with midazolam alone and is considered safe under adequate patient monitoring. It is also associated with a faster postprocedural recovery [34]. During the last decade, the use of propofol has been proven to be superior to the use of benzodiazepines for sedation during ERCP. In one study, complete ERCP was possible in >90% of patients compared to 80% of patients on midazolam [35]. Because propofol has a narrow therapeutic window, close patient monitoring is essential [35]. Berzin et al. [36], in a prospective cohort study of sedation-related adverse events, evaluated patient- and procedure-related risk factors associated with sedation, as well as endoscopist and patient satisfaction with anesthesiologist-administered sedation. The study showed that the anesthesiologist-administered sedation for ERCP patients is safe and effective although it is less cost-effective.

Propofol Alone and with Combinations

Effective sedation includes the control of anxiety, analgesia, and temporary amnesia. Anxiety is allayed through preprocedural education of the patient regarding the procedure and administration of anxiolytics if needed. In addition to analgesia, post-procedure amnesia plays an equally important role in patient comfort.

Propofol sedation is preferred over traditionally used benzodiazepines. Propofol use has faster induction times and recovery times and leads to improved patient tolerance of the procedure [15]. Despite the short half-life, propofol should be administered by individuals credentialed and trained in advance airway monitoring and management. Since it has a very narrow therapeutic index, it can result in profound respiratory depression and inhibit gag and cough reflexes and has no specific antagonist that may be used to reverse its effects [37]. However, propofol sedation during diagnostic and therapeutic ERCP is found to be more effective than midazolam/meperidine sedation and can be administered safely under adequate patient monitoring even in elderly high-risk patients [38].

Propofol in intermittent boluses or continuous infusion can be used, and the choice is typically left to the discretion of the anesthesia provider. In our experience, a continuous infusion supplemented by additional boluses of propofol as needed during the course of the procedure seems to provide the best outcome. This protocol however has not shown to be effective over anesthesiologist-controlled or patient-controlled intermittent boluses [15]. Propofol infusion causes pain; it is recommended to use a cannula placed in larger veins. Lidocaine dosing administered just prior to initiating propofol infusion can help reduce the pain.

Dexmedetomidine alone was not as effective as propofol combined with fentanyl for providing conscious sedation during ERCP. Furthermore, dexmedetomidine was associated with greater hemodynamic instability and a prolonged recovery [39]. Midazolam, when used with propofol, was shown to reduce the requirement for propofol, but this regimen was not superior to propofol alone in terms of sedation and was associated with longer recovery times [40].

In complex ERCP procedures which are often associated with pain (especially if pancreatic intervention is required), the addition of analgesic agents, also known as "sedato-analgesic cocktail," potentially reduces the overall requirement for propofol. This is due to the additive and synergistic effects of the cocktail, hence improving the safety of routine propofol administration in ERCP [41]. It is also proposed that a decreased variability in patient depth of sedation with this combination improves patient tolerance. However, concomitant use of propofol with narcotics amplifies the respiratory depressant effects, and thus, continuous patient monitoring is essential [42]. Cohen et al. concluded that propofol in small bolus doses, combined with midazolam and an opioid, can maximize its safety profile while maintaining efficacy [43, 44].

Ketamine, when used in conjunction with propofol, has been shown to maintain better mean arterial pressures and is associated with less apnea compared with fentanyl and propofol [45]. In a study that compared the analgesic and sedative effects of propofol-ketamine versus propofol-fentanyl in patients undergoing ERCP, the results showed equal sedative effects in both groups [46].

Caution during sedation is advised with the elderly, very ill, or debilitated patients, in whom the respiratory depressant effect is more pronounced. Small doses of intravenous propofol alone are often adequate in sedating such patients during ERCP [41].

The majority of ERCP and EUS procedures can be safely performed with monitored anesthesia care. A standard sedation protocol that is superior to all others has not been described. Choice of sedative agents and deep sedation or general anesthesia for patients should be individualized keeping in mind risk factors of the patient, indication, and complexity of the procedure. We propose using propofol and fentanyl with or without an anxiolytic under MAC for most of the ERCP cases. General anesthesia with intubation is to be considered on a case-by-case basis according to the patient and ERCP specifics.

Special Cases in ERCP

Pregnancy and Lactating Women

Hormonal changes during pregnancy can increase bile lithogenicity, decrease gallbladder emptying, and predispose to gallstone formation. Cholangitis and pancreatitis carry significant morbidity and can be fatal for the mother and fetus [47]. The use of ERCP during pregnancy was introduced in 1990 [48] and since then has been studied in several small-case series and large cohort studies [49]. Second trimester has been suggested as the optimal safe window for a non-emergent ERCP [47]. In a large study of 3052 patients undergoing endoscopy during pregnancy, risk during ERCP was similar to risk of upper or lower endoscopy during pregnancy; the risk may be independent of trimester [49]. Reported adverse fetal outcomes include spontaneous abortion, anomalous development, premature labor, and fetal demise as complications of endoscopy. Whether fetal complications were related to procedure versus sedation, a clear relationship has not been established. When ERCP is performed during pregnancy, every effort should be made to reduce radiation exposure. Additional protection for the fetus is achieved with placement of lead shield underneath the pelvis and lower abdomen of the pregnant patient.

Caution is advised with sedation using propofol and midazolam in the third trimester with greater than 3-hour procedure or repeated use as there is a concern for dose-dependent transient neonatal depression. Propofol and meperidine are classified as category B and Fentanyl is category C, while midazolam is category D. Midazolam and propofol have been used during ERCP with no differences in efficacy or safety [47]. An additional concern during pregnancy is the position of the patient undergoing ERCP. The suggested position is a left lateral position instead of the more commonly practiced prone position.

For lactating women, ASGE guidelines suggest that breastfeeding may be continued after maternal fentanyl administration [50]. The American Academy of Pediatrics (AAP) considers fentanyl to be compatible with breastfeeding [51].

Propofol is excreted in breast milk with maximum concentrations at 4–5 hours [52]. Breastfeeding may be resumed after maternal propofol administration as soon as the mother awakes and has sufficiently recovered from general anesthesia or deep sedation. AAP considers the effects of midazolam on the nursing infant unknown [51]. It is recommended to withhold nursing of the infant for at least 4 hours following maternal administration of midazolam. The safety of reversal agents like naloxone and flumazenil in this setting is unknown. Naloxone is not orally bioavailable, so it is unlikely to affect the infant [50].

Elderly Patients

Elderly patients, especially those who are 80 years or above, require significantly less sedation compared to younger adults undergoing ERCP [53]. Even with less sedation, elderly patients have a higher risk of sedation-related complications during ERCP including hypoxia, asystole, and bradycardia. Minimal effective sedation medications and careful observation of cardiovascular status and oxygen saturation are suggested in this population.

Post-procedure Care

Once ERCP is completed, the medication effect can extend for hours post the procedure; it is critical that patients get monitored until they are fully awake and able to maintain an open airway, ventilate spontaneously, and have adequate oxygenation. Continued oxygen supply is recommended until the patient shows signs of full recovery. Before discharge, the patient should be alert, hemodynamically stable, responding purposefully to commands, verbally communicating, and able to tolerate oral fluids [54]. Analgesics especially opioids can cause nausea; antiemetics as needed can be administered.

Case Outcome

A nasogastric tube was placed overnight and left to low intermittent suction for decompression of the stomach. ERCP was performed the next morning with general anesthesia with intubation. Narrowing was noted in the duodenum secondary to tumor invasion through which the duodenoscope could not be traversed to the second part of the duodenum. Large ulcerations were noted in the second part of the duodenum with tumor erosion adjacent to the major papilla. A wire was advanced under fluoroscopic and endoscopic guidance across the duodenal stent into the third portion of the duodenum.

A 22 mm × 9 cm uncovered duodenal stent was deployed across the strictured area with the proximal end located in the duodenal bulb. Patient was discharged to home with plans to attempt ERCP via the duodenal stent in a few days after allowing for stent expansion. If this was unsuccessful, a percutaneous approach would be required for establishing adequate biliary drainage.

Pearls and Key Points

- Optimized pre-anesthesia care can identify and prevent many intra- and post-ERCP complications. This includes a focused review of patient's history, ERCP indication, and focused physical exam. ASA class identification should be assessed in every patient. Screening for OSA can help prevent hypoventilation with proactive measures including use of LMA or nasal trumpet proactively if recognized prior to the procedure.
- In patients who are high risk for aspiration, nasogastric tube suctioning and the option for general anesthesia and intubation for airway protection should be readily available and done by specialized anesthesia personnel.
- MAC sedation is widely used for ERCP. General anesthesia should be considered in complex cases and in patients who are at risk of aspiration.
- Propofol use increases patient satisfaction and comfort, allowing the endoscopist to complete the ERCP successfully. Adding an analgesic provides synergistic effect. Close monitoring is indicated when propofol is used alone or in combination.
- Monitoring during MAC sedation is critical to detect early complications, especially hypoxemia and respiratory depression.
- Supplemental oxygen helps to maintain oxygenation prior to, during, and after ERCP procedures.
- Monitoring CO_2 allows for early detection of respiratory depression.

- Medication doses should be titrated to effect. Always consider dose adjustment for age, kidney, or liver function if indicated.
- Intra-procedural medication effect can last for hours beyond the procedure; hence, post-anesthesia care is a must. Patient needs to be alert, hemodynamically stable, and spontaneously breathing before discharge.
- Regular communication between the endoscopist and the anesthesia team is critical to ensure patient safety, satisfaction, and early recovery. It also helps with early detection and prompt management of complications.
- Special consideration needs to be taken in elderly, pregnant and lactating women.

References

1. Hu L, Sun X, Hao J, et al. Long-term follow-up of therapeutic ERCP in 78 patients aged 90 years or older. Sci Rep. 2014;4:4918.
2. Practice advisory for preanesthesia evaluation: an updated report by the American Society of Anesthesiologists Task Force on Preanesthesia Evaluation. Anesthesiology. 2012;116:522–38.
3. Practice guidelines for moderate procedural sedation and snalgesia 2018A report by the American Society of Anesthesiologists Task Force on Moderate Procedural Sedation and Analgesia, the American Association of Oral and Maxillofacial Surgeons, American College of Radiology, American Dental Association, American Society of Dentist Anesthesiologists, and Society of Interventional Radiology. Anesthesiology. 2018;128:437–79.
4. Apfelbaum JL, Hagberg CA, Caplan RA, et al. Practice guidelines for management of the difficult airway: an updated report by the American Society of Anesthesiologists Task Force on Management of the Difficult Airway. Anesthesiology. 2013;118:251–70.
5. For more information visit www.uptodate.com.
6. Coté GA, Hovis CE, Hovis RM, Waldbaum L, Early DS, Edmundowicz SA, Azar RR, Mullady DK, Jonnalagadda SS. A screening instrument for sleep apnea predicts airway maneuvers

in patients undergoing advanced endoscopic procedures. Clin Gastroenterol Hepatol. 2010;8:660–665.e1.
7. Coté GA, Hovis RM, Ansstas MA, Waldbaum L, Azar RR, Early DS, Edmundowicz SA, Mullady DK, Jonnalagadda SS. Incidence of sedation-related complications with propofol use during advanced endoscopic procedures. Clin Gastroenterol Hepatol. 2010;8:137–42.
8. Patel S, Vargo JJ, Khandwala F, Lopez R, Trolli P, Dumot JA, Conwell DL, Zuccaro G. Deep sedation occurs frequently during elective endoscopy with meperidine and midazolam. Am J Gastroenterol. 2005;100:2689–95.
9. Raymondos K, Panning B, Bachem I, Manns MP, Piepenbrock S, Meier PN. Evaluation of endoscopic retrograde cholangiopancreatography under conscious sedation and general anesthesia. Endoscopy. 2002;34:721–6.
10. Etzkorn KP, Diab F, Brown RD, Dodda G, Edelstein B, Bedford R, Venu RP. Endoscopic retrograde cholangiopancreatography under general anesthesia: indications and results. Gastrointest Endosc. 1998;47:363–7.
11. Cotton P, Romagnuolo J. A new comprehensive scale for ranking complexity of endoscopic procedures. Gut. 2011;60:A14.
12. Barnett SR, Berzin T, Sanaka S, Pleskow D, Sawhney M, Chuttani R. Deep sedation without intubation for ERCP is appropriate in healthier, non-obese patients. Dig Dis Sci. 2013;58:3287–92.
13. Thosani N, Banerjee S. Deep sedation or general anesthesia for ERCP? Dig Dis Sci. 2013;58:3061–3.
14. Atkins JH, Mandel JE. Recent advances in patient-controlled sedation. Curr Opin Anaesthesiol. 2008;21:759–65.
15. Mazanikov M, Udd M, Kylänpää L, Lindström O, Aho P, Halttunen J, Färkkilä M, Pöyhiä R. Patient-controlled sedation with propofol and remifentanil for ERCP: a randomized, controlled study. Gastrointest Endosc. 2011;73:260–6.
16. Crepeau T, Poincloux L, Bonny C, Lighetto S, Jaffeux P, Artigue F, Walleckx P, Bazin JE, Dapoigny M, Bommelaer G. Significance of patient-controlled sedation during colonoscopy. Results from a prospective randomized controlled study. Gastroenterol Clin Biol. 2005;29:1090–6.
17. Wehrmann T, Grotkamp J, Stergiou N, Riphaus A, Kluge A, Lembcke B, Schultz A. Electroencephalogram monitoring facilitates sedation with propofol for routine ERCP: a randomized, controlled trial. Gastrointest Endosc. 2002;56:817–24.

18. Soehle M, Ellerkmann RK, Grube M, Kuech M, Wirz S, Hoeft A, Bruhn J. Comparison between bispectral index and patient state index as measures of the electroencephalographic effects of sevoflurane. Anesthesiology. 2008;109:799–805.
19. Al-Sammak Z, Al-Falaki MM, Gamal HM. Predictor of sedation during endoscopic retrograde cholangiopancreatography--bispectral index vs clinical assessment. Middle East J Anaesthesiol. 2005;18:141–8.
20. Qadeer MA, Vargo JJ, Dumot JA, Zuccaro G, Stevens T, Parsi MA, Sanaka MR, Jang S, Lopez R. Capnography prevents hypoxemia during ERCP and EUS: a randomized controlled trial. Gastrointest Endosc. 2008;67:AB84.
21. Schlag C, Wörner A, Wagenpfeil S, Kochs EF, Schmid RM, von Delius S. Capnography improves detection of apnea during procedural sedation for percutaneous transhepatic cholangiodrainage. Can J Gastroenterol. 2013;27:582–6.
22. Bell GD, Quine A, Antrobus JH, Morden A, Burridge SM, Coady TJ, Lee J. Upper gastrointestinal endoscopy: a prospective randomized study comparing continuous supplemental oxygen via the nasal or oral route. Gastrointest Endosc. 1992;38:319–25.
23. Training Committee. American Society for Gastrointestinal Endoscopy. Training guideline for use of propofol in gastrointestinal endoscopy. Gastrointest Endosc. 2004;60:167–72.
24. Spoletini G, Alotaibi M, Blasi F, Hill NS. Heated humidified high-flow nasal oxygen in adults: mechanisms of action and clinical implications. Chest. 2015;148:253–61.
25. Chanques G, Constantin J-M, Sauter M, Jung B, Sebbane M, Verzilli D, Lefrant J-Y, Jaber S. Discomfort associated with underhumidified high-flow oxygen therapy in critically ill patients. Intensive Care Med. 2009;35:996–1003.
26. Kallstrom TJ, American Association for Respiratory Care (AARC). AARC Clinical Practice Guideline: oxygen therapy for adults in the acute care facility--2002 revision and update. Respir Care. 2002;47:717–20.
27. Tiruvoipati R, Lewis D, Haji K, Botha J. High-flow nasal oxygen vs high-flow face mask: a randomized crossover trial in extubated patients. J Crit Care. 2010;25:463–8.
28. Schumann R, Natov NS, Rocuts-Martinez KA, Finkelman MD, Phan TV, Hegde SR, Knapp RM. High-flow nasal oxygen availability for sedation decreases the use of general anesthesia

during endoscopic retrograde cholangiopancreatography and endoscopic ultrasound. World J Gastroenterol. 2016;22:10398–405.
29. Daşkaya H, Uysal H, Çiftçi T, Baysal B, İdin K, Karaaslan K. Use of the gastro-laryngeal tube in endoscopic retrograde cholangiopancreatography cases under sedation/analgesia. Turk J Gastroenterol. 2016;27:246–51.
30. Fabbri C, Luigiano C, Cennamo V, Polifemo AM, Maimone A, Jovine E, D'Imperio N, Zanello M. The Gastro-Laryngeal Tube for interventional endoscopic biliopancreatic procedures in anesthetized patients. Endoscopy. 2012;44:1051–4.
31. Osborn IP, Cohen J, Soper RJ, Roth LA. Laryngeal mask airway--a novel method of airway protection during ERCP: comparison with endotracheal intubation. Gastrointest Endosc. 2002;56:122–8.
32. Terblanche NCS, Middleton C, Choi-Lundberg DL, Skinner M. Efficacy of a new dual channel laryngeal mask airway, the LMA®Gastro™ Airway, for upper gastrointestinal endoscopy: a prospective observational study. Br J Anaesth. 2018;120:353–60.
33. LMA Gastro Airway Photos copyright to Dr. Sreeni Jonnalagadda.
34. Wehrmann T, Kokabpick S, Lembcke B, Caspary WF, Seifert H. Efficacy and safety of intravenous propofol sedation during routine ERCP: a prospective, controlled study. Gastrointest Endosc. 1999;49:677–83.
35. Jung M, Hofmann C, Kiesslich R, Brackertz A. Improved sedation in diagnostic and therapeutic ERCP: propofol is an alternative to midazolam. Endoscopy. 2000;32:233–8.
36. Berzin TM, Sanaka S, Barnett SR, Sundar E, Sepe PS, Jakubowski M, Pleskow DK, Chuttani R, Sawhney MS. A prospective assessment of sedation-related adverse events and patient and endoscopist satisfaction in ERCP with anesthesiologist-administered sedation. Gastrointest Endosc. 2011;73:710–7.
37. Byrne MF, Baillie J. Propofol for conscious sedation? Gastroenterology. 2002;123:373–5.
38. Riphaus A, Stergiou N, Wehrmann T. Sedation with propofol for routine ERCP in high-risk octogenarians: a randomized, controlled study. Am J Gastroenterol. 2005;100:1957–63.
39. Muller S, Borowics SM, Fortis EA, Stefani LC, Soares G, Maguilnik I, Breyer HP, Hidalgo MPL, Caumo W. Clinical efficacy of dexmedetomidine alone is less than propofol for conscious sedation during ERCP. Gastrointest Endosc. 2008;67:651–9.

40. Seifert H, H Schmitt T, Gültekin T, F Caspary W, Wehrmann T. Sedation with propofol plus midazolam versus propofol alone for interventional endoscopic procedures: a prospective, randomized study. Aliment Pharmacol Ther. 2000;14:1207–14.
41. Ong WC, Santosh D, Lakhtakia S, Reddy N. A randomized controlled trial on use of propofol alone versus propofol with midazolam, ketamine, and pentazocine "sedato-analgesic cocktail" for sedation during ERCP. Endoscopy. 2007;39:807–12.
42. Graber RG. Propofol in the endoscopy suite: an anesthesiologist's perspective. Gastrointest Endosc. 1999;49:803–6.
43. Cohen LB, Dubovsky AN, Aisenberg J, Miller KM. Propofol for endoscopic sedation: a protocol for safe and effective administration by the gastroenterologist. Gastrointest Endosc. 2003;58:725–32.
44. Cohen LB, Hightower CD, Wood DA, Miller KM, Aisenberg J. Moderate level sedation during endoscopy: a prospective study using low-dose propofol, meperidine/fentanyl, and midazolam. Gastrointest Endosc. 2004;59:795–803.
45. Goh PK, Chiu CL, Wang CY, Chan YK, Loo PL. Randomized double-blind comparison of ketamine-propofol, fentanyl-propofol and propofol-saline on haemodynamics and laryngeal mask airway insertion conditions. Anaesth Intensive Care. 2005;33:223–8.
46. Bahrami Gorji F, Amri P, Shokri J, Alereza H, Bijani A. Sedative and analgesic effects of propofol-fentanyl versus Propofol-Ketamine during endoscopic retrograde cholangiopancreatography: a double-blind randomized clinical trial. Anesthesiol Pain Med. 2016; https://doi.org/10.5812/aapm.39835.
47. Akcakaya A, Koc B, Adas G, Kemik O. The use of ERCP during pregnancy: is it safe and effective? Hepato-Gastroenterology. 2014;61:296–8.
48. Basso L, McCollum PT, Darling MR, Tocchi A, Tanner WA. A study of cholelithiasis during pregnancy and its relationship with age, parity, menarche, breast-feeding, dysmenorrhea, oral contraception and a maternal history of cholelithiasis. Surg Gynecol Obstet. 1992;175:41–6.
49. Ludvigsson JF, Lebwohl B, Ekbom A, Kiran RP, Green PHR, Höijer J, Stephansson O. Outcomes of pregnancies for women undergoing endoscopy while they were pregnant: a nationwide cohort study. Gastroenterology. 2017;152:554–563.e9.

50. Shergill AK, Ben-Menachem T, Chandrasekhara V, et al. Guidelines for endoscopy in pregnant and lactating women. Gastrointest Endosc. 2012;76:18–24.
51. Drugs C on. The transfer of drugs and other chemicals into human Milk. Pediatrics. 2001;108:776–89.
52. Dailland P, Cockshott ID, Lirzin JD, Jacquinot P, Jorrot JC, Devery J, Harmey JL, Conseiller C. Intravenous propofol during cesarean section: placental transfer, concentrations in breast milk, and neonatal effects. A preliminary study. Anesthesiology. 1989;71:827–34.
53. Finkelmeier F, Tal A, Ajouaou M, Filmann N, Zeuzem S, Waidmann O, Albert J. ERCP in elderly patients: increased risk of sedation adverse events but low frequency of post-ERCP pancreatitis. Gastrointest Endosc. 2015;82:1051–9.
54. Amornyotin S. Sedation and monitoring for gastrointestinal endoscopy. World J Gastrointest Endosc. 2013;5:47–55.

Chapter 3
Difficult Biliary Cannulation

Rajesh N. Keswani

Case Presentations

Case 1

A 60-year-old female presents for an ambulatory ERCP for abnormal imaging of the bile duct suggesting a distal common bile duct mass. Endoscopic ultrasound is performed which identifies a distal biliary filling defect in an otherwise nondilated bile duct and a normal pancreas.

Initially, ventral pancreatic duct access is obtained with a guidewire. Contrast is not injected. To facilitate biliary cannulation, a guidewire is left in the pancreas duct, and biliary cannulation is attempted over the guidewire (Video 3.1).

Electronic Supplementary Material The online version of this chapter (https://doi.org/10.1007/978-3-030-12741-1_3) contains supplementary material, which is available to authorized users.

R. N. Keswani (✉)
Division of Gastroenterology, Northwestern Memorial Hospital, Chicago, IL, USA
e-mail: raj-keswani@northwestern.edu

D. K. Mullady (ed.), *Dilemmas in ERCP*,
https://doi.org/10.1007/978-3-030-12741-1_3

Case 2

A 75-year-old female presents for ambulatory ERCP for jaundice and suspected bile duct stricture on cross-sectional imaging. Endoscopic ultrasound is performed which identifies a distal biliary stricture with upstream bile duct dilation and a normal pancreas. ERCP is requested for tissue acquisition and palliation of jaundice.

Initially, only pancreatic duct access is obtained. The pancreas duct is nondilated. Guidewire access to the ventral duct is easily achieved. However, deep guidewire access past the head of the pancreas is not possible due to preferential advancement of the guidewire through a pancreatic side branch. Thus, we proceeded with freehand needle knife sphincterotomy for biliary access (Video 3.2).

Assessment

What Is a Difficult Biliary Cannulation?

When considering the best approach to a difficult biliary cannulation, it is important to acknowledge that even the definition of "difficult" cannulation is not standardized. In most research protocols, a cannulation is considered difficult if the endoscopist unsuccessfully attempts cannulation for at least 5–6 minutes and/or when there are more than 8–10 "attempts" (i.e., touches of the papilla) at cannulation [1, 2]. In the clinical trial setting, endoscopists may then consider some of the adjunctive measures detailed below to facilitate cannulation. However, in practice, many endoscopists may simply persist with standard cannulation techniques past 6 minutes before "trying something new."

Treatment/Management Options

Approach to Difficult Biliary Cannulation

We present a potential schematic approach to difficult biliary cannulation (Fig. 3.1). As can be seen by reviewing the algorithm, there are a finite number of endoscopic options to manage difficult biliary cannulation – the main difference for each individual situation is *when* each option is considered. In other words, while a needle knife sphincterotomy/fistulotomy can always be considered, the endoscopist might consider it at different timepoints/after trying different things based on the individual patient, endoscopist expertise, and endoscopic characteristics. Thus, the expert ERCP endoscopist should be familiar with each option as they may be periodically required to achieve cannulation.

The first major branchpoint in considering difficult biliary cannulation is whether or not the papilla is reached. Patients with altered anatomy (see Chap. 17) are considered separately. However, the papilla may also be inaccessible due to gastric or duodenal obstruction, often related to malignancy. In these patients, if expertise is available, the endoscopist has two options. Traditionally, these patients may be referred directly for percutaneous biliary drainage with an interventional radiologist; the main downside of this approach is the need for a percutaneous drain, at least temporarily. However, if requisite therapeutic EUS expertise is available, the endoscopist can consider EUS-guided drainage (see below).

Use of Optimal Technique, a Different Device and/or Changing Endoscope Position

Prior to switching devices, the endoscopist should consider whether they have implemented all reasonable interventions to facilitate cannulation. Of critical importance, the endoscopist should ensure that the papilla is fully visualized. When a transverse duodenal fold is obscuring the papilla, the endoscopist can utilize the cannulating device to lift that fold out of

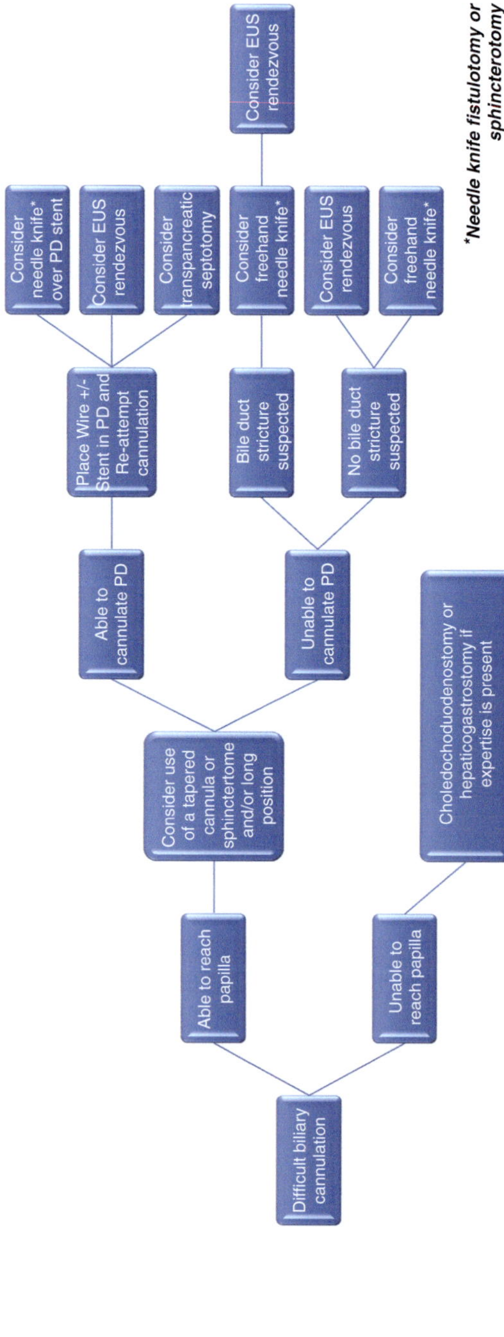

FIGURE 3.1 An algorithmic approach to difficult biliary cannulation

the way. This allows the endoscopist to better visualize the suspected trajectory of the bile duct. In some cases, the bile duct impression on the duodenal wall may inform the endoscopist that the direction of the bile duct is not the direction initially suspected. Finally, there should be careful adherence to best ERCP practice, including practices such as gently engaging the papilla, generally trying to access the bile duct at the 11 o'clock position, and beginning the approach to the bile duct from "below" the papilla [3].

If cannulation fails despite best practices, the endoscopist can consider switching cannulation devices [4] and/or changing position. However, there is limited data on switching cannulation devices or endoscope positions during ERCP to facilitate cannulation. Most recommendations are based on anecdotal experience and expert recommendations. Broadly, two types of cannulation devices are traditionally utilized during ERCP [4]. Cannulas are devices with at least one port (for guidewire or contrast injection) but no cutting wire for sphincterotomy. These devices tend to be smaller in caliber, which may aid in cannulation, but often do not allow the assistant to control the angulation of the device. In contrast, sphincterotomes can change their "bow" via tensing the cutting wire and thus changing the approach to the papilla. Based on the available data, most experts feel that a device that can "bow" (i.e., change direction/angle of approach) is superior to a straight cannula, and this is the general "first" approach [4].

As noted, most sphincterotomes are slightly larger caliber than most cannulas. Thus, there is a potential benefit in patients with small papillae to "trade" the ability of the sphincterotome to bow for the narrower profile of a tapered cannula. Thus, prior to considering a more "advanced" technique for biliary cannulation, the endoscopist should consider whether an alternate device would be useful. If a sphincterotome is being utilized without successful cannulation of either the bile duct or pancreas duct, consider the use of a tapered cannula. Alternatively, if a cannula is being utilized, consider use of a bowed sphincterotome to approach the bile duct at a more preferred angle.

In select cases, cannulation may be difficult for anatomic reasons including atypical position of the papilla (at the duodenal apex or in the distal duodenum) or intradiverticular position of the papilla. When the papilla is proximal (closer to the apex of the duodenum), the duodenoscope position may be very unstable. In these cases, changing the duodenoscope position from the short position to the long position can stabilize the duodenoscope and change the angle of approach to the papilla.

When the papilla is on the rim of diverticula, cannulation can generally be achieved in standard fashion. However, when cannulating the bile duct in a papilla adjacent to a diverticulum, it is important to consider that the bile duct generally traverses away from the diverticulum. Furthermore, due to the peridiverticular location of the papilla, the papilla tends to be "floppy." In our experience, simply engaging the superior aspect of the papilla with a lower profile cannula achieves biliary access in these cases. In contrast, when the papilla is entirely intradiverticular, simply identifying the papilla can be challenging. When the diverticulum is very large, the duodenoscope can almost always safely enter the diverticula to precisely identify the location of the papilla. Once the papilla is located, cannulation can be achieved in a standard fashion, generally with a more tapered cannulating device. If pancreatic access is achieved, consider immediate placement of a pancreatic stent as this may evert the papilla a bit, aiding in cannulation (see below).

Use of Inadvertent Pancreatic Cannulation to Facilitate Biliary Cannulation

During attempts at biliary cannulation, the endoscopist may inadvertently cannulate the pancreas duct. Although the natural inclination is to immediately remove the guidewire/device, the endoscopist should pause at this point to consider options. Specifically, if cannulation has persisted for several minutes, the endoscopist should strongly consider one of two advanced cannulation techniques at this point – cannulation over a guidewire ("double-guidewire technique") [5] or cannulation over a pancreas stent [5, 6]. The concept inherent to both techniques is that a guidewire or stent within the pancreas duct "straightens" the bile duct, thereby reducing the angulation required to achieve biliary cannulation. Moreover, the guidewire or stent provides an anatomical landmark to facilitate biliary cannulation.

There are several important considerations when trying to determine whether pancreatic duct access should be used to facilitate biliary cannulation, and if so, which technique should be utilized. First, it is important to consider whether or not deep guidewire access is easily achievable. Patients with pancreas divisum have a very short ventral duct, and attempts to place a deep guidewire or short pancreas stent are likely to be unsuccessful. Thus, most endoscopists reserve these techniques for conventional pancreatic ductal anatomy. Beyond this, some patients may have a very tortuous or looped pancreas duct in the head. Attempts at deep guidewire advancement may be traumatic in these cases, and the endoscopist may want to terminate further attempts. Second, the endoscopist should consider whether or not they ultimately would like to place a pancreas stent to reduce the risk of post-ERCP pancreatitis (see Chap. 14). Thus, if a stent is ultimately going to be placed anyway, the endoscopist may choose to cannulate over the pancreatic stent instead of the double-guidewire technique; this approach also reduces cost as a second guidewire is not needed. Additionally, it is reasonable to subjectively consider the size of the papillary orifice. Anecdotally, if the orifice is very small, the double-guidewire technique is preferred; in these cases, after placement of a pancreas stent, there is generally little room to cannulate "above" the stent. As it is much easier to cross over from double-guidewire technique to cannulating over a pancreas stent than vice versa, we will often begin with a double-guidewire technique in the setting of a very small papillary orifice. Finally, it is more challenging to securely maintain pancreatic duct guidewire access during cannulation attempts; with extensive duodenoscope manipulation, the guidewire may fall out. Thus, if achieving deep guidewire access is challenging, we prefer to immediately place a pancreas stent rather than attempt double-guidewire cannulation.

The initial approach to cannulation is similar for both techniques. Once pancreatic access is secured, the endoscopist engages the papilla at the 11 o'clock position – above and to the left – relative to the guidewire/stent. In our experience, the bile duct can often be accessed without bowing of the sphincterotome once a pancreas duct stent or guidewire is in place. If a bowed sphincterotome is required, it may be helpful to initially very superficially engage the papilla and then bow the sphincterotome. In cases where a pancreas stent has been placed and there is little room for engagement of the papilla, two techniques may be useful. First, we can advance the guidewire a few millimeters outside of the sphincterotome or cannula. This creates a much narrower profile leading edge of the cannulating device, facilitating engagement of the papilla above the stent. Alternatively, the endoscopist can switch to a more tapered cannulating device [5].

Use of a Needle Knife

When an endoscopist cannot place a deep pancreas guidewire/stent *or* placement of the guidewire/stent does not aid in biliary cannulation, the endoscopist might consider use of a needle knife [7]. A needle knife is a straight cutting wire that facilitates incision of the papillary tissue to achieve cannulation. A needle knife can be utilized over a pancreas stent or "free hand." Placement of the pancreas stent is valuable whenever possible to provide an anatomical landmark and to reduce the risk of post-ERCP pancreatitis (see Chap. 14). In our experience, a needle knife is felt to be a safer option – and potentially utilized before EUS access – when a pancreas stent is present.

Regardless of whether a pancreas stent is present, there are two main approaches to use of a needle knife – a needle knife sphincterotomy and a needle knife fistulotomy. A sphincterotomy, as the name implies, begins with the knife at the papillary orifice, and the goal is to replicate the typical pull-type sphincterotomy but without deep guidewire access into the bile duct. The main downside of this approach is that the endoscopist is working adjacent to the pancreas duct, and, especially when a pancreas stent is not present, the risk of pancreatitis is significant. Alternatively, the needle knife fistulotomy begins closer to the apex of the ampulla, distant from the papillary orifice. The main advantage of this approach is avoiding the pancreatic duct orifice. In fact, some endoscopists advocate a needle knife fistulotomy as an *initial* approach in cannulation for this reason, though this is very speculative based on available data [8].

Our general approach to use of a needle knife is to carefully dissect the tissue in layers and ideally ultimately identifying a "blush" of bile that identifies the precise location of the bile duct. Careful attention should be paid to the direction of the incision to avoid a retroperitoneal perforation. In some cases, biliary cannulation is not achieved after needle knife sphincterotomy/fistulotomy due to swelling or obscured landmarks. If ERCP is not urgent and no contrast has been injected into the bile duct, terminating the procedure and returning another day for a repeat attempt may facilitate biliary cannulation on a subsequent procedure.

Other Advanced ERCP Techniques

There are a variety of other ERCP techniques described in the literature when the above techniques have been unsuccessful. The appropriateness of these techniques must be considered in the context of the patient. Among the factors most important to consider is the risk of post-ERCP pancreatitis. Specifically, patients with pancreatic malignancy are less likely to develop severe post-ERCP pancreatitis with pancreatic duct manipulation. In patients with pancreas malignancy where deep pancreatic duct cannulation is achieved – but cannulation over a guidewire or stent is not possible – our preference is to consider endoscopic transpancreatic septotomy [9], often prior to needle knife sphincterotomy or fistulotomy. There appears to be little long-term harm to performing a pancreatic sphincterotomy in patients with advanced pancreas malignancy, and the deep pancreatic access allows for a more controlled cut than many achieve with a needle knife. In contrast, we do not advocate for this approach above EUS techniques in patients with a normal pancreas due to the risk of pancreatitis and unclear long-term risks of the pancreatic sphincterotomy.

Alternatively, suprapapillary puncture of the bile duct has been described in the literature but not widely adopted due to a lack of widely available tools [10]. This technique utilizes a needle to access the bile duct just above the papillary orifice. After guidewire access is achieved in the suspected biliary direction, a cholangiogram is performed to confirm biliary access. Once access is confirmed, the tract is dilated and utilized for further therapy. Similar to pure endoscopic suprapapillary access, EUS-guided suprapapillary access has been described, but limited data is available [11].

EUS-Guided Biliary Access

In select patients where basic and/or advanced ERCP techniques are unsuccessful in achieving bile duct access, EUS-guided biliary access may be considered [12]. While this is an important adjunctive technique to achieve biliary access, it is infrequently needed when ERCP is performed by expert endoscopists. Although a full assessment of EUS-guided biliary access is beyond the scope of this review, it is important for the endoscopist to have a basic understanding of its use and complexities. EUS-guided biliary access can be broadly categorized into three modalities:

1. EUS can be utilized to directly achieve biliary drainage, creating a fistula between the stomach and the left intrahepatic ducts (hepaticogastrostomy) or duodenal bulb and main bile duct (choleodochoduodenostomy) [13]. In cases where access to the papilla is not possible (e.g., malignant

duodenal obstruction), this may be the only endoscopic way to achieve biliary drainage. However, both hepatico-gastrostomy and choleodochoduodenostomy remain technically challenging. As tools evolve, this therapeutic modality may become more frequent [14].

2. Alternatively, after biliary access is achieved, the guidewire can be passed antegrade through the papilla. All endoscopic therapy is then performed in an antegrade fashion using the echoendoscope. For example, if a malignant distal CBD stricture is present, a metal stent is advance antegrade over the guidewire and placed transpapillary. This technique is generally only performed when antegrade access is achieved through the liver and may be of most use in altered anatomy (see Chap. 17).
3. Finally, and most commonly, EUS can be utilized to pass a wire antegrade through the papilla to facilitate standard ERCP, the so-called rendezvous technique. For this technique, endoscopic access to the papilla is mandatory. After the wire is passed antegrade through the papilla, the endoscopist exchanges the duodenoscope off the wire and then reintroduces the duodenoscope adjacent to the guidewire. The endoscopist can then cannulate the bile duct adjacent to the existing transpapillary wire or, instead, grasp the wire and backload it into the duodenoscope to facilitate cannulation. When considering rendezvous ERCP, the endoscopist has two choices – transgastric access via the intrahepatic ducts or transduodenal access to the main duct. Each option has its advantages and disadvantages. With transduodenal access, the risk of bile leak is greater, and antegrade advancement of the guidewire is challenging especially in the presence of a stricture; however, the main duct is generally a larger target making initial access easier. Alternatively, the transhepatic approach has a much lower risk of bile leak (due to surrounding liver parenchyma), and antegrade wire passage is easier, though the intrahepatic ducts are frequently less dilated making initial access more challenging.

Conclusions

Achieving initial biliary access is the essential first step to successfully provide biliary therapy. While careful attention to optimal technique will successfully achieve bile duct cannulation in the majority of cases, advanced techniques – most frequently double guidewire or cannulating over a pancreas stent – will be useful to cannulate the bile duct in more challenging cases. With the use of adjunctive techniques, bile duct cannulation success rates of well over 90% in native papillae are expected [15].

Pearls and Pitfalls

- Take time to obtain optimal position to visualize the ampulla and to understand the trajectory of the duct of interest before attempting cannulation.
- Develop a step-wise approach to cannulation, and know *when* to progress through the algorithm.
- Be comfortable with pancreatic duct wire and stent placement which may be necessary to facilitate biliary cannulation.
- In non-urgent ERCPs, it may be better to stop and try again another day rather than persist at biliary cannulation which may increase the risk for complications.

References

1. Cote GA, Mullady DK, Jonnalagadda SS, et al. Use of a pancreatic duct stent or guidewire facilitates bile duct access with low rates of precut sphincterotomy: a randomized clinical trial. Dig Dis Sci. 2012;57:3271–8.
2. Elmunzer BJ, Scheiman JM, Lehman GA, et al. A randomized trial of rectal indomethacin to prevent post-ERCP pancreatitis. N Engl J Med. 2012;366:1414–22.
3. Reddy DN, Nabi Z, Lakhtakia S. How to improve cannulation rates during endoscopic retrograde cholangiopancreatography. Gastroenterology. 2017;152:1275–9.

4. Committee AT, Kethu SR, Adler DG, et al. ERCP cannulation and sphincterotomy devices. Gastrointest Endosc. 2010;71:435–45.
5. Dumonceau JM, Deviere J, Cremer M. A new method of achieving deep cannulation of the common bile duct during endoscopic retrograde cholangiopancreatography. Endoscopy. 1998;30:S80.
6. Goldberg E, Titus M, Haluszka O, et al. Pancreatic-duct stent placement facilitates difficult common bile duct cannulation. Gastrointest Endosc. 2005;62:592–6.
7. Siegel JH. Precut papillotomy: a method to improve success of ERCP and papillotomy. Endoscopy. 1980;12:130–3.
8. Jin YJ, Jeong S, Lee DH. Utility of needle-knife fistulotomy as an initial method of biliary cannulation to prevent post-ERCP pancreatitis in a highly selected at-risk group: a single-arm prospective feasibility study. Gastrointest Endosc. 2016;84:808–13.
9. Goff JS. Long-term experience with the transpancreatic sphincter pre-cut approach to biliary sphincterotomy. Gastrointest Endosc. 1999;50:642–5.
10. Artifon EL, Sakai P, Ishioka S, et al. Suprapapillary puncture of the common bile duct for selective biliary access: a novel technique (with videos). Gastrointest Endosc. 2007;65:124–31.
11. Matsushita M, Uchida K, Okazaki K. EUS-guided suprapapillary puncture for safe selective biliary access. Gastrointest Endosc. 2007;66:865–6; author reply 866-7.
12. Khashab MA, Levy MJ, Itoi T, et al. EUS-guided biliary drainage. Gastrointest Endosc. 2015;82:993–1001.
13. Giovannini M, Moutardier V, Pesenti C, et al. Endoscopic ultrasound-guided bilioduodenal anastomosis: a new technique for biliary drainage. Endoscopy. 2001;33:898–900.
14. Paik WH, Lee TH, Park DH, et al. EUS-guided biliary drainage versus ERCP for the primary palliation of malignant biliary obstruction: a multicenter randomized clinical trial. Am J Gastroenterol. 2018;113(7):987.
15. Holt BA, Hawes R, Hasan M, et al. Biliary drainage: role of EUS guidance. Gastrointest Endosc. 2016;83:160–5.

Chapter 4
Difficult Bile Duct Stones

Rizwan Mahmood and Neil Gupta

Case 1

A 37-year-old female with a history of Billroth II gastrectomy, diabetes mellitus, hypertension, and hypercholesterolemia presents to the hospital emergency department with complaint of severe epigastric pain. Her onset of pain was 2 weeks ago, but it was on and off. The patient endorses nausea and two episodes of vomiting. On physical examination, the patient was seen to have yellow discoloration of the eyes and skin. Abdominal exam was normal, with no guarding or organomegaly. Vitals taken in the emergency department showed a fever of 100.3F. Laboratory results obtained showed elevated serum bilirubin and alkaline phosphatase.

R. Mahmood · N. Gupta (✉)
Department of Gastroenterology, Loyola University Medical Center, Maywood, IL, USA
e-mail: negupta@lumc.edu

D. K. Mullady (ed.), *Dilemmas in ERCP*,
https://doi.org/10.1007/978-3-030-12741-1_4

Transabdominal ultrasound was performed showing a dilated bile duct. A CT scan confirmed multiple stones in the common bile duct.

Diagnosis/Assessment

Often clinical evaluation and laboratory testing are not sufficient tools to diagnose choledocholithiasis. Imaging like transabdominal ultrasound and computed tomography is generally the first step to reaching a diagnosis. In patients with ascites or obesity, transabdominal ultrasound may not be sufficient to assess if stones are present in the common bile duct. Contrast agents administered during CT scanning may also cause unwanted side effects. When choledocholithiasis is equivocal, endoscopic ultrasonography (EUS) is a highly accurate modality to confirm the presence of stones prior to ERCP without the risk for complications such as pancreatitis. However, due to the anatomical changes after Billroth II gastrectomy or Roux-en-Y reconstruction, EUS may not be as accurate. ERCP is the first-line treatment for patients with confirmed, or high probability for, choledocholithiasis. In patients with altered anatomy, performing ERCP with therapeutic maneuvers can become difficult. In patients with a Billroth II gastrectomy, one option is to use a forward-viewing endoscope with a distal cap instead of a duodenoscope (Figs. 4.1 and 4.2).

Treatment/Management

The first step in common bile duct stone removal is an endoscopic sphincterotomy (EST). This has been the standard first-line therapy since it was first described in 1973. The main goal is to cut the sphincter of Oddi which may be the main obstruction to passage of the stone. Once the sphincter has been widened, the stone can be captured in a basket or removed with the help of a balloon tip catheter inflated

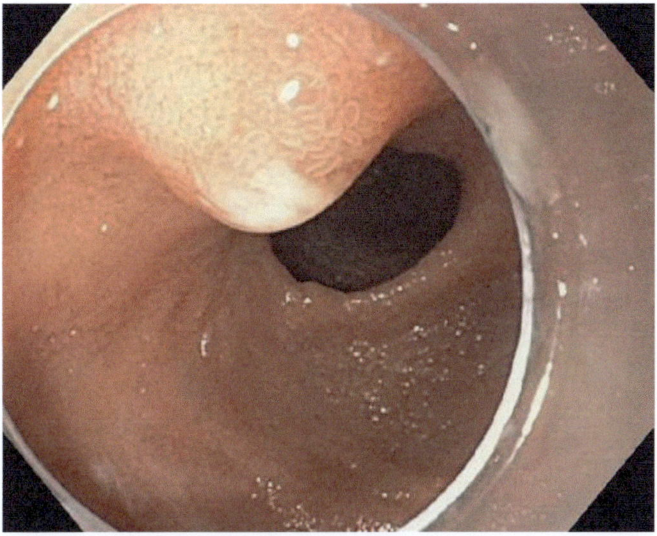

FIGURE 4.1 Pus emerging from the major papilla

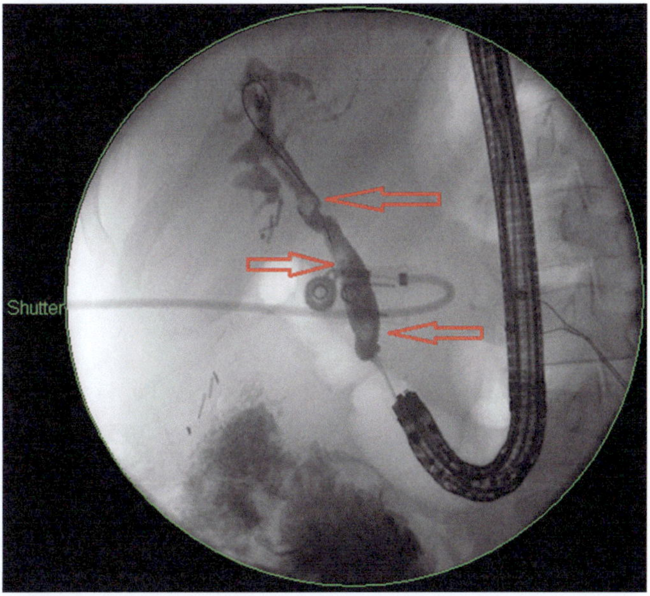

FIGURE 4.2 Fluoroscopic imaging showing multiple stones (red arrows) throughout the biliary tree

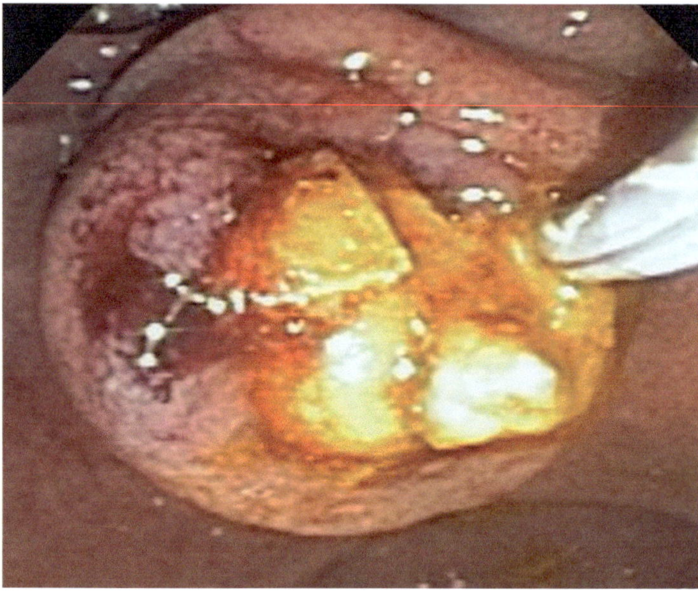

FIGURE 4.3 Extraction of biliary stone after sweeping the duct with a balloon

above the stone (Fig. 4.3). For standard stones, up to a 90% extraction rate can be achieved with EST. However, for larger stones (>15 mm), the extraction rate is much lower [1].

Stones that cannot be extracted after endoscopic sphincterotomy are often categorized as difficult bile duct stones. Endoscopic papillary balloon dilation (EPBD) or sphincteroplasty (without sphincterotomy) has recently been advocated as a first-line intervention for patients with difficult bile stones (Fig. 4.4a, b). The goal here is to dilate the papilla using a dilation balloon so that the biliary orifice is larger than the diameter of the stone. The exact duration of inflation is not standardized, but generally, the balloon is left inflated at least until there is obliteration of the waist on the balloon. Then the stone can be extracted from the bile duct using a standard basket or extraction balloon. A randomized control trial done by Liao et al. found that increasing the time of dilation from

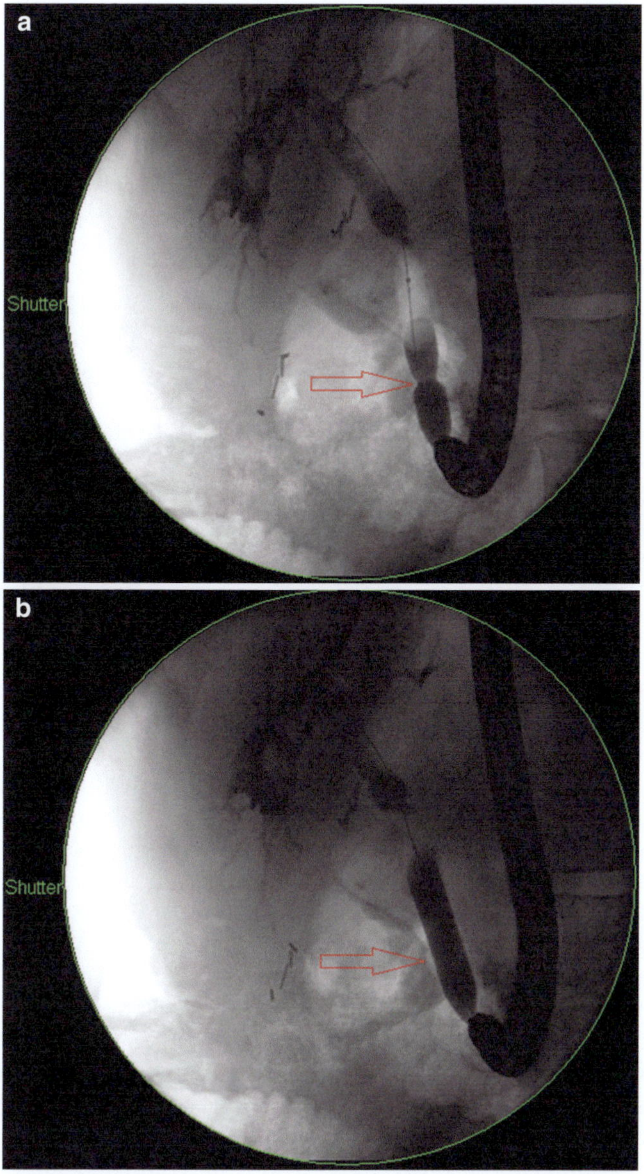

FIGURE 4.4 (**a**) Intraoperative fluoroscopic view from ERCP showing "waist" of sphincter (red arrow). (**b**) Intraoperative fluoroscopic view from ERCP demonstrating disappearance of sphincter "waist"

1 minute to 5 minutes improved efficacy and decreased the risk of pancreatitis [2]. This result is counterintuitive since pancreatitis would be expected to be higher the longer the pancreatic orifice is occluded. In fact, some studies have revealed an increased risk for pancreatitis with balloon dilation without EST compared to EST. Fujita et al. reported 100% and 99.3% clearance rate for EST and EPBD, respectively. They also found a rate of acute pancreatitis of 10.9% in the EPBD group compared to 2.8% in the EST group. Similarly, Ochi et al. found clearance rates of 98.17% and 92.7% in EST and EPBD groups, respectively [3, 4].

Multiple randomized controlled trials have assessed the safety and efficacy of EPBD vs EST. A majority of these trials found that though the rate of success for both procedures was similar, EPBD has a higher rate of pancreatitis when compared to EST [5–7]. In patients with a previous Billroth II gastrectomy, a standard EST may be difficult due to the inverted anatomy of the Billroth II state, and the design of the sphincterotome and cases where EST is attempted have an increased risk of bleeding [8]. EPBD has shown to have similar success rates but the rates of the bleeding are lower compared to EST [4, 5, 8]. In cases other than previous Billroth II gastrectomy and patients with increased bleeding risk, EST is still considered to be the gold standard due to the decreased risk of pancreatitis.

In cases of large stones, EST can be combined with large balloon dilation. A partial EST with large balloon dilation (ESLBD) was shown to be safe and has very good outcomes. A randomized trial by Heo et al. compared large stone removal in an ESLBD group and in an EST alone group. Successful stone removal was recorded in 94.4% of ESLBD group patients compared to 96.7% for the EST alone group [9]. Performing only a partial EST helps in reducing the overall bleeding risk, and the separation of the pancreatic and biliary orifices reduces the risk pancreatitis due to EPBD. Randomized controlled trials comparing ESLBD to EST alone found that though the success rate was relatively similar in both groups, the complication rates were lower in combined therapy patients. Teoh et al. also compared patients undergoing ESLBD to patients undergoing EST alone. They showed a clearance rate of 89% in both groups and complication rate of 10.3% in the EST alone group and 6.8% in the ESLBD group [3, 10]. Another study compared a group of patients subjected to ESLBD with a group subjected to EST followed by mechanical lithotripsy and found a success rate of 98% in the ESLBD group and 91% the EST plus mechanical lithotripsy group. Complications were reported at 4.4% and 20% for the ESLBD and EST group, respectively [11]. Complications for these procedures can be divided into short-term and long-term complications as shown in Table 4.1.

The success rate of EST, EPBD, and ESLBD is high, but it is not 100%. There are cases when multiple attempts are still unable to extract the stone in the common bile duct. The most common are patients where the diameter of the biliary orifice and distal CBD cannot be made large enough to accommodate the size of the stone. Biliary endoprosthesis/stenting is often performed to prevent impaction of the stone, to decompress the biliary tree to alleviate jaundice and cholangitis, and to act as a bridge for future curative therapy (Fig. 4.5). These also provide a mechanism for the stone to be gradually softened and fragmented over time due to the constant pressure of the stent on the stone. In many studies, a stent placement for 3–6 months resulted in the subsequent reduction in size of large stones, fragmentation into smaller stones, or complete clearance of the stone from the duct [12–14]. The stent is then removed, the bile duct is dilated and cleaned out to remove any stones that may be remaining. These stents can be either plastic or fully covered metal stents. However, in our experience, plastic stents are more effective in these cases.

Table 4.1 Complications of EST and ESLBD procedures

Early complications	Late complications
Pancreatitis	Recurrence of bile duct stones
Bleeding	Acute cholecystitis
Perforation	Bleeding
Cholangitis	

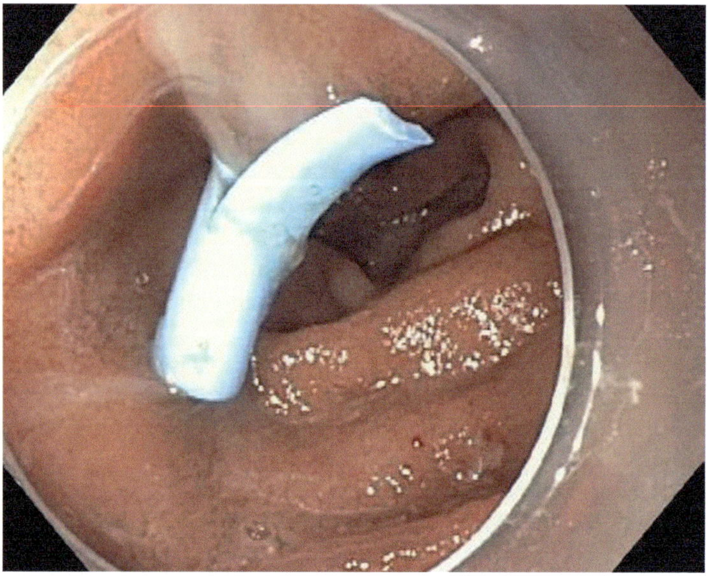

FIGURE 4.5 Plastic biliary stent with a single external flap and a single internal flap. Pus can be seen flowing from the stent

Case 2

A 66-year-old male has a 2-month history of intermittent right upper quadrant pain. He has a history of alcohol abuse and chronic pancreatitis. He is ill appearing and jaundiced. On examination, there is tenderness on palpation of the right upper quadrant. Laboratory results show hyperbilirubinemia, elevated alkaline phosphatase, and an elevated white cell count with left shift. Temperature was 101.1F. Transabdominal ultrasound showed dilated gallbladder with stones along with a dilated common bile duct. ERCP performed outlined a 15 mm stone in the common hepatic duct with a narrow intrapancreatic CBD without overt stricture. At the time of ERCP, ESLBD was performed but was unsuccessful in removing the stone due to the large size of the stone and inability to dilate the distal CBD.

When these methods of extraction fail, lithotripsy is the next best option. There are three main types of lithotripsy therapy:

- Mechanical lithotripsy.
- Electrohydraulic lithotripsy (EHL).
- Laser lithotripsy.

Mechanical lithotripsy involves capturing a stone in a lithotripter compatible metal basket and advancing a metal cable to the center of the stone by cranking a handle to apply pressure on and fragment the stone (Figs. 4.6 and 4.7). The

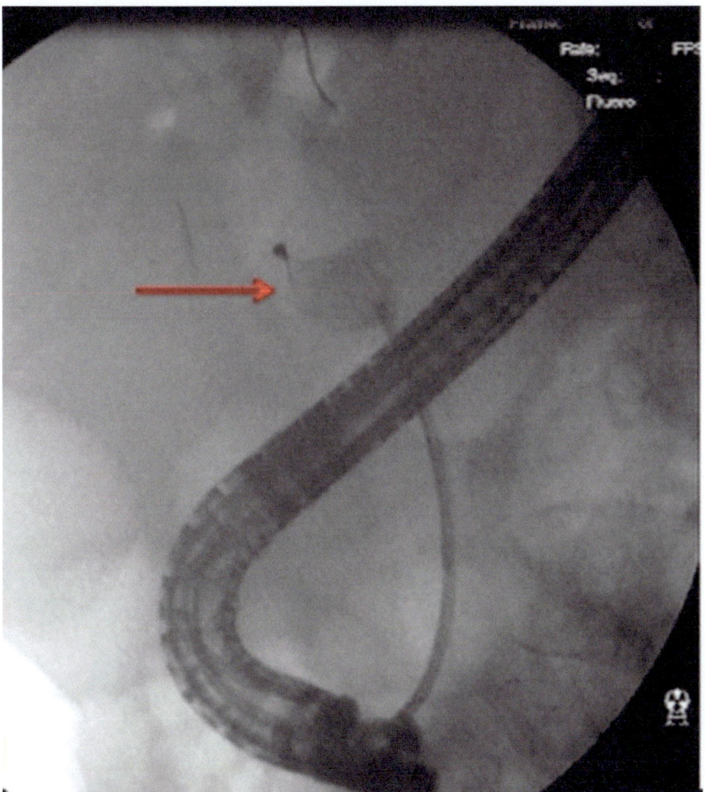

FIGURE 4.6 Fluoroscopic view of basket (red arrow) encapsulating stone

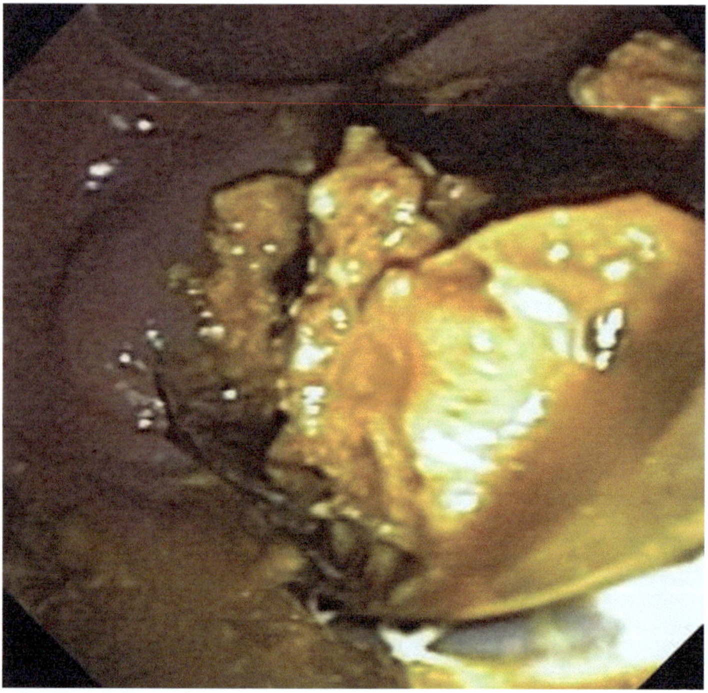

FIGURE 4.7 Extraction of biliary stone using a basket

stone fragments can then be retrieved with standard extraction techniques. In cases of excessively large stones, mechanical lithotripsy may need to be repeated several times to achieve complete extraction. The success rates of mechanical lithotripsy are about 80–90%; however, multiple attempts may be required. [15–17] The major complication associated with this procedure is basket impaction. Other complications include pancreatitis, cholangitis, and bleeding but at lower rates.

Electrohydraulic lithotripsy and laser lithotripsy are most useful for stones too large to be captured in a basket for mechanical lithotripsy. The preferred option for laser lithotripsy has become pulsed solid-state lasers like the holmium:YAG and q-switched neodymium:YAG. Less commonly used are the flashlamp-pumped pulsed dye lasers containing coumarin dye or rhodamine 6G dye. This procedure involves advancing an EHL or laser fiber through a cholangioscope as close as possible to the stone. A preset wattage pulse is then delivered for 1–2 seconds until the stone fragments. Constant saline irrigation is required for this procedure, as this helps in visualization and clearing of debris and in EHL it aids transmission of the shock wave. The fragments are then removed using standard extraction techniques. Successful fragmentation is achieved in about 75–80% of EHL cases, but combination of EHL with laser lithotripsy achieves stone clearance rates of up to 90% [18, 19]. The main complication of EHL and laser lithotripsy is perforation of the bile duct. Extra care should be used to prevent the EHL and laser probes from touching the wall of the bile duct. However, the rate of perforation is only about 1%.The underlying principle and indications for laser lithotripsy are similar to EHL. Laser lithotripsy provides a focused high-energy shock wave to fragment stones through pulsed laser systems. The fragmented stones are then extracted through standard techniques. Trials comparing laser lithotripsy with conventional lithotripsy show that laser lithotripsy achieves higher rate of clearance of large bile duct stones. However, there is an extra cost to this procedure, and it is not readily available. Hemobilia due to tissue damage during the laser pulse is one of the main complications of this procedure. Other complications include cholangitis and pancreatitis, but to a lesser extent.

Outcomes

- Case 1: This patient presented with multiple large stones in the bile duct on CT imaging and was admitted for stone removal. Following an unsuccessful ESLBD for stone removal, a plastic stent was placed and the patient was discharged. The patient was reevaluated after 3 months with repeat ERCP confirming resolution of stones, and the stents were successfully removed.

- Case 2: This patient was diagnosed with a large (15 mm) stone in the common hepatic duct by ERCP at which time ESLBD was attempted but unsuccessful due to the large stone size. Mechanical lithotripsy was utilized to fragment the stone, and fragments were removed with basket retrieval and the patient was discharged.

Once stones have been successfully removed, any stents that were placed are also removed and not replaced. We do not use ursodiol for stone dissolution. The patient's liver function is evaluated 2–4 weeks post procedure to ensure normal levels of liver enzymes. Recurrence of choledocholithiasis following an endoscopic bile duct clearance ranges between 4% and 25% [20, 21]. Thus, the patient is counseled on the risk of recurrence and the monitor for any signs and symptoms of recurrence. The patients are also asked to follow up in the clinic to ensure that they are asymptomatic. We do not use regular surveillance, blood testing, or imaging for follow-up with patients.

Pearls and Pitfalls

- To remove a bile duct stone, the endoscopist must either make the biliary orifice and distal CBD diameter larger than the stone (through EST, EPBD, or ESLBD) or make the stone smaller than the diameter of the biliary orifice/distal CBD (through lithotripsy).
- Our practice is to perform EST (even partial EST) prior to balloon dilation of the papilla (i.e., ESLBD) in patients with difficult bile duct stones to reduce the risk of pancreatitis associated with EPBD alone.
- Biliary endoprosthesis has shown to reduce the size of and fragment large stones and can be utilized as bridging therapy.
- In patients with a narrow/strictured distal CBD, lithotripsy (EHL and/or laser lithotripsy) should be considered early.

References

1. Lauri A, Horton RC, Davidson BR, Burroughs AK, Dooley JS. Endoscopic extraction of bile duct stones: management related to stone size. Gut. 1993;34(12):1718–21.
2. Liao WC, Lee CT, Chang CY, Leung JW, Chen JH, Tsai MC, et al. Randomized trial of 1-minute versus 5-minute endoscopic balloon dilation for extraction of bile duct stones. Gastrointest Endosc. 2010;72(6):1154–62.
3. Fujita N, Maguchi H, Komatsu Y, Yasuda I, Hasebe O, Igarashi Y, et al. Endoscopic sphincterotomy and endoscopic papillary balloon dilatation for bile duct stones: a prospective randomized controlled multicenter trial. Gastrointest Endosc. 2003;57(2):151–5.
4. Ochi Y, Mukawa K, Kiyosawa K, Akamatsu T. Comparing the treatment outcomes of endoscopic papillary dilation and endoscopic sphincterotomy for removal of bile duct stones. J Gastroenterol Hepatol. 1999;14(1):90–6.
5. Disario JA, Freeman ML, Bjorkman DJ, Macmathuna P, Petersen BT, Jaffe PE, et al. Endoscopic balloon dilation compared with sphincterotomy for extraction of bile duct stones. Gastroenterology. 2004;127(5):1291–9.
6. Arnold JC, Benz C, Martin WR, Adamek HE, Riemann JF. Endoscopic papillary balloon dilation vs. sphincterotomy for removal of common bile duct stones: a prospective randomized pilot study. Endoscopy. 2001;33(7):563–7.
7. Weinberg BM, Shindy W, Lo S. Endoscopic balloon sphincter dilation (sphincteroplasty) versus sphincterotomy for common bile duct stones. Cochrane Database Syst Rev. 2006;18(4):CD004890.
8. Bergman JJ, van Berkel AM, Bruno MJ, Fockens P, Rauws EA, Tijssen JG, et al. A randomized trial of endoscopic balloon dilation and endoscopic sphincterotomy for removal of bile duct stones in patients with a prior Billroth II gastrectomy. Gastrointest Endosc. 2001;53(1):19–26.
9. Heo JH, Kang DH, Jung HJ, et al. Endoscopic sphincterotomy plus large-balloon dilation versus endoscopic sphincterotomy for removal of bile-duct stones. Gastrointest Endosc. 2007;66(4):720–6; quiz 768, 771.
10. Teoh AY, Cheung FK, Hu B, Pan YM, Lai LH, Chiu PW, et al. Randomized trial of endoscopic sphincterotomy with balloon dilation versus endoscopic sphincterotomy alone for removal of bile duct stones. Gastroenterology. 2013;144(2):341–345.e1.

11. Stefanidis G, Viazis N, Pleskow D, Manolakopoulos S, Theocharis L, Christodoulou C, Kotsikoros N, et al. Large balloon dilation vs. mechanical lithotripsy for the management of large bile duct stones: a prospective randomized study. Am J Gastroenterol. 2011;106(2):278–85.
12. Horiuchi A, Nakayama Y, Kajiyama M, Kato N, Kamijima T, Graham DY, et al. Biliary stenting in the management of large or multiple common bile duct stones. Gastrointest Endosc. 2010;71(7):1200–1203.e2.
13. Aslan F, Arabul M, Celik M, Alper E, Unsal B. The effect of biliary stenting on difficult common bile duct stones. Prz Gastroenterol. 2014;9(2):109–15.
14. Chan AC, Ng EK, Chung SC, Lai CW, Lau JY, Sung JJ, et al. Common bile duct stones become smaller after endoscopic biliary stenting. Endoscopy. 1998;30(4):356–9.
15. Chang WH, Chu CH, Wang TE, Chen MJ, Lin CC. Outcome of simple use of mechanical lithotripsy of difficult common bile duct stones. World J Gastroenterol. 2005;11(4):593–6.
16. Garg PK, Tandon RK, Ahuja V, Makharia GK, Batra Y. Predictors of unsuccessful mechanical lithotripsy and endoscopic clearance of large bile duct stones. Gastrointest Endosc. 2004;59(6):601–5.
17. Shaw MJ, Mackie RD, Moore JP, Dorsher PJ, Freeman ML, Meier PB, et al. Results of a multicenter trial using a mechanical lithotripter for the treatment of large bile duct stones. Am J Gastroenterol. 1993;88(5):730–3.
18. Adamek HE, Maier M, Jakobs R, Wessbecher FR, Neuhauser T, Riemann JF. Management of retained bile duct stones: a prospective open trial comparing extracorporeal and intracorporeal lithotripsy. Gastrointest Endosc. 1996;44(1):40–7.
19. Adamek HE, Schneider AR, Adamek MU, Jakobs R, Buttmann A, Benz C, et al. Treatment of difficult intrahepatic stones by using extracorporeal and intracorporeal lithotripsy techniques: 10 years' experience in 55 patients. Scand J Gastroenterol. 1999;34(11):1157–61.
20. Konstantakis C, Triantos C, Theopistos V, Theocharis G, Maroulis I, Diamantopoulou G, Thomopoulos K. Recurrence of choledocholithiasis following endoscopic bile duct clearance: long term results and factors associated with recurrent bile duct stones. World J Gastrointest Endosc. 2017;9(1):26–33.
21. Tanaka S, Sawayama T, Yoshioka T. Endoscopic papillary balloon dilation and endoscopic sphincterotomy for bile duct stones: long-term outcomes in a prospective randomized controlled trial. Gastrointest Endosc. 2004;59(6):614–8.

Chapter 5
Indeterminate Biliary Strictures

Motaz H. Ashkar and Natalie Cosgrove

Case Presentation

A 73-year-old male with abdominal pain was found to have cholelithiasis and underwent a cholecystectomy. He presented 7 months later with continued abdominal pain and new onset jaundice with total bilirubin elevated at 7.4 mg/dL. MRI/MRCP demonstrated a 4 cm long stricture of the common bile duct extending to the hilum and involving the distal right intrahepatic bile ducts with resulting intrahepatic duct dilation (Fig. 5.1), as well as amorphous soft tissue filling the hepatic hilum and surrounding the common duct concerning for malignancy. ERCP at that time showed a 40 mm stricture from the mid common bile duct to common hepatic duct (Fig. 5.2). Cytology from ERCP brushings revealed scattered atypical cells. EUS demonstrated a dilated common hepatic duct to 14 mm with an abrupt tapering of the bile duct

---

Electronic Supplementary Material The online version of this chapter (https://doi.org/10.1007/978-3-030-12741-1_5) contains supplementary material, which is available to authorized users.

M. H. Ashkar · N. Cosgrove (✉)
Division of Gastroenterology, Washington University in St. Louis, School of Medicine, St. Louis, MO, USA
e-mail: motaz.ashkar@wustl.edu; ncosgrove@wustl.edu

D. K. Mullady (ed.), *Dilemmas in ERCP*,
https://doi.org/10.1007/978-3-030-12741-1_5

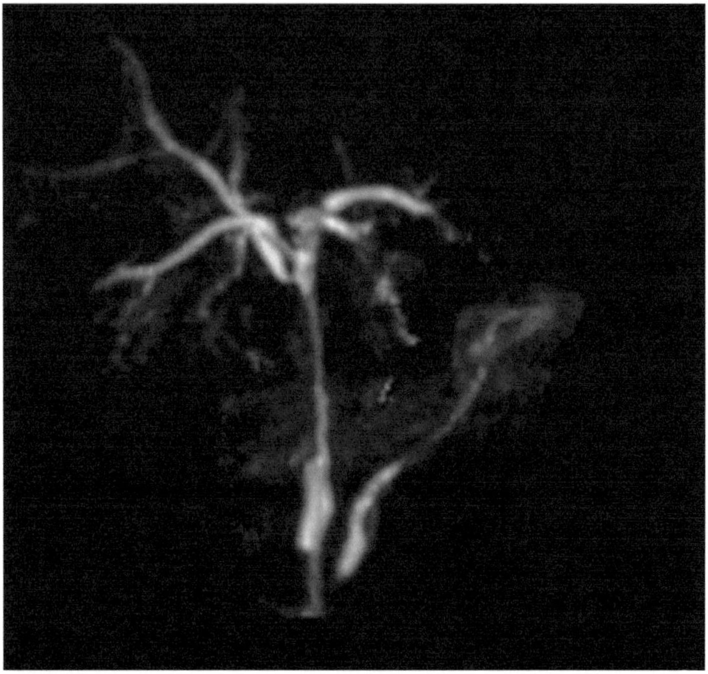

FIGURE 5.1 Long common bile duct stricture with hilar and distal right intrahepatic bile duct involvement causing intrahepatic duct dilation (***MRCP***)

as it was traced toward the hilum. No adenopathy or mass lesion was seen. CA 19-9 was normal at <0.8 units/mL, while CEA was elevated at 7.2 ng/mL (ULN 3).

Diagnosis and Assessment

Clinical History and Differential Diagnosis

The clinical history of a patient presenting with an indeterminate biliary stricture may be helpful in suggesting a diagnosis. The patient's medical comorbidities, surgical history, and pre-

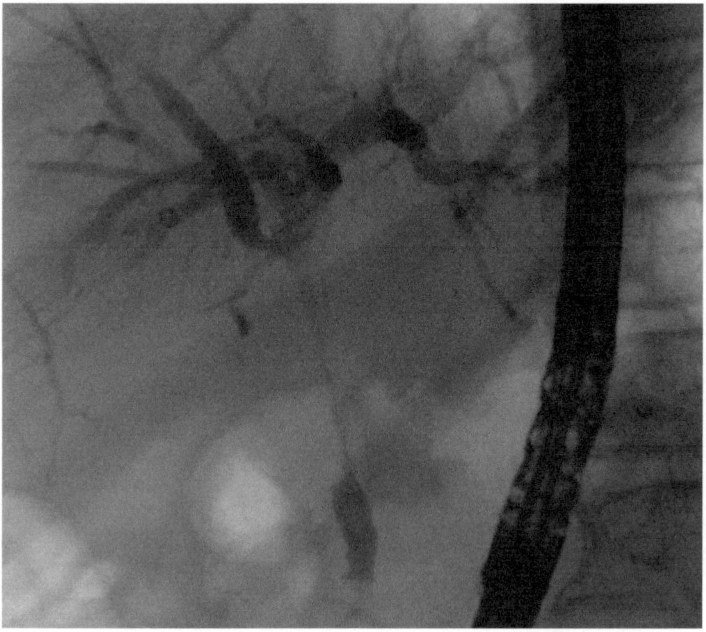

FIGURE 5.2 Long (4 cm) stricture extending from mid common bile duct to common hepatic duct (***ERCP***)

senting symptoms may aid in increasing the pretest probability of either benign or malignant etiology (Table 5.1). Specifically, a history of inflammatory bowel disease, PSC, chronic pancreatitis, elevated IgG4, and acuity of presenting symptoms is useful. Often, however, the diagnosis is still unclear. While symptoms such as weight loss are classically associated with malignancy, this can be seen in both benign and malignant disease [1]. Benign conditions, notably primary sclerosing cholangitis (PSC) and IgG4-related sclerosing cholangitis, can often mimic malignant disease. Iatrogenic biliary injury post cholecystectomy and liver transplant are responsible for the majority of benign biliary strictures. In primary sclerosing cholangitis (PSC), the typical cholangiographic pattern of intra- or extrahepatic ductal beading in the presence or absence of inflammatory bowel disease is fairly diagnostic, but

Table 5.1 Causes of biliary strictures (1, 2)

Benign causes
Primary sclerosing cholangitis
IgG4-mediated cholangiopathy
Iatrogenic biliary injury with fibrotic or ischemic strictures (i.e., post cholecystectomy and liver transplant)
HIV-related cholangiopathy
Pancreatitis (acute and chronic)
Pancreatic cysts
Mirizzi syndrome
Eosinophilic cholangitis
Infiltrative hepatic sarcoidosis
Radiation induced strictures
Portal bilopathy
Malignant causes
Cholangiocarcinoma
Primary pancreatic adenocarcinoma
Hepatocellular carcinoma
Ampullary cancer
Lymphoma
Metastatic cancer (i.e., regional lymphadenopathy)

the higher association with cholangiocarcinoma (30%) creates a dilemma when a single dominant stricture is the initial presentation of PSC. IgG4-related sclerosing cholangitis may present similarly to cholangiocarcinoma with obstructive cholestasis, enlargement of the pancreas, and regional lymphadenopathy. The likelihood of an underlying malignancy is usually associated with higher direct hyperbilirubinemia, elevated serum CA 19-9 levels, normal to high-normal serum IgG4 levels, and complete ductal obstruction on cholangiogram.

Malignancy accounts for approximately 70% of biliary strictures, most commonly due to pancreatic adenocarcinoma and cholangiocarcinoma. In contrast, only up to 30% of biliary strictures are secondary to benign causes [1, 2]. Therefore, in approaching patients with an indeterminate biliary stricture, it is prudent to presume malignancy until definitive evidence of a benign cause is apparent.

Tumor Markers

Many serum tumor biomarkers offer good diagnostic value to delineate the malignant potential of biliary strictures, most notably carbohydrate antigen 19-9 (CA 19-9) and carcinoembryonic antigen (CEA). CEA has diagnostic sensitivity of (33–68%) and specificity of (79–95%) for cholangiocarcinoma. CA 19-9 is the most commonly used circulating marker for both cholangiocarcinoma and exocrine pancreatic cancer. At levels above 37 U/mL, CA 19-9 achieves a median diagnostic sensitivity of 79% and a median specificity of 82% for pancreatic adenocarcinoma. CA 19-9 diagnostic performance must be interpreted with caution at a cutoff point of 100 U/mL, which increases specificity to 98% at the expense of a sensitivity reduction to 68%. The rate of false-positive results is also increased in the setting of cholestasis, cholangitis, and other non-cancerous conditions including hepatic cirrhosis, cholecystitis, pancreatitis, thyroiditis, cystic fibrosis, and non-pancreaticobiliary neoplasia (i.e., colorectal, gastric, and ovarian cancer) [1, 2].

Several circulating biomarkers have been studied for the diagnosis of cholangiocarcinoma including transthyretin (TTR), interleukin-6 (IL-6), mucin-5AC (MUC5AC), and matrix metalloproteinase-7 (MMP-7). However, these tests remain with limited utility due to insufficient validation and are therefore not used routinely during the workup of indeterminate biliary strictures.

Cross-Sectional Imaging

Transabdominal ultrasound (US) is readily available, noninvasive, and safe, which makes it a useful utility as an initial screening imaging modality for patients with new onset cholestasis. However, while this test is highly sensitive in detecting intrahepatic biliary dilatation, it has significant limitations in exploring for downstream biliary obstruction and accurate evaluation for biliary strictures or masses. Abdominal CT offers better diagnostic sensitivity (69%) for neoplastic biliary strictures compared with routine abdominal ultrasound (47%), and the use of new scanners (i.e., multi-detector CT) provides detailed characteristics of malignant strictures which can determine surgical resectability based on tumor spread and vascular invasion. On contrast CT, ductal infiltrating cholangiocarcinoma manifests as a hypo-attenuating pathology on the arterial phase in the absence of a mass lesion with delayed phase enhancement. While the specificity reaches 80% in diagnosing biliary strictures, CT cannot accurately distinguish between cancerous and non-cancerous strictures in the absence of focal mass lesions [3]. MRI/MRCP is the imaging modality of choice for suspected biliary strictures. Compared to CT, MRI lacks ionizing radiation and offers a noninvasive alternative to ERCP with high test sensitivity and specificity in determining the level and type of obstructive cholestasis. In a meta-analysis, MRCP sensitivity and specificity was 98% in identifying the biliary obstruction level and diagnosed malignant strictures with 88% sensitivity and 95% specificity. MRCP is limited however by high cost, motion artifact, and inability to perform tissue acquisition [1, 2].

Endoscopy

Endoscopy with ERCP or EUS-FNA helps facilitate obtaining a tissue diagnosis, while ERCP allows concurrent palliation of any jaundice. There is no approved algorithmic approach in choosing one or more endoscopic techniques in the evaluation of indeterminate biliary strictures; it is largely dependent on availability, diagnostic accuracy in evaluating distal versus proximal biliary strictures, presence of mass lesions, and low pretest probability for benign causes of biliary obstruction.

Endoscopic Retrograde Cholangiopancreatography (ERCP)

ERCP is a widely used intervention in evaluating biliary strictures as it provides both diagnostic and therapeutic options for biliary obstruction. Contrast injection during ERCP delineates biliary strictures to determine their location and approximate length. On interpretation of the fluoroscopic images, certain cholangiographic morphologies suggestive of malignancy include longer stricture length, irregular margins, shelf-like morphology, asymmetrical narrowing, presence of nodularity, and dual simultaneous dilation in the common bile duct and main pancreatic duct (double duct sign). Exclusively, the cholangiographic appearance of a biliary stricture has low and variable sensitivities (11–74%) in diagnosing malignancy with accuracy ranging between 72% and 80%. Therefore, cholangiography must be coupled with either conventional (i.e., bile aspirate cytology, removed plastic stents cytology, direct brush cytology, fluoroscopy-guided forceps biopsy) or advanced methods (i.e., fluorescent in situ hybridization) of tissue acquisition in establishing a diagnosis for indeterminate biliary strictures [1–4]. Multiple methods of obtaining tissue should be utilized to improve diagnostic yield. A prospective series that combined both routine brush cytology and fluoroscopy-guided forceps biopsy yielded diagnostic accuracy of 63% versus individual sensitivities of 43% and 35%, respectively. This was replicated in a second study reporting dual modality sensitivity of 70% compared to separate brush cytology sensitivity of 47% and 65% for biopsy sampling [3–6].

Brush Cytology

Brush cytology performed during ERCP is safe, cost-effective, and easy to perform. For this reason, it is the first-line and most preferred diagnostic method for tissue acquisition in biliary strictures. Abundant cellularity on cytology samples is an essential component of diagnosing neoplasia; however, this is an uncommon feature of indeterminate biliary strictures, likely in part due to the presence of firm desmoplastic reactions in biliary malignancies that create insufficient cellularity. This leads to high false-negative and low-yield cytological examinations. In general, brush cytology offers high specificity in sampling malignant biliary strictures approaching 95%. However, sensitivity is low at 30–57% [7–9]. Many factors are responsible for the variability and poor diagnostic yield of this modality, primarily related to the stricture type, cytology analysis interpretation, and endoscopist expertise. Indeterminate brush cytology results are more common in hilar and severely narrow lesions and in strictures with neoplastic involvement of the medial walls of the bile ducts [2, 6]. Gross cancer characteristics of surface mucosal ulceration can also impact the degree of cellularity sampled by brushing. Diagnosing an intrinsic biliary stricture secondary to cholangiocarcinoma by brush cytology offers cancer detection rates ranging between 44% and 80% compared to detection rates of 15–65% for extrinsic strictures related to pancreatic adenocarcinoma.

To perform brush cytology, the stricture is first delineated on cholangioscopy. A cytology brush is then advanced through the sheath proximal to the stricture then moved back and forth across the narrowed segment approximately five to 10 times. The brush is then withdrawn into the sheath, and both are withdrawn from the endoscope as one unit. The brush end is then cut and placed in a preservative solution for cytopathological analysis. This technique was shown to improve diagnostic accuracy for malignancy. Modifications to the brush cytology technique for better cellularity by disrupting the epithelial ductal surface of biliary strictures using balloon dilation, catheter dilators, and the use of longer or stiffer brushes have not been shown to improve diagnostic accuracy [3, 4, 6].

Bile Aspirate and Biliary Stents Cytology

Although safe and simple, the diagnostic accuracy for both isolated intraductal bile aspiration and retrieved biliary stents cytology is low at 11.5% and 13%, respectively. Both techniques can however be coupled with routine brush cytology to improve yield. To perform intraductal bile aspiration, aspiration of at least 20 mL of bile through a catheter at the proximal end of a biliary stricture is done following brush cytology. Biliary stents exfoliate ductal epithelium by repeated trauma and cause adherence of neoplastic cells; hence, removed stent surface may be smeared and washed into cytology solution for analysis [6].

Fluoroscopy-Guided Forceps Biopsy

Fluoroscopy-guided forceps biopsy allows for direct tissue acquisition from biliary strictures under fluoroscopic guidance in an attempt to overcome the low diagnostic yield of brush cytology. Theoretically, it samples the biliary ducts subepithelial stroma and hence can sample tumors that are limited to the subepithelial layer and not projecting into the ductal lumen. Unfortunately, various studies comparing ERCP intraductal biopsy performance to brush cytology found no significant difference between the two techniques with pooled sensitivity of 48% and 45%, respectively, while both modalities remain highly specific at 99%. This shared limitation is probably secondary to the variability in tumors characteristics. As expected, the diagnostic accuracy in cancer detection is higher with visualized ampullary tumors (up to 88%), followed by infiltrative cholangiocarcinoma (44–89%) and lowest with extrinsic compression by pancreatic adenocarcinoma (33–74%) [3, 4, 6].

Intraductal biopsy offers the ability to sample both proximal and distal biliary strictures but remains technically difficult. The technique is fairly standard, involving the passage of biopsy forceps through the papilla, usually facilitated by biliary sphincterotomy, up to the level of the biliary stricture; under fluoroscopic guidance, the forceps are opened pushed against the strictured region and then closed and pulled to acquire tissue. Diagnostic sensitivity is maximized if three or more specimens are collected, but additional attempts will likely increase the rate of post biopsy complications including hemobilia or biliary perforation [3, 4, 6]. Reports of patients with direct hyperbilirubinemia (more than 10 mg/dl) or circumferential biliary strictures demonstrated higher diagnostic accuracy when sampled by intraductal biopsy forceps. Immediate and cost-effective cytopathologic analysis can be achieved by adopting the "smash protocol" in handling the collected specimens. This approach requires smearing samples between two glass slides after staining with rapid Papanicolaou to allow for immediate interpretation by an on-site pathologist. In one study, the immediate diagnostic sensitivity reached 72% using this technique [3, 4, 6].

Advanced Cytology Techniques

Aneuploidy (abnormal number of chromosomes) is expressed in approximately 80% of pancreaticobiliary malignancies. Several adjunct molecular techniques were introduced in the past decade to examine genetic variations (i.e., chromosomal deletions, duplications, and polysomy) in cholangiocarcinoma and aid in establishing a diagnosis for malignant-appearing indeterminate biliary strictures [6].

Fluorescent In Situ Hybridization (FISH)

FISH is a cytogenic method which utilizes fluorescent-labeled DNA probes complimentary to the DNA sequence to assess for genetic alterations in known chromosomal loci. It first highlights aneuploidy then quantifies cells containing nuclei with abnormal probe signal numbers. Commercially available FISH kits use DNA probes to hybridize to regions of chromosomes 3, 7, 17, and INK4 (9p21) locus on chromosome 9, which are known genetic variants in cholangiocarcinoma. FISH is considered positive when polysomy is detected or if trisomy of chromosome 3 or 7 is identified in at least five cells. FISH has the advantage of analyzing cells sampled by routine brush cytology without requiring additional tissue acquisition techniques. FISH is limited by center availability with high technical expertise and long processing time and is subject to interpretation errors. Additionally, FISH performance in detecting neoplasia in indeterminate biliary strictures with negative routine cytology is variable. Several factors contribute to the suboptimal diagnostic sensitivity of FISH, including the inconsistent expression of aneuploidy in cholangiocarcinoma (see in only 80% cases). Additionally, benign biliary strictures such as those in PSC can manifest with chromosomal alterations in up to 80% of cases, which leads to false-positive results. An earlier prospective trial reported 62% sensitivity and 79% specificity in surgically proven malignant biliary strictures. Later studies reported improved test sensitivity from 5–20% to 35–60% compared to brush cytology but lower specificity ranging from 67% to 88%. A combined modality approach of routine brush cytology, intraductal biopsy, and FISH improves the overall diagnostic yield of indeterminate biliary strictures with sensitivity of 82%, specificity of 100%, positive predictive value of 100%, and negative predictive value of 87% [1, 3, 4, 6, 10].

Digital Image Analysis (DIA) and Flow Cytometry

The DIA technique assesses for cellular aneuploidy and neoplastic characteristics by quantifying the DNA content via special stains. It incorporates the conversion of transmitted light through the acquired specimen into captured digital images of the cell nucleus and other cellular contents (i.e., DNA, chromatin). The resulting images are analyzed for neoplastic characteristics. In non-PSC strictures, the diagnostic sensitivity for DIA is 30% compared to FISH sensitivity of 63%, while the combined sensitivity and specificity of both cytogenic modalities reach 70% and 82%, respectively. Flow cytometry identifies tumor cells in collected cytology specimens by detecting hyperploidy. This requires collecting samples with high degree of cellularity and malignant cells. Compared to brush cytology, it has similar diagnostic sensitivity of 42% but inferior specificity of 77%. Neither of these molecular techniques is routinely used in the evaluation of indeterminate biliary strictures due to their many limitations [3, 4, 6].

Endoscopic Ultrasonography (EUS)

Endoscopic ultrasonography (EUS) aids in diagnosis and staging of malignant biliary strictures and can be a useful modality for establishing a malignant diagnosis in patients with indeterminate biliary strictures. EUS imaging itself may reveal or suggest a diagnosis, such as varices, Mirizzi's syndrome, chronic pancreatitis, or a previously unappreciated mass lesion [11], while FNA allows diagnostic tissue to be obtained from lesions or lymph nodes. One advantage of performing EUS for indeterminate biliary strictures is the ability to identify biliary masses that were not appreciated on previous imaging [12]. In a small study, patients with proximal biliary strictures who underwent EUS-FNA following negative/nondiagnostic ERCP brush cytology, a mass lesion was visualized in 96% patients, 57% of whom did not have a mass lesion detected on previous imaging [13]. EUS may also identify pancreatic masses that were not noted on previous imaging, allowing direct targeted biopsy of a pancreatic lesion. In a retrospective study of patients with suspected pancreaticobiliary malignancy who had indeterminate results on contrast-enhanced multi-detector row CT, EUS-FNA had 87.3%

sensitivity, 98.3% specificity, and 92.1% accuracy in diagnosing pancreatic neoplasm [14]. The presence of pancreatic duct dilation was significantly associated with EUS detection of pancreatic adenocarcinoma ($p < 0.001$). In addition to identifying a lesion of interest, EUS allows evaluation of the relationship of the lesion to the hepatic parenchyma, portal vasculature, and hepatic arteries for staging and assessment of resectability [12]. Indwelling biliary stents at the time of EUS may produce significant acoustic shadowing that interferes with tumor imaging, and consideration should be made for their removal prior to performing EUS. However, indwelling stents in patients with indeterminate biliary strictures may also provide a point of reference and help facilitate tumor identification if left in place during EUS [12].

Endoscopic Ultrasound Fine Needle Aspiration (EUS-FNA)

The reported sensitivity of EUS-FNA for diagnosing pancreaticobiliary malignancy is high at 85–93% [15]. A recent systematic review and meta-analysis reported a sensitivity of 79% (95% CI 72–86%) and a specificity of 99% (95% CI 95–100%) for diagnosing biliary malignancies with EUS-FNA in patients with extrahepatic biliary strictures in the absence of extrinsic compression of pancreatic head cancer [16]. The reported negative predictive value, however, is low at 29% (95% CI 4–71%), emphasizing that a high clinical suspicion for malignancy should be maintained following negative EUS-FNA [12].

EUS-FNA has been shown in several studies to be superior to ERCP tissue sampling in evaluating suspected malignant biliary obstruction. In a prospective single-blind study of patients who underwent same session EUS and ERCP, EUS-FNA was significantly more sensitive than ERCP (94 vs 50%, respectively), with significantly higher accuracy (94 vs 53%, respectively) [15]. However, on subanalysis, a significant difference was only seen for patients with pancreatic masses, as the reported sensitivity for biliary masses (79 vs 79%) and indeterminate strictures (80 vs 67%, respectively) were statistically comparable. This intuitively makes sense, as EUS-FNA of a pancreatic mass directly samples the mass itself, while ERCP with brushings obtains tissue from the location of extrinsic biliary compression by the mass [15]. Despite the utility of EUS-FNA in diagnosing pancreaticobiliary malignancy, EUS shares the limitation of ERCP of a low negative predictive value and the inability to safely rule out malignancy with a negative test. In a recent meta-analysis of EUS versus ERCP for tissue diagnosis of malignant biliary stricture, the negative predictive values of EUS and ERCP were similarly poor at 47% and 34%, respectively [17].

While EUS typically images extrahepatic bile duct strictures well, imaging common hepatic and hilar strictures can be difficult [18]. This is because the distal portion of the common bile duct lies close to the duodenal wall, while the proximal ducts course further from the duodenal wall and are more difficult to visualize with EUS. Despite this limitation, EUS-FNA appears to have the ability to diagnose malignancy in both proximal and distal biliary strictures in some studies. In a study of patients with suspected malignant biliary obstruction, EUS-FNA correctly identified malignancy in 71% of distal and 86% proximal cholangiocarcinoma, with 2 of the 15 patients establishing a diagnosis by FNA of non-primary sites [15]. However, a single-center study of patients with cholangiocarcinoma did note a significantly higher sensitivity of EUS-FNA for distal versus proximal cholangiocarcinoma (81 vs 59%) [19].

Studies of FNA of biliary strictures report low adverse events, at 0–1% [15, 16]. However, peritoneal metastases due to needle tract seeding may occur after FNA of cholangiocarcinoma [20]. While some studies have shown that preoperative EUS-FNA may be safely performed in patients with cholangiocarcinoma without adversely affecting overall or progression-free survival [21], posttransplant immunosuppression may increase the chance of tumor recurrence in patients with peritoneal tumor seeding. Because of this, in many centers previous FNA of cholangiocarcinoma is a contraindication to liver transplantation [12]. For this reason, FNA of primary biliary lesions should not be performed in patients who are potential candidates for curative surgery or transplantation. In these cases, performing imaging with EUS alone without FNA may still be beneficial. In a retrospective study of patients with unexplained common bile duct strictures after ERCP and intraductal tissue sampling, EUS imaging alone was superior to FNA in establishing a malignant diagnosis [22]. Bile duct wall thickness ≥3 mm had a sensitivity for malignancy of 79% and specificity of 79%. The finding of a pancreatic head mass and/or irregular bile duct wall had sensitivity of 88% and NPV of 84%. In contrast, the sensitivity of EUS-FNA was only 47% with NPV low at 50%. However, EUS without FNA did not note a significant difference in the echo features of malignant versus benign lesions in another study of potentially operable patients with suspected hilar CCA and negative brush cytology [23]. Despite the controversy of performing EUS-FNA of primary biliary lesions, FNA of lymph nodes may safely be performed in this setting, as this is not a contraindication to liver transplantation for cholangiocarcinoma. Typical EUS features used for determining malignant nodal involvement are not predictive of malignant nodes in CCA, and no specific EUS morphology predicts the presence of malignancy, so routine FNA of regional lymph nodes should be considered in patients under consideration for liver transplantation to assess for metastatic disease [24].

Intraductal Ultrasonography (IDUS)

Intraductal ultrasonography (IDUS) is performed using a small radial 20 MHz ultrasound miniprobe (about 2 mm) that is passed through a standard duodenoscope or percutaneously over a guidewire to directly image the biliary or pancreatic ducts. IDUS imaging is generally obtained during catheter withdrawal to limit trauma to the mechanical drive of the probe. Ultrasonographic features suggestive of malignancy include disruption of the normal three-layer sonographic pattern of the bile duct wall, a hypoechoic mass with irregular margins, and heterogenous echo-poor areas invading surrounding tissue, while benign features include preservation of the normal wall pattern, homogenous hyperechoic echo patterns, smooth margins, and absence of mass lesion, lymphadenopathy, or vascular invasion [25]. Bile duct wall thickness ≤7 mm at the stricture site, in the absence of extrinsic compression, had a NPV of 100% in a retrospective study of patients without an identifiable mass on cross-sectional imaging [26]. Background inflammation in the setting of PSC or prolonged stenting can make IDUS interpretation difficult. Additionally, due to a shallow depth of penetration, IDUS is not suitable for imaging structures greater than 1 cm from the bile duct and is therefore not beneficial for nodal staging [25, 27]. Despite these limitations, IDUS has been shown to have superior accuracy in preoperative diagnosing and T-staging of malignant biliary strictures compared to EUS [25, 28] and is significantly more specific and accurate than ERCP with tissue sampling. In a prospective study of patients including patients with known or suspected biliary strictures who underwent ERCP with IDUS, combining IDUS with ERCP plus tissue sampling increased accuracy from 73.3% to 91.6%, sensitivity from 48.4% to 90.3%, and NPV from 64% to 90% [25]. Fourteen of the 16 false-negative diagnoses based on the ERCP with tissue sampling were correctly diagnosed as malignant strictures by IDUS. ERCP with IDUS was significantly better at detecting malignancy than endoscopic transpapillary forceps biopsies, EUS, and CT in a cohort study of patients with indeterminate biliary strictures [29].

Peroral Cholangioscopy (POC)

Peroral cholangioscopy (POC), or direct visualization of the biliary tree, allows direct visualization and targeted biopsies of indeterminate strictures. Cholangioscopy was historically performed with mother-daughter systems, where one endoscopist controlled a mother duodenoscope and a second endoscopist controlled the cholangioscope, or with slim gastroscopes. More recently, a digital-imaging single-operator single-use digital scope has become available (SpyGlass™ DS System, Boston Scientific) which attaches to the head of the duodenoscope and advances through the accessory channel. The scope may be passed over a wire or via fluoroscopic guidance. A biopsy cable (SpyBite) is passed through the digital scope to take targeted biopsies. Dilated tortuous vasculature coursing through the epithelium and variable degrees of exophytic mass protrusion into the lumen of the bile duct are suspicious for malignancy [30]. Stent association changes and trauma from stricture dilation may make visual diagnosis with POC challenging. Despite this limitation, the ability to perform targeted biopsies has significantly increased accuracy of POC over other methods of intraductal sampling.

The pooled sensitivity and specificity of cholangioscopy-guided biopsies in the diagnosis of indeterminate malignant biliary strictures were 60.1% (95% CI 54.9–65.2%) and 98% (95% CI 96–99%), respectively, in a meta-analysis [31]. For patients who had undergone prior ERCPs with indeterminate and/or negative brushing or biopsy results, the sensitivity of cholangioscopy-guided biopsies was even higher at 74.7%. Cholangioscopy-guided targeted biopsies with mini forceps appear to be superior to ERCP brushings and standard forceps biopsies. In a prospective cohort study where patients underwent triple sampling during ERCP with cholangioscopy-guided mini forceps, brushing, and standard ERCP forceps, mini forceps biopsy achieved significantly higher sensitivity and accuracy than the other methods [32]. The use of intraprocedural rapid onsite evaluation with touch imprint cytology during cholangioscopy-guided biopsy may further improve its sensitivity, with one study reporting 100% sensitivity in diagnosing malignancy after mean 3.3 biopsies performed (30). Despite the added expense of using a single-use disposable catheter, a recent cost-effective analysis of ERCP-based modalities for the diagnosis of CCA in the setting of PSC which compared ERCP with brushings, FISH, intraductal biopsy, and POC with targeted biopsy noted that POC with targeted biopsy was the most cost-effective modality [33].

A large amount of continuous flushing is often required during cholangioscopy to clear the visual field of bile or debris. For this reason, patients should generally be intubated, or the stomach frequently aspirated. Aggressive irrigation may also increase bacterial translocation in the biliary tree, as high rates of bacteremia following ERCP with cholangioscopy have been reported [34]. Periprocedural antibiotics should therefore be given routinely.

Confocal Laser Endomicroscopy (CLE)

Confocal laser endomicroscopy (CLE) allows high-resolution real-time assessment of mucosal histology at the cellular level to provide an "optical biopsy." A low-power laser is focused on tissue at a specific depth, and fluorescent light that is reflected back is detected. This is done following administration of intravenous fluorescein. Endoscope-based CLE is too large for biliary examination. To perform biliary CLE, probe-based CLE (pCLE) is done, which utilizes a flexible reusable miniprobe (CholangioFlex; Mauna Kea Technologies) that is passed through the duodenoscope channel. A classification system called the Miami classification system was developed based on a consensus of pCLE users to differentiate benign from malignant disease [35]. A multicenter registry of patients with indeterminate pancreaticobiliary strictures using the Miami classification showed 98% sensitivity and 97% NPV for pCLE for detecting cancerous strictures [36] with overall accuracy of 81% compared to 75% for index pathology. The accuracy of ERCP increased significantly when combined with pCLE (73 vs 90%). The Miami classification was revised to the Paris classification in an attempt to improve accuracy for diagnosing benign inflammatory strictures [11, 37]. In practice, the use of pCLE to ERCP does not seem to consistently improve accuracy. In a prospective international multicenter study of patients with indeterminate biliary strictures which evaluated the diagnostic performance of ERCP, pCLE, and tissue sampling, diagnostic accuracy was 81% for ERCP alone, 82% for ERCP with pCLE, and 88% for ERCP with pCLE when tissue sampling results were available [38]. However, the use of pCLE may have an impact on overall clinical impression. The sensitivity of the clinical impression during ERCP with pCLE was significantly higher than the sensitivity of tissue sampling alone with a trend toward improved accuracy of combined ERCP, pCLE, and tissue sampling versus ERCP with tissue sampling alone.

Use of pCLE is limited by false positives and resulting poor specificity. This is likely due to variability in imaging interpretation and learning curves. A meta-analysis of pCLE performed for undetermined biliary stenoses showed a pooled sensitivity of 0.9 (0.84–0.94) and specificity of 0.75 (0.66–0.83), with significant heterogeneity seen in reported specificity [39]. As endomicroscopy interpretation is examiner dependent, varying learning curves are seen, and discrepancies in the interpretation of pCLE findings have been reported with poor to fair interobserver agreement [35, 40]. While this may be improved with specialized training [41], this remains a significant barrier to more widespread use of pCLE.

Treatment/Management

No standard algorithm or guideline exists for managing indeterminate biliary stricture. In evaluating indeterminate biliary strictures, a multimodality approach is crucial. Patient-specific considerations should be made based on the clinical history and presentation to assess for potential benign etiologies. Adequate cross-sectional imaging (ideally multi-detector CT or MRI/MRCP) should be obtained. This may identify a mass lesion (notably pancreatic or ampullary) or malignant-appearing adenopathy that will help guide the diagnosis and provide a target for obtaining a tissue diagnosis via EUS-FNA. Due to limitations of cross-sectional imaging in identifying smaller mass lesions, performing routine EUS even in the absence of a mass lesion is recommended. Tumor markers, including CA 19-9 and CEA, should additionally be obtained on all patients. Performing repeat ERCP with multiple methods of tissue acquisition, such as brush cytology, intraductal biopsy, and cholangioscopic-directed biopsy, should be done to improve diagnostic sensitivity. Additional techniques such as IDUS and CLE may be considered based on center experience and expertise. In cases where a definitive diagnosis remains unclear, repeat interval ERCP, EUS, and/or cross-sectional imaging is necessary to establish stability or progression and provide additional opportunity for obtaining a tissue diagnosis. As the majority of indeterminate biliary strictures are later determined to be malignant, a high sustained clinical suspicion for malignancy is crucial. For this reason, a multi-disciplinary approach is also necessary, and eligible patients should be referred for consideration of surgical resection even in the absence of a tissue diagnosis [42].

Special Considerations for PSC

PSC carries a known increased risk of cholangiocarcinoma, and the diagnosis of early localized cancer is often challenging, especially in the presence of a dominant biliary stricture. Features suggestive of malignancy include stricture length over 1 cm, location at the bifurcation versus common bile duct, and irregular margins; however, the reported sensitivity and specificity of cholangiography for malignancy in the setting of PSC are low at 66% and 51%, respectively [43]. Compared to non-PSC biliary strictures, the utility of conventional endoscopic brush cytology carries similar specificity of >95% and a modest sensitivity of 43% in detecting cholangiocarcinoma [44]. The presence of false-positive chromosomal alterations in up to 80% of benign biliary strictures in PSC patients impacts FISH performance. In a meta-analysis, the reported sensitivity and specificity of FISH in diagnosing cholangiocarcinoma were 68% and 70%, respectively [45]. Direct tissue acquisition by peroral cholangioscopy carries a better diagnostic yield with 82% test sensitivity and 91% specificity [46]. Although the data is limited, the addition of confocal laser endomicroscopy to cholangioscopy can help to improve the diagnostic sensitivity [42, 47]. A multimodality approach must be used to improve the diagnostic yield of indeterminate biliary strictures in PSC.

Endoscopic management is recommended to manage symptomatic benign dominant PSC strictures, mainly by ERCP-guided balloon or catheter dilation with or without temporary stent placement to prevent from cholangitis, jaundice, and decline in liver function. In a prospective study, such interventions preserved the common bile duct function in PSC patients with a 10-year survival rate of 52% without liver transplantation [42, 48].

Case Outcome

Due to indeterminate cytology and clinical concerns for cholangiocarcinoma, repeat ERCP with cholangioscopy was performed. Repeat ERCP again showed a 40 mm stricture of the common hepatic duct. Cholangioscopy using Spyglass™ DS (Boston Scientific) demonstrated neovascularization and abnormal-appearing biliary epithelium suspicious for malignancy at the level of the stricture (Fig. 5.3a, b, Video 5.1). Targeted biopsies of the abnormal-appearing biliary epithelium were taken using SpyBite™ miniature forceps. Pathology showed invasive moderate to poorly differentiated adenocarcinoma, confirming the suspected diagnosis of cholangiocarcinoma.

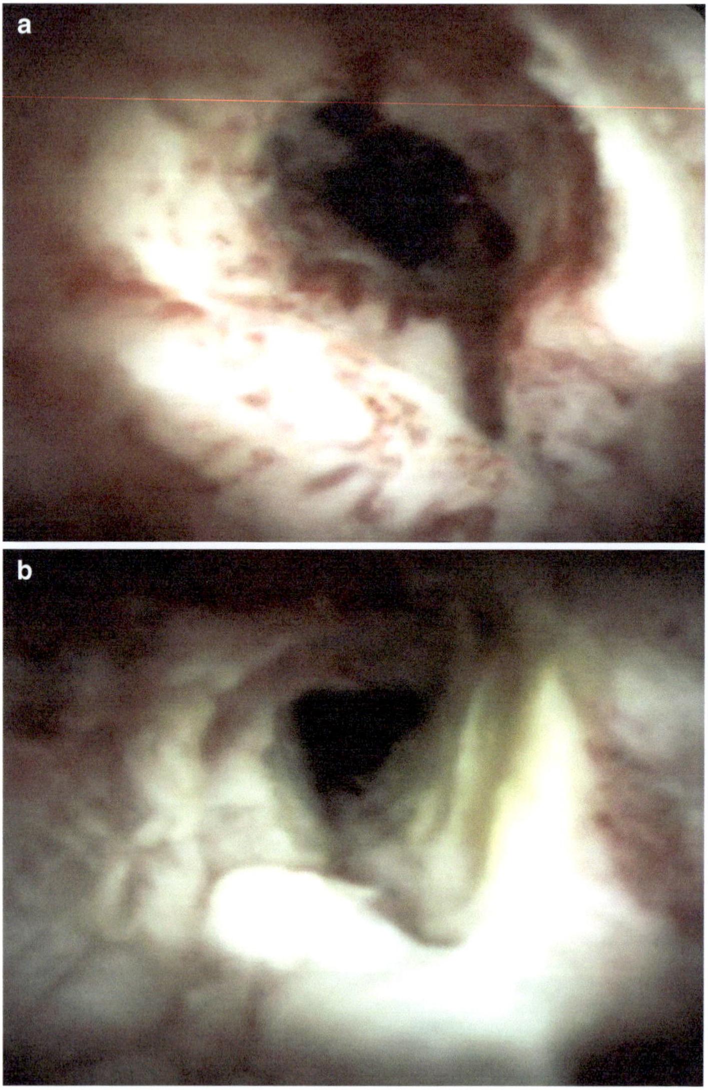

FIGURE 5.3 (**a**) Neovascularization with abnormal-appearing biliary epithelium by cholangioscopy using Spyglass™ DS (Boston Scientific). (**b**) Abnormal biliary epithelial surface at the stricture level by cholangioscopy using Spyglass™ DS (Boston Scientific)

Pearls and Pitfalls

- Utilizing multiple modalities of tissue acquisition during ERCP should be done to increase diagnostic yield.
- Routine EUS should be performed as mass lesions not previously seen on cross-sectional imaging are often identified.
- FNA of primary biliary lesions should not be performed in patients who are potential candidates for curative surgery or transplantation due to theoretical risks of tumor seeding.
- The majority of indeterminate biliary strictures are malignant, so a high clinical suspicion is warranted and consideration should be made for surgical referral even in the absence of a tissue diagnosis.

References

1. Bowlus CL, Olson KA, Gershwin ME. Evaluation of indeterminate biliary strictures. Nat Rev Gastroenterol Hepatol. 2016;13(1):28–37.
2. Singh A, Gelrud A, Agarwal B. Biliary strictures: diagnostic considerations and approach. Gastroenterol Rep (Oxf). 2015;3(1):22–31.
3. Victor DW, Sherman S, Karakan T, Khashab MA. Current endoscopic approach to indeterminate biliary strictures. World J Gastroenterol. 2012;18(43):6197–205.
4. Tabibian JH, Visrodia KH, Levy MJ, Gostout CJ. Advanced endoscopic imaging of indeterminate biliary strictures. World J Gastrointest Endosc. 2015;7(18):1268–78.
5. Navaneethan U, Njei B, Lourdusamy V, Konjeti R, Vargo JJ, Parsi MA. Comparative effectiveness of biliary brush cytology and intraductal biopsy for detection of malignant biliary strictures: a systematic review and meta-analysis. Gastrointest Endosc. 2015;81(1):168–76.
6. Korc P, Sherman S. ERCP tissue sampling. Gastrointest Endosc. 2016;84(4):557–71.

7. Parsi MA, Li A, Li CP, Goggins M. DNA methylation alterations in endoscopic retrograde cholangiopancreatography brush samples of patients with suspected pancreaticobiliary disease. Clin Gastroenterol Hepatol. 2008;6(11):1270–8.
8. Govil H, Reddy V, Kluskens L, Treaba D, Massarani-Wafai R, Selvaggi S, et al. Brush cytology of the biliary tract: retrospective study of 278 cases with histopathologic correlation. Diagn Cytopathol. 2002;26(5):273–7.
9. Selvaggi SM. Biliary brushing cytology. Cytopathology. 2004;15(2):74–9.
10. Singhi AD, Slivka A. Evaluation of indeterminate biliary strictures: is it time to FISH or cut bait? Gastrointest Endosc. 2016;83(6):1236–8.
11. Caillol F, Filoche B, Gaidhane M, Kahaleh M. Refined probe-based confocal laser endomicroscopy classification for biliary strictures: the Paris Classification. Dig Dis Sci. 2013;58(6):1784–9.
12. Khashab MA, Fockens P, Al-Haddad MA. Utility of EUS in patients with indeterminate biliary strictures and suspected extrahepatic cholangiocarcinoma (with videos). Gastrointest Endosc. 2012;76(5):1024–33.
13. DeWitt J, Misra VL, Leblanc JK, McHenry L, Sherman S. EUS-guided FNA of proximal biliary strictures after negative ERCP brush cytology results. Gastrointest Endosc. 2006;64(3):325–33.
14. Wang W, Shpaner A, Krishna SG, Ross WA, Bhutani MS, Tamm EP, et al. Use of EUS-FNA in diagnosing pancreatic neoplasm without a definitive mass on CT. Gastrointest Endosc. 2013;78(1):73–80.
15. Weilert F, Bhat YM, Binmoeller KF, Kane S, Jaffee IM, Shaw RE, et al. EUS-FNA is superior to ERCP-based tissue sampling in suspected malignant biliary obstruction: results of a prospective, single-blind, comparative study. Gastrointest Endosc. 2014;80(1):97–104.
16. Sadeghi A, Mohamadnejad M, Islami F, Keshtkar A, Biglari M, Malekzadeh R, et al. Diagnostic yield of EUS-guided FNA for malignant biliary stricture: a systematic review and meta-analysis. Gastrointest Endosc. 2016;83(2):290–8 e1.
17. De Moura DTH, Moura EGH, Bernardo WM, De Moura ETH, Baraca FI, Kondo A, et al. Endoscopic retrograde cholangiopancreatography versus endoscopic ultrasound for tissue diagnosis of malignant biliary stricture: systematic review and meta-analysis. Endosc Ultrasound. 2018;7(1):10–9.

18. Topazian M. Endoscopic ultrasonography in the evaluation of indeterminate biliary strictures. Clin Endosc. 2012;45(3):328–30.
19. Mohamadnejad M, DeWitt JM, Sherman S, LeBlanc JK, Pitt HA, House MG, et al. Role of EUS for preoperative evaluation of cholangiocarcinoma: a large single-center experience. Gastrointest Endosc. 2011;73(1):71–8.
20. Heimbach JK, Sanchez W, Rosen CB, Gores GJ. Trans-peritoneal fine needle aspiration biopsy of hilar cholangiocarcinoma is associated with disease dissemination. HPB (Oxford). 2011;13(5):356–60.
21. El Chafic AH, Dewitt J, Leblanc JK, El H II, Cote G, House MG, et al. Impact of preoperative endoscopic ultrasound-guided fine needle aspiration on postoperative recurrence and survival in cholangiocarcinoma patients. Endoscopy. 2013;45(11):883–9.
22. Lee JH, Salem R, Aslanian H, Chacho M, Topazian M. Endoscopic ultrasound and fine-needle aspiration of unexplained bile duct strictures. Am J Gastroenterol. 2004;99(6):1069–73.
23. Fritscher-Ravens A, Broering DC, Knoefel WT, Rogiers X, Swain P, Thonke F, et al. EUS-guided fine-needle aspiration of suspected hilar cholangiocarcinoma in potentially operable patients with negative brush cytology. Am J Gastroenterol. 2004;99(1):45–51.
24. Gleeson FC, Rajan E, Levy MJ, Clain JE, Topazian MD, Harewood GC, et al. EUS-guided FNA of regional lymph nodes in patients with unresectable hilar cholangiocarcinoma. Gastrointest Endosc. 2008;67(3):438–43.
25. Farrell RJ, Agarwal B, Brandwein SL, Underhill J, Chuttani R, Pleskow DK. Intraductal US is a useful adjunct to ERCP for distinguishing malignant from benign biliary strictures. Gastrointest Endosc. 2002;56(5):681–7.
26. Krishna NB, Saripalli S, Safdar R, Agarwal B. Intraductal US in evaluation of biliary strictures without a mass lesion on CT scan or magnetic resonance imaging: significance of focal wall thickening and extrinsic compression at the stricture site. Gastrointest Endosc. 2007;66(1):90–6.
27. Tamada K, Kanai N, Ueno N, Ichiyama M, Tomiyama T, Wada S, et al. Limitations of intraductal ultrasonography in differentiating between bile duct cancer in stage T1 and stage T2: in-vitro and in-vivo studies. Endoscopy. 1997;29(8):721–5.
28. Menzel J, Poremba C, Dietl KH, Domschke W. Preoperative diagnosis of bile duct strictures--comparison of intraductal ultrasonography with conventional endosonography. Scand J Gastroenterol. 2000;35(1):77–82.

29. Heinzow HS, Kammerer S, Rammes C, Wessling J, Domagk D, Meister T. Comparative analysis of ERCP, IDUS, EUS and CT in predicting malignant bile duct strictures. World J Gastroenterol. 2014;20(30):10495–503.
30. Varadarajulu S, Bang JY, Hasan MK, Navaneethan U, Hawes R, Hebert-Magee S. Improving the diagnostic yield of single-operator cholangioscopy-guided biopsy of indeterminate biliary strictures: ROSE to the rescue? (with video). Gastrointest Endosc. 2016;84(4):681–7.
31. Navaneethan U, Hasan MK, Lourdusamy V, Njei B, Varadarajulu S, Hawes RH. Single-operator cholangioscopy and targeted biopsies in the diagnosis of indeterminate biliary strictures: a systematic review. Gastrointest Endosc. 2015;82(4):608–14 e2.
32. Draganov PV, Chauhan S, Wagh MS, Gupte AR, Lin T, Hou W, et al. Diagnostic accuracy of conventional and cholangioscopy-guided sampling of indeterminate biliary lesions at the time of ERCP: a prospective, long-term follow-up study. Gastrointest Endosc. 2012;75(2):347–53.
33. Njei B, McCarty TR, Varadarajulu S, Navaneethan U. Cost utility of ERCP-based modalities for the diagnosis of cholangiocarcinoma in primary sclerosing cholangitis. Gastrointest Endosc. 2017;85(4):773–81 e10.
34. Othman MO, Guerrero R, Elhanafi S, Davis B, Hernandez J, Houle J, et al. A prospective study of the risk of bacteremia in directed cholangioscopic examination of the common bile duct. Gastrointest Endosc. 2016;83(1):151–7.
35. Wallace M, Lauwers GY, Chen Y, Dekker E, Fockens P, Sharma P, et al. Miami classification for probe-based confocal laser endomicroscopy. Endoscopy. 2011;43(10):882–91.
36. Meining A, Chen YK, Pleskow D, Stevens P, Shah RJ, Chuttani R, et al. Direct visualization of indeterminate pancreaticobiliary strictures with probe-based confocal laser endomicroscopy: a multicenter experience. Gastrointest Endosc. 2011;74(5):961–8.
37. Taunk P, Singh S, Lichtenstein D, Joshi V, Gold J, Sharma A. Improved classification of indeterminate biliary strictures by probe-based confocal laser endomicroscopy using the Paris Criteria following biliary stenting. J Gastroenterol Hepatol. 2017;32(10):1778–83.
38. Slivka A, Gan I, Jamidar P, Costamagna G, Cesaro P, Giovannini M, et al. Validation of the diagnostic accuracy of probe-based confocal laser endomicroscopy for the characterization of indeterminate biliary strictures: results of a prospective multicenter international study. Gastrointest Endosc. 2015;81(2):282–90.

39. Liu Y, Lu Y, Sun B, Zhang WM, Zhang ZZ, He YP, et al. Probe-based confocal laser endomicroscopy for the diagnosis of undetermined biliary stenoses: a meta-analysis. Clin Res Hepatol Gastroenterol. 2016;40(6):666–73.
40. Peter S, Council L, Bang JY, Neumann H, Monkemuller K, Varadarajulu S, et al. Poor agreement between endoscopists and gastrointestinal pathologists for the interpretation of probe-based confocal laser endomicroscopy findings. World J Gastroenterol. 2014;20(47):17993–8000.
41. Talreja JP, Turner BG, Gress FG, Ho S, Sarkaria S, Paddu N, et al. Pre- and post-training session evaluation for interobserver agreement and diagnostic accuracy of probe-based confocal laser endomicroscopy for biliary strictures. Dig Endosc. 2014;26(4):577–80.
42. Hu B, Sun B, Cai Q, Wong Lau JY, Ma S, Itoi T, et al. Asia-Pacific consensus guidelines for endoscopic management of benign biliary strictures. Gastrointest Endosc. 2017;86(1):44–58.
43. Petersen BT. Indeterminate biliary stricture. In: Baron TH, Kozarek RA, Carr-Locke DL, editors. ERCP. 3rd ed. Philadelphia: Elsevier; 2019. p. 394–404.
44. Trikudanathan G, Navaneethan U, Njei B, Vargo JJ, Parsi MA. Diagnostic yield of bile duct brushings for cholangiocarcinoma in primary sclerosing cholangitis: a systematic review and meta-analysis. Gastrointest Endosc. 2014;79(5):783–9.
45. Navaneethan U, Njei B, Venkatesh PG, Vargo JJ, Parsi MA. Fluorescence in situ hybridization for diagnosis of cholangiocarcinoma in primary sclerosing cholangitis: a systematic review and meta-analysis. Gastrointest Endosc. 2014;79(6):943–50 e3.
46. Siiki A, Rinta-Kiikka I, Koivisto T, Vasama K, Sand J, Laukkarinen J. Spyglass single-operator peroral cholangioscopy seems promising in the evaluation of primary sclerosing cholangitis-related biliary strictures. Scand J Gastroenterol. 2014;49(11):1385–90.
47. Heif M, Yen RD, Shah RJ. ERCP with probe-based confocal laser endomicroscopy for the evaluation of dominant biliary stenoses in primary sclerosing cholangitis patients. Dig Dis Sci. 2013;58(7):2068–74.
48. Gotthardt DN, Rudolph G, Kloters-Plachky P, Kulaksiz H, Stiehl A. Endoscopic dilation of dominant stenoses in primary sclerosing cholangitis: outcome after long-term treatment. Gastrointest Endosc. 2010;71(3):527–34.

Chapter 6
Hilar Biliary Strictures

Anna Tavakkoli and Richard S. Kwon

Case One

A 45-year-old female presents to our clinic with pruritus and elevated transaminases. Three weeks prior, she was admitted to an outside hospital for acute right upper quadrant pain and abnormal liver function tests: ALT 432 U/L, AST 207 U/L, alkaline phosphatase 742 mg/dL, and total bilirubin of 1.8 mg/dL. An ultrasound showed choledocholithiasis, and she underwent an ERCP, sphincterotomy, and stone extraction. She underwent a cholecystectomy without complication 1 week later. In our clinic, she denied pain or jaundice but reported persistent pruritus. Her liver enzymes remained elevated (AST 121, ALT 300, alkaline phosphatase 666 mg/dL, and total bilirubin 1.3 mg/dL). Abdominal ultrasound showed dilated intrahepatic ducts with a 5 mm common bile duct. A subsequent MRCP showed obstruction of the right and left hepatic ducts at the level of the right/left hepatic duct confluence with extension into the proximal common bile duct (1–2 cm). Her CA19-9

A. Tavakkoli
Division of Gastroenterology, University of Texas, Southwestern, Dallas, TX, USA

R. S. Kwon (✉)
Division of Gastroenterology, University of Michigan, Ann Arbor, MI, USA
e-mail: rskwon@med.umich.edu

D. K. Mullady (ed.), *Dilemmas in ERCP*,
https://doi.org/10.1007/978-3-030-12741-1_6

was 18 U/ml. The patient was referred for endoscopic retrograde cholangiopancreatography (ERCP) for evaluation and treatment of her hilar stricture.

Diagnosis of Hilar Strictures

Distinguishing between malignant and benign strictures involving the hilum of the liver is often difficult and can require multiple procedures to obtain a diagnosis [1]. Malignant hilar strictures include cholangiocarcinoma or metastatic disease causing extrinsic compression. Benign biliary strictures include postoperative injuries, particularly following cholecystectomy, or intrinsic liver disease such as primary sclerosing cholangitis (PSC) or autoimmune cholangiopathy. ERCP, in combination with laboratory values and cross-sectional imaging, plays an important role in determining the etiology of these strictures since tissue can be obtained either through brushings for cytology, biopsy, or cholangioscopy.

Cross-Sectional Imaging and Laboratory Values

Bloodwork, including alkaline phosphatase isoenzyme, serum bilirubin, and CA19-9, in combination with imaging findings on computed tomography (CT) or magnetic resonance imaging (MRI), can be used to suggest benign or malignant causes of hilar strictures [1]. Laboratory values that have been reported to distinguish malignant strictures include increased alkaline phosphatase (>200 U/L), total bilirubin (>8.4 mg/dl), and CA 19-9 levels (>100 U/L) [2, 3]. Imaging findings associated with malignancy include increased thickness of bile duct wall to ≥5 mm, regional lymphadenopathy, and the appearance of an abrupt cutoff and separation of biliary ductal system on cholangiogram [2, 3]. Between imaging modalities, MRI has been shown to differentiate benign and malignant causes of biliary obstruction more accurately than CT [1, 2]. Our imaging study of choice to evaluate hilar strictures and to identify hilar masses is MRI/MRCP. In a multidisciplinary approach, we use imaging findings in conjunction with elevations in serum bilirubin and alkaline phosphatase and CA 19-9 to determine our suspicion for malignancy.

Brushings

One of the most common ways to obtain tissue during ERCP is with cytologic brushing. The reported sensitivity of cytology brushings varies between 35% and 70%, and reported specificity is usually greater than 90% [4–32]. In 1 study of 58 patients with confirmed hilar cholangiocarcinoma, malignancy was found in only 40% of patients with brush cytology alone [33]. Fluorescence in situ hybridization (FISH), which uses fluorescence-labeled probes to evaluate chromosomal abnormalities in cells obtained during biliary brushings, has been shown to increase the sensitivity of cytology brushings, with one study showing an increase from 35% to 44% while maintaining a specificity of 99% [34–36].

The accuracy of brush cytology may vary based on technique. The majority of the literature describes brushing over the stricture at least ten times and immediately cutting the brush off and placing it into fixative as soon as the catheter have been withdrawn from the patient [36]. Stricture dilation prior to brushing has been reported to increase the diagnostic yield [37–40].

In our own practice, we typically dilate hilar strictures before performing brushings for cytology. However, we have found that cytology brushings alone are often insufficient to make a diagnosis among patients with hilar strictures and have implemented the addition of FISH analysis in the presence of atypical cells when noted by our cytologists. A second dedicated brush should be used for FISH analysis and can be sent when malignancy is not diagnosed by brush cytology alone.

Biopsy

The sensitivity of biopsies using standard forceps advanced into the bile duct ranges from 43% to 88% with a specificity of greater than 90% [4–32]. However, based on the current literature, it is unclear how the combination of biopsy forceps and brush cytology may increase the sensitivity of obtaining a diagnosis. While some studies have shown an incremental increase in sensitivity of up to 15–25% by combining brush cytology and biopsy forceps, others have shown that increase in sensitivity was too small to routinely use both techniques [11, 41]. Furthermore, the use of standard forceps requires a biliary sphincterotomy and wire-free cannulation and includes a possible increased risk of bile duct perforation. Our general practice is to use biopsy forceps in combination with cytology brushings among patients who have had a previous negative brush cytology alone.

Cholangioscopy

Cholangioscopy allows for direct visualization and assessment of biliary strictures, including hilar strictures. Findings that are concerning for malignancy include tumor vessels, described as irregularly dilated and tortuous blood vessels, intraductal nodules, or papillary/villous mucosal projections [42, 43]. A meta-analysis of eight studies found that visual inspection with cholangioscopy alone was 90% sensitive and 87% specific for diagnosing a bile duct malignancy [44–48]. The added benefit of cholangioscopy is the ability to take targeted biopsies which can achieve tissue diagnosis in as high as 86% of patients with malignancy [44–47]. Biopsy taken through a cholangioscope is often quite small and may lack adequate depth for accurate histologic assessment, so it is imperative to take multiple biopsies. It is also important to note that cholangioscopy has been associated with higher adverse events, including cholangitis, so periprocedural antibiotics should be administered. In our experience, visual inspection among patients with previous biliary stent can be difficult to interpret due to stent-induced changes to the bile duct [49]. The use of cholangioscopy varies based on the availability of the equipment and endoscopists with appropriate expertise. For patients with hilar strictures, we typically reserve cholangioscopy for patients who have previously undergone ERCP with a negative work-up, but some endoscopists prefer to perform cholangioscopy at the first ERCP in patients highly suspicious for malignancy. This is part to visualize the duct before stent-induced changes which may obfuscate image interpretation.

Intraductal Ultrasonography

Intraductal ultrasonography (IDUS) is a method to help further characterize hilar strictures. Using a wire-guided approach, a high-frequency ultrasound probe is advanced into the bile duct to obtain images of the bile duct and periductal tissue [50]. The probe is radiopaque and may require a sphincterotomy to pass into the bile duct [50]. Findings on IDUS that differentiate benign from malignant strictures include disruption of the normal triple layer wall architecture, eccentric wall thickening, presence of a hypoechoic mass with irregular margins or invasion of adjacent structures, and/or the identification of malignant-appearing periductal lymph nodes [50–54]. The sensitivity of IDUS ranges between 80% and 90% with a specificity of 83% [50–54]. IDUS requires a separate processor, and IDUS probes are quite fragile and easy to damage [50]. As such, the use of IDUS is often limited by the availability and the experience of the endoscopist.

Diagnostic Dilemma and Outcome of Case

Hilar strictures that are concerning for cholangiocarcinoma are often clinically challenging since the current means of diagnosing bile duct malignancies are imperfect. Among patients with a clinical history that may explain their stricture, such as postsurgical patients, an exhaustive work-up may not be necessary. However, among patients with an indeterminate biliary stricture (see Chap. 5) or with primary sclerosing cholangitis (PSC), which is a known risk factor for cholangiocarcinoma, multiple ERCPs may be required in order to secure a diagnosis. Of note, EUS with fine needle aspiration or CT-guided biopsy are additional options to obtain diagnostic tissue, but the concern for seeding the tract with malignant tumor cells has made these diagnostic methods fall out of favor.

As described above, our initial preference for diagnosis of hilar strictures is to perform dilation to at least 4–6 mm prior to obtaining both cytology brushings. If atypical cells appear on brushings, we perform FISH analysis to hopefully increase the diagnostic yield of malignancy. If the endoscope position allows for easy cannulation, we will advance biopsy forceps into the duct to biopsy the stricture. In general, we reserve cholangioscopy for patients with negative cytology brushings and/or biopsies. However, if our concern for cholangiocarcinoma is high enough (based on imaging, labs, and clinical background), we will proceed to cholangioscopy on the initial ERCP.

Outcomes of the Case

The patient underwent ERCP, and her cholangiogram revealed a tight hilar stricture (Fig. 6.1). We were concerned this stricture may be malignant since there were no reported operative complications, nor any adjacent errant surgical clips to explain her stricture. As such, we proceeded with cholangioscopy revealed a pinpoint stricture in the hilum without abnormal vessels and villous-/frond-like projections (Fig. 6.2). Brushings and targeted biopsies by cholangioscopy were obtained but were nondiagnostic. The stricture persisted on repeat ERCPs despite repeat balloon dilations and the placement of multiple plastic stents (Fig. 6.3). Due to a lack of response to dilations, the development of weight loss, and new finding of a possible mass on a repeat MRCP, she was taken to the operating room for a hepaticojejunostomy. She was found to have T3N1 cholangiocarcinoma. She underwent adjuvant chemotherapy and radiation and is doing well 4 years afterward.

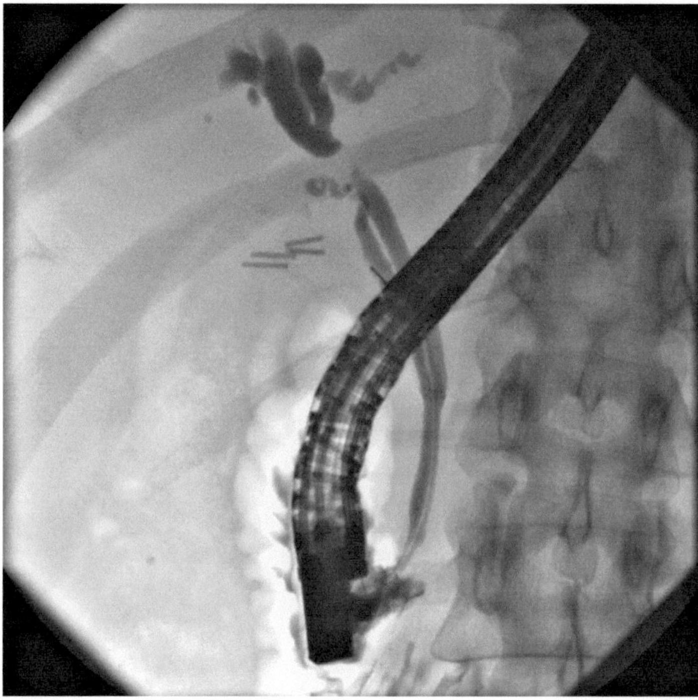

FIGURE 6.1 Cholangiogram with a tight hilar stricture in a patient with elevated transaminases and pruritus postcholecystectomy

Case Two

A 72-year-old female with stage IV colon cancer and metastasis to the liver presents to our hospital for a second opinion on management of her cancer. At the time of presentation, her bilirubin was 37 mg/dL. Cross-sectional imaging revealed enlarged hilar lymph nodes and markedly dilated intrahepatic biliary dilatation. The patient was admitted and underwent ERCP, which was notable for diffuse intrahepatic irregularities and a hilar stricture (Fig. 6.4), which was stented with one plastic stent into the right main hepatic duct. She was discharged the next day. However, less than a week later,

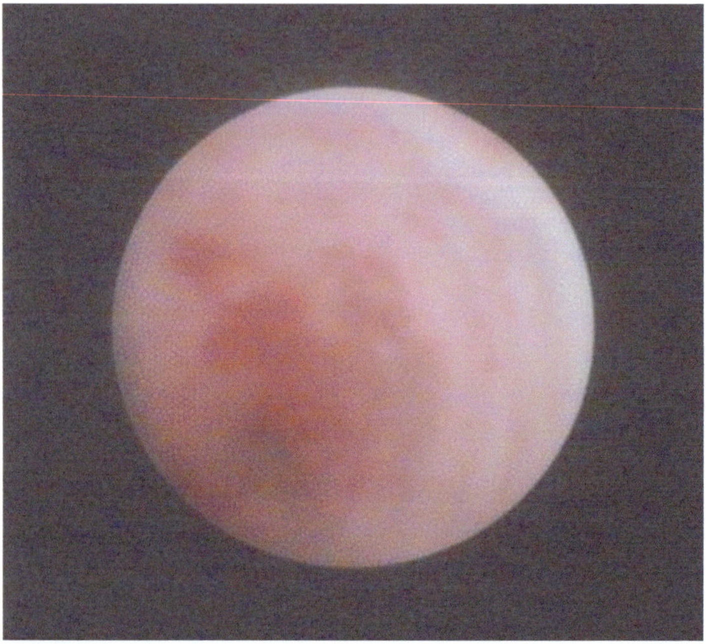

FIGURE 6.2 Fiber-optic cholangioscopy notable for pinpoint stricture within the common hepatic duct. There was no obvious intraluminal mass or growth

she was readmitted to the hospital with lethargy and persistent hyperbilirubinemia (bilirubin 32 mg/dL). Her imaging showed stable position of the previously placed plastic stent, as well as persistent intrahepatic biliary dilatation (Fig. 6.5). The patient was admitted for a repeat ERCP.

Management: Biliary Drainage of Hilar Strictures

The optimal approach for biliary drainage of hilar strictures is somewhat controversial. While both percutaneous transhepatic biliary drainage (PTBD) and ERCP are accepted

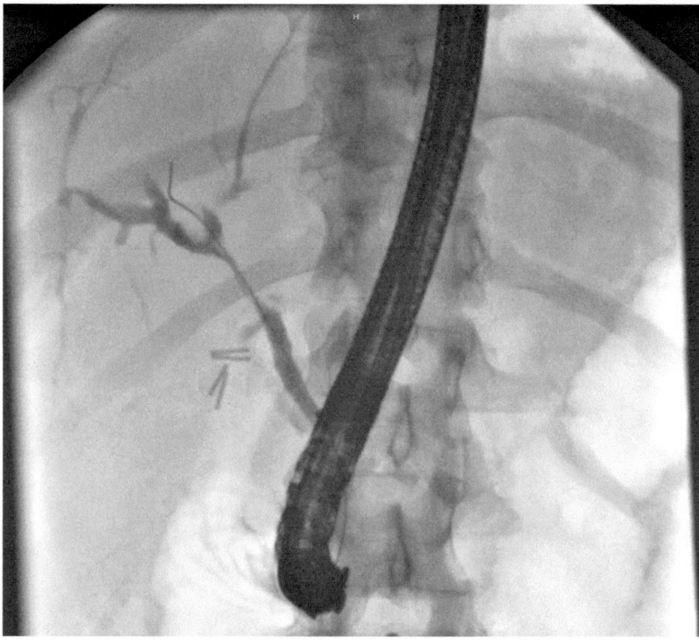

FIGURE 6.3 Cholangiogram with a persistently abnormal hilar stricture despite multiple balloon dilations and plastic stent placement. Her CA 19-9 was normal

approaches for drainage of hilar strictures, ERCP is often preferred due to a number of factors, including improved quality of life with endoscopic stents rather than an external drain [55–57]. When ERCP is pursued for the management of these strictures, endoscopists must then decide whether to pursue unilateral or bilateral drainage, the use of plastic or self-expanding metal stents (SEMS), and if bilateral drainage with SEMS is pursued, what configuration of SEMS is optimal for the patient's disease. These decisions involve several factors, such as the resectability of the malignant obstruction, as well as the availability and expertise of endoscopists, and should be made in a multidisciplinary fashion.

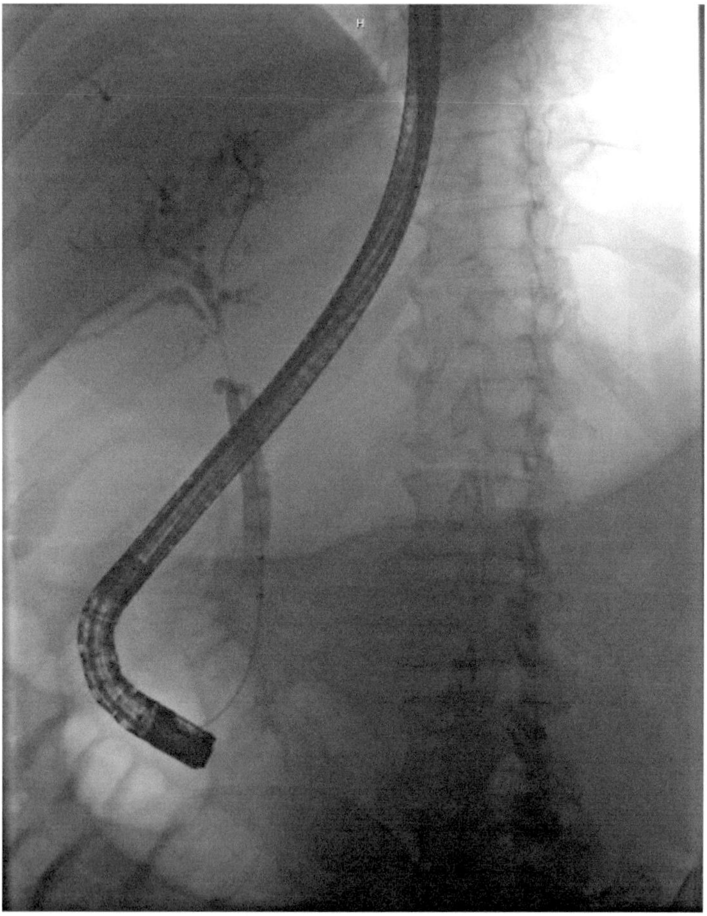

Figure 6.4 Cholangiogram with hilar stricture and rarefaction of intrahepatic bile ducts. (Courtesy of Ryan Law, DO, University of Michigan)

Unilateral Versus Bilateral Biliary Drainage

Unilateral versus bilateral biliary drainage among hilar malignancies is a highly debated question in the current literature. Bilateral drainage typically involves the placement of

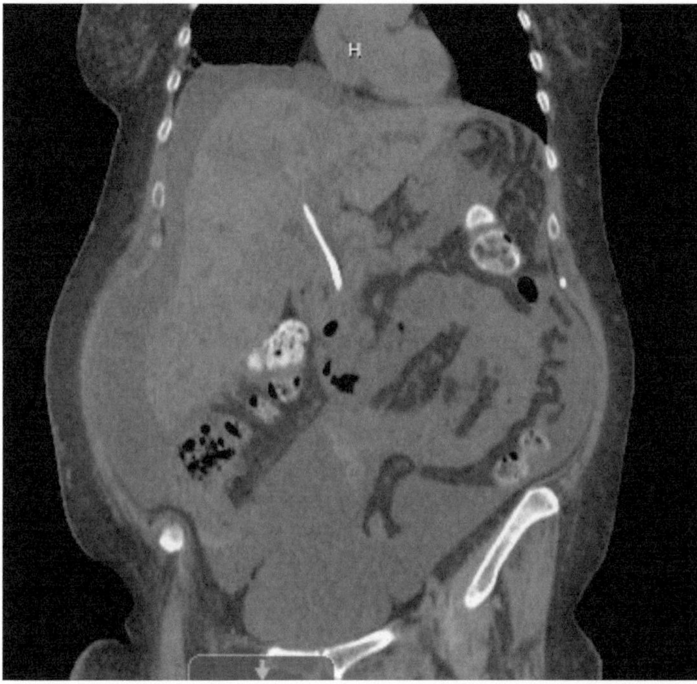

FIGURE 6.5 CT abdomen with previously placed plastic biliary stent and intrahepatic biliary dilation from metastatic colon cancer. (Courtesy of Ryan Law, DO, University of Michigan)

two stents across the right and left intrahepatic biliary systems to achieve drainage of both lobes of the liver [56]. Liver volume is often a marker to assist in determining whether unilateral versus bilateral drainage is necessary since drainage of >50% of viable liver volume seems to correlate with better outcomes [56, 58–60]. However, implementing this in practice can be difficult since complex hilar tumors may sequester individual liver sectors and bilateral placement of stents is often technically more challenging [56, 60–62]. Unilateral drainage alone may not relieve jaundice completely and may leave the patient at risk for cholangitis. Studies have found that the use of two or more stents improved survival as compared with one stent and reduced procedure-related mortality and cholangitis [63]. Furthermore, a retrospective study of 480 patients with hilar cholangiocarcinoma found superior cumulative stent patency rates for bilateral metal or plastic stents compared with unilateral metal or plastic stents [64]. Lastly, one of the most recent randomized trials evaluated unilateral versus bilateral SEMs for patients with malignant hilar strictures and found similar clinical success rates among both groups but that the proportion of patients whose bilirubin decreased to <2.0 mg/dL was higher among those with bilateral drainage and that primary reintervention occurred less often in the bilateral SEMS group [3].

In our own clinical practice, we try to achieve bilateral biliary drainage whenever possible to help maximize drainage and reduce adverse events associated with unilateral drainage. However, it is important to note that some patient's anatomy does not allow for bilateral drainage, so review of imaging prior to ERCP is important to determine the dominant biliary system that should be prioritized for drainage.

Plastic Versus Metal Stent Placement

The majority of the data available suggests that SEMS are preferable to plastic stents among patients with malignant hilar strictures. Randomized trials and retrospective studies have found that SEMS are associated with lower occlusion rates, less need for reintervention, and lower rates of adverse events, such as cholangitis, stent migration, or stent occlusion [65–68]. Although a recent meta-analysis did not find a statistically significant difference between SEMS in terms of reintervention, they did confirm prior findings that SEMS had lower occlusion rates and less frequent episodes of cholangitis [61]. The benefits of SEMS over plastic stents were attributed to the smaller caliber introducer of SEMS, greater flexibility of SEMS which allows for easier insertion, and the open mesh interstices in SEMS that allow improved drainage [61]. Although the cost of metal stents is higher than plastic stents, the overall cost burden may be significantly less given the complication rates associated with plastic stents.

Even within our own institution, practice patterns vary by endoscopists. We prefer to use plastic stents first to assess whether we can establish adequate drainage. If we are able to normalize the bilirubin, we then will switch the stent to uncovered open-cell designed SEMS. In patients who may have resectable disease (<30% of all hilar malignancies) or who may be candidates for liver transplantation, we continue to use plastic stents with targeted drainage of liver segments contralateral to the region of resection (often referred to as the functional liver remnant) to optimize postoperative liver function [56, 57, 69, 70]. Again, these clinical decisions should be made in a multidisciplinary fashion.

SEMS Placement: Side-by-Side Versus Stent-in-Stent

Two techniques have been described for the placement of bilateral SEMS among patients with malignant hilar strictures: side-by-side stenting and stent-in-stent deployment.

Side-by-side stenting is defined by placing two SEMS in parallel in the common bile duct [59]. The proximal ends of the SEMS are positioned in the left and right intrahepatic bile ducts, and the distal ends of the SEMS would ideally be transpapillary to allow for easier access to the biliary system at subsequent procedures. In order to achieve this, typically a 10–12-cm-long SEMS is required. Side-by-side stenting can be performed simultaneously, with a 6-Fr delivery system or serially, with a 7-Fr or 8-Fr delivery system. If serial deployment is performed, it is recommended to deploy the first SEMS in the most difficult biliary anatomy and the second SEMS in the straighter, less angulated intrahepatic duct [59].

Stent-in-stent placement is defined by placing a second SEMS through the interstices of the first SEMS. Two wires are placed into the left and right intrahepatic system, and the first SEMS is deployed in the most angulated or most difficult biliary anatomy. After deployment of the first SEMS, a wire is used to cannulate through the stent interstices of the first stent, using the second guidewire as a landmark. It can be difficult to place a wire through the stent interstices especially when the stent is newly deployed and not yet fully expanded. Therefore, balloon dilation can be performed to make the stent interstices larger, which helps to facilitate wire and stent placement. Stent-in-stent deployment can be technically difficult, especially when open-cell SEMS are not available [59]. Reintervention of the biliary system can be more difficult with the stent-in-stent model because it may require traversing through the interstices of the second SEMS [59].

In general, a stent-in-stent technique is considered more technically difficult as compared to stent-by-stent technique since advancing a second wire through the mesh interstices can be challenging. However, some endoscopists believe that stent-in-stent is preferred over stent-by-stent because it allows full expansion of the stents in the common bile duct and may be more anatomically compliant. There have been no prospective studies comparing stent-in-stent versus stent-by-stent. A few retrospective studies comparing these two techniques have been performed, but there is no consensus for the superiority of one technique over another to relieve jaundice. There does not seem to be any statistical difference in complications including cholecystitis, cholangitis, and liver abscess [71]. Additionally, there is no difference in the need for reintervention or procedure time between the two techniques [72].

PTC Versus ERCP for Biliary Decompression in Hilar Stricture

Currently, ERCP is the preferred method of biliary decompression among patients with hilar strictures. However, some observational studies have found that PTBD is superior in achieving complete biliary drainage as compared to ERCP and that many patients who undergo an initial ERCP for malignant hilar strictures require subsequent PTBD for adequate drainage [55, 57, 73–75]. Although some studies have found that the risk of adverse events is higher among patients with PTBD versus ERCP, there have been no randomized studies that have evaluated the preferred modality of drainage among patients with malignant hilar strictures [55]. The INTerventional Radiology vs. ERC for Perihilar Tumors (INTERCPT) trial is an ongoing multicenter, randomized trial comparing ERCP vs. PTBD for decompression of malignant hilar obstruction that will hopefully clarify the optimal modality of biliary decompression among patients with malignant hilar obstruction [55].

Diagnostic Dilemma and Outcomes of Case

The endoscopic management of malignant hilar strictures is often technically difficult. Endoscopists must determine whether to pursue unilateral vs. bilateral drainage or plastic or metal stent placement, and if bilateral SEMS are pursued, what the optimal configuration of SEMS is for the patient's disease in order to provide the maximal amount of biliary drainage. The initial approach for management of these strictures includes a multidisciplinary review of cross-sectional imaging to help establish resectability and to delineate the anatomy prior to their procedure. If a patient is a surgical candidate, our approach is to place bilateral plastic stents to allow for optimal preoperative biliary drainage. If a patient is not a surgical candidate, then placement of bilateral SEMS, in either a stent-in-stent or stent-by-stent approach, should be pursued based on the endoscopists' experience with these two methods.

Outcomes of Case

Given that this patient had a hilar stricture from metastatic disease, and incomplete biliary drainage with unilateral plastic stent placement, the decision was made to place bilateral SEMS in a stent-by-stent orientation. These stents have a 6-Fr delivery system and can be deployed simultaneously (Fig. 6.6). Since deployment of her stents, her bilirubin normalized, and she was able to receive chemotherapy.

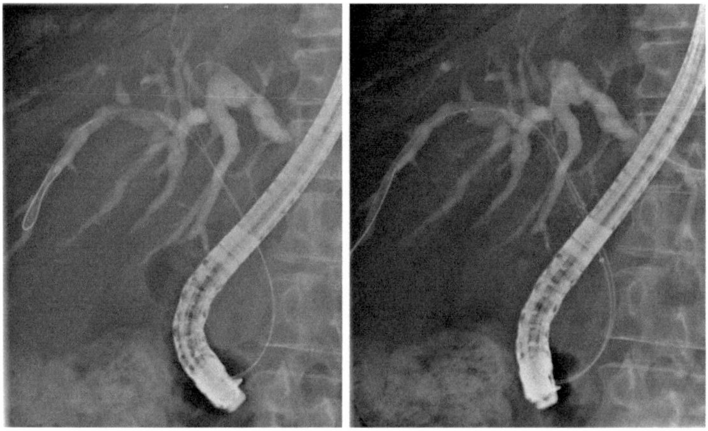

FIGURE 6.6 Cholangiogram with bilateral guidewire placement and two metal stents deployed simultaneously within the bile duct. (Courtesy of Ryan Law, DO, University of Michigan)

Pearls and Pitfalls

- The diagnosis and endoscopic management of hilar strictures are complex and require a multidisciplinary approach with radiologists and surgery.
- Obtaining a diagnosis of a hilar malignancy often requires multiple ERCPs. Our preference is to start with cytology brushings and biopsy forceps and to obtain brushings after dilation to increase diagnostic yield.
- If samples obtained are negative, the endoscopist should consider cholangioscopy, which can directly visualize the stricture and allow targeted biopsies.
- Drainage of hilar strictures can be complex because of the decisions that need to be made endoscopically including unilateral vs. bilateral drainage, plastic stents versus SEMS, and the configuration of SEMS if used.

- Although the current evidence is conflicting, our preference is to pursue bilateral drainage whenever possible in order to maximize drainage and minimize delays in treatment due to persistent jaundice.
- Given the difficulty in diagnosing hilar strictures, if malignancy is not confirmed and/or staging has not been completed, we place plastic stents.
- If the diagnosis of malignancy is confirmed and a patient is considered to be resectable or a transplant candidate after multidisciplinary review, we place plastic stents and aim to achieve bilateral drainage when possible.
- If the diagnosis is confirmed and the patient is not a surgical candidate, we attempt to place SEMS since they have been associated with lower rates of stent occlusion and cholangitis.
- If SEMS are placed, we prefer to use open-cell designed metal stents.
- Stent-in-stent versus stent-by-stent configurations can be used for bilateral metal stent placement. Although stent-in-stent seems more anatomically correct, it is often more technically challenging. The decision should be based on the endoscopists experience and the patient's anatomy.
- PTBD may allow for more optimal biliary drainage but has been associated with an increase in adverse events.

References

1. Singh RR, Singh V. Endoscopic management of hilar biliary strictures. World J Gastrointest Endosc. 2015;7:806–13.
2. Saluja SS, Sharma R, Pal S, et al. Differentiation between benign and malignant hilar obstructions using laboratory and

radiological investigations: a prospective study. HPB (Oxford). 2007;9:373–82.

3. Kim HJ, Lee KT, Kim SH, et al. Differential diagnosis of intrahepatic bile duct dilatation without demonstrable mass on ultrasonography or CT: benign versus malignancy. J Gastroenterol Hepatol. 2003;18:1287–92.
4. Kurzawinski TR, Deery A, Dooley JS, et al. A prospective study of biliary cytology in 100 patients with bile duct strictures. Hepatology. 1993;18:1399–403.
5. Schöfl R. Diagnostic endoscopic retrograde cholangiopancreatography. Endoscopy. 2001;33:147–57.
6. Trent V, Khurana KK, Pisharodi LR. Diagnostic accuracy and clinical utility of endoscopic bile duct brushing in the evaluation of biliary strictures. Arch Pathol Lab Med. 1999;123:712–5.
7. Lee JG, Leung JW, Baillie J, et al. Benign, dysplastic, or malignant--making sense of endoscopic bile duct brush cytology: results in 149 consecutive patients. Am J Gastroenterol. 1995;90:722–6.
8. Logrono R, Kurtycz DF, Molina CP, et al. Analysis of false-negative diagnoses on endoscopic brush cytology of biliary and pancreatic duct strictures: the experience at 2 university hospitals. Arch Pathol Lab Med. 2000;124:387–92.
9. Rumalla A, Baron TH, Leontovich O, et al. Improved diagnostic yield of endoscopic biliary brush cytology by digital image analysis. Mayo Clin Proc. 2001;76:29–33.
10. Pugliese V, Antonelli G, Vincenti M, et al. Endoductal tissue sampling of biliary strictures through endoscopic retrograde cholangiopan creatography (ERCP). Tumori. 1997;83:698–702.
11. Schoefl R, Haefner M, Wrba F, et al. Forceps biopsy and brush cytology during endoscopic retrograde cholangiopancreatography for the diagnosis of biliary stenoses. Scand J Gastroenterol. 1997;32:363–8.
12. Parasher VK, Huibregtse K. Endoscopic retrograde wire-guided cytology of malignant biliary strictures using a novel scraping brush. YMGE. 1998;48:288–90.
13. Fogel EL, Sherman S. How to improve the accuracy of diagnosis of malignant biliary strictures. Endoscopy. 1999;31:758–60.
14. Foutch PG. Diagnosis of cancer by cytologic methods performed during ERCP. YMGE. 1994;40:249–52.
15. Howell DA, Beveridge RP, Bosco J, et al. Endoscopic needle aspiration biopsy at ERCP in the diagnosis of biliary strictures. YMGE. 1992;38:531–5.

16. Mohandas KM, Swaroop VS, Gullar SU, et al. Diagnosis of malignant obstructive jaundice by bile cytology: results improved by dilating the bile duct strictures. YMGE. 1994;40:150–4.
17. Ponsioen CY, Vrouenraets SM, van Milligen de Wit AW, et al. Value of brush cytology for dominant strictures in primary sclerosing cholangitis. Endoscopy. 1999;31:305–9.
18. Stewart CJ, Burke GM. Value of p53 immunostaining in pancreatico-biliary brush cytology specimens. Diagn Cytopathol. 2000;23:308–13.
19. Morales CP, Burdick JS, Saboorian MH, et al. In situ hybridization for telomerase RNA in routine cytologic brushings for the diagnosis of pancreaticobiliary malignancies. YMGE. 1998;48:402–5.
20. Itoi T, Shinohara Y, Takeda K, et al. Detection of telomerase activity in biopsy specimens for diagnosis of biliary tract cancers. YMGE. 2000;52:380–6.
21. Patel AH, Harnois DM, Klee GG, et al. The utility of CA 19-9 in the diagnoses of cholangiocarcinoma in patients without primary sclerosing cholangitis. Am J Gastroenterol. 2000;95:204–7.
22. Saurin JC, Joly-Pharaboz MO, Pernas P, et al. Detection of Ki-ras gene point mutations in bile specimens for the differential diagnosis of malignant and benign biliary strictures. Gut. 2000;47:357–61.
23. Ryan ME, Baldauf MC. Comparison of flow cytometry for DNA content and brush cytology for detection of malignancy in pancreaticobiliary strictures. YMGE. 1994;40:133–9.
24. Tamada K, Sugano K. Diagnosis and non-surgical treatment of bile duct carcinoma: developments in the past decade. J Gastroenterol. 2000;35:319–25.
25. Rumalla A, Petersen BT. Diagnosis and therapy of biliary tract malignancy. Semin Gastrointest Dis. 2000;11:168–73.
26. Bain VG, Abraham N, Jhangri GS, et al. Prospective study of biliary strictures to determine the predictors of malignancy. Can J Gastroenterol. 2000;14:397–402.
27. Adamsen S, Olsen M, Jendresen MB, et al. Endobiliary brush biopsy: intra- and interobserver variation in cytological evaluation of brushings from bile duct strictures. Scand J Gastroenterol. 2006;41:597–603.
28. Glasbrenner B, Ardan M, Boeck W, et al. Prospective evaluation of brush cytology of biliary strictures during endoscopic retrograde cholangiopancreatography. Endoscopy. 1999;31:712–7.

29. Yamaguchi T, Shirai Y, Nakamura N, et al. Usefulness of brush cytology combined with pancreatic juice cytology in the diagnosis of pancreatic cancer: significance of pancreatic juice cytology after brushing. Pancreas. 2012;41:1225–9.
30. Vandervoort J, Soetikno RM, Montes H, et al. Accuracy and complication rate of brush cytology from bile duct versus pancreatic duct. YMGE. 1999;49:322–7.
31. Ferrari Júnior AP, Lichtenstein DR, Slivka A, et al. Brush cytology during ERCP for the diagnosis of biliary and pancreatic malignancies. YMGE. 1994;40:140–5.
32. Weber A, Gaa J, Rosca B, et al. Complications of percutaneous transhepatic biliary drainage in patients with dilated and nondilated intrahepatic bile ducts. Eur J Radiol. 2009;72:412–7.
33. Weber A, Weyhern v C, Fend F, et al. Endoscopic transpapillary brush cytology and forceps biopsy in patients with hilar cholangiocarcinoma. World J Gastroenterol. 2008;14:1097–101.
34. Moreno Luna LE, Kipp B, Halling KC, et al. Advanced cytologic techniques for the detection of malignant pancreatobiliary strictures. YGAST. 2006;131:1064–72.
35. Levy MJ, Baron TH, Clayton AC, et al. Prospective evaluation of advanced molecular markers and imaging techniques in patients with indeterminate bile duct strictures. Am J Gastroenterol. 2008;103:1263–73.
36. Brooks C, Gausman V, Kokoy-Mondragon C, et al. Role of fluorescent in situ hybridization, cholangioscopic biopsies, and EUS-FNA in the evaluation of biliary strictures. Dig Dis Sci. 2018;63:636–44.
37. Farrell RJ, Jain AK, Brandwein SL, et al. The combination of stricture dilation, endoscopic needle aspiration, and biliary brushings significantly improves diagnostic yield from malignant bile duct strictures. YMGE. 2001;54:587–94.
38. de Bellis M, Fogel EL, Sherman S, et al. Influence of stricture dilation and repeat brushing on the cancer detection rate of brush cytology in the evaluation of malignant biliary obstruction. YMGE. 2003;58:176–82.
39. Ornellas LC, Santos GDC, Nakao FS, et al. Comparison between endoscopic brush cytology performed before and after biliary stricture dilation for cancer detection. Arq Gastroenterol. 2006;43:20–3.
40. de Bellis M, Sherman S, Fogel EL, et al. Tissue sampling at ERCP in suspected malignant biliary strictures (Part 2). YMGE. 2002;56:720–30.

41. Pugliese V, Conio M, Nicolò G, et al. Endoscopic retrograde forceps biopsy and brush cytology of biliary strictures: a prospective study. YMGE. 1995;42:520–6.
42. Seo DW, Lee SK, Yoo KS, et al. Cholangioscopic findings in bile duct tumors. YMGE. 2000;52:630–4.
43. Kim HJ, Kim MH, Lee SK, et al. Tumor vessel: a valuable cholangioscopic clue of malignant biliary stricture. YMGE. 2000;52:635–8.
44. Shah RJ, Langer DA, Antillon M-R, et al. Cholangioscopy and cholangioscopic forceps biopsy in patients with indeterminate pancreaticobiliary pathology. YJCGH. 2006;4:219–25.
45. Fukuda Y, Tsuyuguchi T, Sakai Y, et al. Diagnostic utility of peroral cholangioscopy for various bile-duct lesions. YMGE. 2005;62:374–82.
46. Williamson JB, Draganov PV. The usefulness of SpyGlass™ choledochoscopy in the diagnosis and treatment of biliary disorders. Curr Gastroenterol Rep. 2012;14:534–41.
47. Siddiqui AA, Mehendiratta V, Jackson W, et al. Identification of cholangiocarcinoma by using the Spyglass Spyscope system for peroral cholangioscopy and biopsy collection. Clin Gastroenterol Hepatol. 2012;10:466–71. quiz e48.
48. Sun X, Zhou Z, Tian J, et al. Is single-operator peroral cholangioscopy a useful tool for the diagnosis of indeterminate biliary lesion? A systematic review and meta-analysis. Gastrointest Endosc. 2015;82:79–87.
49. Sethi A, Chen YK, Austin GL, et al. ERCP with cholangiopancreatoscopy may be associated with higher rates of complications than ERCP alone: a single-center experience. Gastrointest Endosc. 2011;73:251–6.
50. Chandrasekhara V, Elmunzer BJ, Khashab M, et al. Clinical gastrointestinal endoscopy. Philadelphia: Elsevier; 2018.
51. Tamada K, Ueno N, Tomiyama T, et al. Characterization of biliary strictures using intraductal ultrasonography: comparison with percutaneous cholangioscopic biopsy. YMGE. 1998;47:341–9.
52. Farrell RJ, Agarwal B, Brandwein SL, et al. Intraductal US is a useful adjunct to ERCP for distinguishing malignant from benign biliary strictures. YMGE. 2002;56:681–7.
53. Stavropoulos S, Larghi A, Verna E, et al. Intraductal ultrasound for the evaluation of patients with biliary strictures and no abdominal mass on computed tomography. Endoscopy. 2005;37:715–21.

54. Vazquez-Sequeiros E, Baron TH, Clain JE, et al. Evaluation of indeterminate bile duct strictures by intraductal US. YMGE. 2002;56:372–9.
55. Al-Kawas F, Aslanian H, Baillie J, et al. Percutaneous transhepatic vs. endoscopic retrograde biliary drainage for suspected malignant hilar obstruction: study protocol for a randomized controlled trial. Trials. 2018;19:108.
56. Easler JJ, Sherman S, Coté GA. Optimizing palliation of malignant hilar strictures by the use of endobiliary stents. Gastrointest Endosc. 2017;86:828–30.
57. Hameed A, Pang T, Chiou J, et al. Percutaneous vs. endoscopic pre-operative biliary drainage in hilar cholangiocarcinoma - a systematic review and meta-analysis. HPB (Oxford). 2016;18:400–10.
58. Vienne A, Hobeika E, Gouya H, et al. Prediction of drainage effectiveness during endoscopic stenting of malignant hilar strictures: the role of liver volume assessment. Gastrointest Endosc. 2010;72:728–35.
59. Moon JH, Rerknimitr R, Kogure H, et al. Topic controversies in the endoscopic management of malignant hilar strictures using metal stent: side-by-side versus stent-in-stent techniques. J Hepatobiliary Pancreat Sci. 2015;22:650–6.
60. Lee TH, Kim TH, Moon JH, et al. Bilateral versus unilateral placement of metal stents for inoperable high-grade malignant hilar biliary strictures: a multicenter, prospective, randomized study (with video). Gastrointest Endosc. 2017;86:817–27.
61. Sawas T, Halabi Al S, Parsi MA, et al. Self-expandable metal stents versus plastic stents for malignant biliary obstruction: a meta-analysis. Gastrointest Endosc. 2015;82:256–267.e7.
62. De Palma GD, Galloro G, Siciliano S, et al. Unilateral versus bilateral endoscopic hepatic duct drainage in patients with malignant hilar biliary obstruction: results of a prospective, randomized, and controlled study. YMGE. 2001;53:547–53.
63. Deviere J, Baize M, de Toeuf J, et al. Long-term follow-up of patients with hilar malignant stricture treated by endoscopic internal biliary drainage. YMGE. 1988;34:95–101.
64. Liberato MJA, Canena JMT. Endoscopic stenting for hilar cholangiocarcinoma: efficacy of unilateral and bilateral placement of plastic and metal stents in a retrospective review of 480 patients. BMC Gastroenterol. 2012;12:103.
65. Perdue DG, Freeman ML, DiSario JA, et al. Plastic versus self-expanding metallic stents for malignant hilar biliary obstruction:

a prospective multicenter observational cohort study. J Clin Gastroenterol. 2008;42:1040–6.
66. Peters RA, Williams SG, Lombard M, et al. The management of high-grade hilar strictures by endoscopic insertion of self-expanding metal endoprostheses. Endoscopy. 1997;29:10–6.
67. Wagner HJ, Knyrim K, Vakil N, et al. Plastic endoprostheses versus metal stents in the palliative treatment of malignant hilar biliary obstruction. A prospective and randomized trial. Endoscopy. 1993;25:213–8.
68. Sangchan A, Kongkasame W, Pugkhem A, et al. Efficacy of metal and plastic stents in unresectable complex hilar cholangiocarcinoma: a randomized controlled trial. Gastrointest Endosc. 2012;76:93–9.
69. Jonas S, Benckert C, Thelen A, et al. Radical surgery for hilar cholangiocarcinoma. Eur J Surg Oncol. 2008;34:263–71.
70. Celotti A, Solaini L, Montori G, et al. Preoperative biliary drainage in hilar cholangiocarcinoma: systematic review and meta-analysis. Eur J Surg Oncol. 2017;43:1628–35.
71. Naitoh I, Hayashi K, Nakazawa T, et al. Side-by-side versus stent-in-stent deployment in bilateral endoscopic metal stenting for malignant hilar biliary obstruction. Dig Dis Sci. 2012;57:3279–85.
72. Law R, Baron TH. Bilateral metal stents for hilar biliary obstruction using a 6Fr delivery system: outcomes following bilateral and side-by-side stent deployment. Dig Dis Sci. 2013;58:2667–72.
73. Paik WH, Park YS, Hwang J-H, et al. Palliative treatment with self-expandable metallic stents in patients with advanced type III or IV hilar cholangiocarcinoma: a percutaneous versus endoscopic approach. Gastrointest Endosc. 2009;69:55–62.
74. Kloek JJ, van der Gaag NA, Aziz Y, et al. Endoscopic and percutaneous preoperative biliary drainage in patients with suspected hilar cholangiocarcinoma. J Gastrointest Surg. 2010;14:119–25.
75. Wiggers JK, Groot Koerkamp B, Coelen RJ, et al. Preoperative biliary drainage in perihilar cholangiocarcinoma: identifying patients who require percutaneous drainage after failed endoscopic drainage. Endoscopy. 2015;47:1124–31.

Chapter 7
Benign Bile Duct Strictures and Bile Leaks

Anand Singla and A. Aziz Aadam

Benign Biliary Strictures

Introduction

The clinical presentation of biliary obstruction can include multiple signs and symptoms depending on etiology and chronicity. Acute biliary obstruction can lead to abdominal pain, infection (cholangitis), and marked elevations in liver transaminases with delayed elevations in bilirubin, as is often seen in pancreaticobiliary lithiasis [1]. Subacute or chronic obstruction can result in varying degrees of abdominal symptoms including pain, nausea, and vomiting, as well as jaundice, pruritus, dark urine, light-colored stools, and significant elevation in bilirubin [2].

Case 1

A 62-year-old man with cirrhosis due to hepatitis C has undergone a liver transplant. Six months after transplant, the

A. Singla
Division of Gastroenterology, University of Washington Medical Center, Seattle, WA, USA

A. A. Aadam (✉)
Division of Gastroenterology, Northwestern Memorial Hospital, Chicago, IL, USA
e-mail: abdul.aadam@northwestern.edu

D. K. Mullady (ed.), *Dilemmas in ERCP*,
https://doi.org/10.1007/978-3-030-12741-1_7

patient presented with elevated transaminases and mildly elevated total bilirubin, with concerns for development of biliary anastomotic stenosis. The patient had undergone a living donor liver transplant and received the right lobe of the donor liver. The right anterior duct was anastomosed to the recipient common bile duct via *a duct-to-duct anastomosis, while the right posterior duct was anastomosed* via *a Roux-en-Y hepaticojejunostomy.*

Diagnosis and Assessment

The clinical presentation of biliary strictures following liver transplant can be highly variable, with some patients remaining asymptomatic, while others presenting with anorexia, pruritus, fever, abdominal pain, and weight loss. In asymptomatic patients, elevated transaminases and total bilirubin should raise suspicion for biliary anastomotic stenosis.

Benign biliary strictures result in biliary obstruction and can lead to all of the above symptoms depending on etiology, which is determined by patient history, comorbid conditions, lab results, and imaging studies [3]. Noninvasive radiographic studies for evaluating the biliary system would include abdominal ultrasonography, computed tomography (CT), and magnetic resonance imaging (MRI) of the abdomen.

Etiologies of benign bile duct strictures are diverse and can be divided into four categories: iatrogenic (postsurgical, post-sphincterotomy, postradiation), inflammatory (pancreatitis, cholangitis, autoimmune), ischemic, and others (papillary stenosis, extrinsic compression, trauma, etc.) [4]. Cholecystectomy and liver transplantation are the most common causes of postsurgical biliary strictures, with a bile duct injury occurring in 0.5% of patients following cholecystectomy and anastomotic stricture occurring in 13–25% of patients following liver transplant [5–8]. The incidence of common bile duct stricture in patients with chronic pancreatitis ranges between 3% and 46% [9, 10].

Treatment and Management

Endoscopic retrograde cholangiopancreatography (ERCP) is considered the first-line treatment option for benign biliary strictures and has been shown to be safe and effective, with excellent long-term results [4, 11, 12]. Techniques used for treatment during ERCP include dilation of the stricture and subsequent stent placement to bridge the stenosis with either multiple plastic biliary stents or a fully covered self-expandable metal stent (FCSEMS).

Balloon dilation followed by stent placement remains the mainstay of treatment for benign biliary strictures [4]. Specifically, for benign biliary strictures, the European Society of Gastrointestinal Endoscopy (ESGE) recommends placing temporary simultaneous plastic stents with re-evaluation and exchange every 3 months for up to 12 months [13]. More recent studies have shown that FCSEMSs are also effective and potentially preferable in certain circumstances.

Endoscopic management with ERCP is considered the first-line management approach to biliary strictures following liver transplant [4]. If a biliary anastomotic stenosis is encountered, a guidewire is advanced past the stricture, and balloon dilation is performed, followed by placement of plastic biliary stents. The stricture should be dilated to the diameter of the donor duct, typically ranging from 4 to 10 mm, progressively increasing in subsequent ERCPs. ERCP is repeated every 3 months to re-examine the stricture site, with greater number of plastic stents placed. Procedures can be stopped once resolution of the stricture is noted, and all stents have been removed [14]. This strategy is safe and effective, with about four ERCPs required, and resolution in 66–100% of patients [4, 12, 15].

Despite the success of endoscopic treatment with multiple plastic stents, fully covered self-expandable metal stents (FCSEMS) have been used in the treatment of posttransplant biliary anastomotic strictures in recent years. One small randomized trial showed similar efficacy of FCSEMS compared to multiple plastic stents resulting in similar success and complication rates, but with fewer overall number of procedures required, leading to cost-effectiveness of the FCSEMS [16]. However, stent migration of FCSEMS is of significant concern, occurring in 33% of patients in a recent prospective, randomized trial [17], and there is potential for a higher number of adverse events [18]. In another study using FCSEMS comparing patients who had failed multiple plastic stents and those who had no previous endoscopic therapy, the rate of stent migration of FCSEMS was still 33%, though stricture resolution was achieved in 72% of patients who had previously failed therapy [19]. Hence, the standard approach of multiple plastic stents is preferred as the primary modality in endoscopic therapy of posttransplant biliary anastomotic strictures, with the use of FCSEMS reserved for when the standard approach fails [14, 19].

Living donor liver transplants (LDLTs) constitute about 5% of all transplants in the United States, with the overall number significantly varying between UNOS regions, and only a few specific centers performing ten or more per year [20]. In the United States, LDLT has been shown to reduce mortality on the transplant waiting list and possibly improve 5-year survival when compared to deceased donor liver transplant (DDLT) [21, 22]. As noted above, biliary complications following liver transplant are common. However, the risk of biliary complications is significantly higher in patients undergoing LDLT when compared to DDLT, a finding that has been observed in multiple studies [23–26].

Patients having undergone LDLT who experience biliary anastomotic stenosis pose additional challenges to the endoscopist. For the typical duct-to-duct anastomosis, the donor duct is typically smaller when compared to DDLT and the biliary system often angulated, resulting in difficulty advancing a wire across the stenosis [27]. Indeed, failure to advance a guidewire through an anastomotic stenosis following LDLT ranges from 16% to 38% [27, 28]. More advanced techniques can be helpful in traversing anastomotic strictures following LDLT, with one case series showing moderate success using cholangioscopy-guided wire passage in those patients who failed initial passage [29].

Long-term outcomes of the treatment of posttransplant biliary anastomotic strictures in patients having undergone LDLT have yet to be studied in detail, but endoscopic therapies seem to be effective. One observational study noted a 21% recurrence rate of strictures, all of which were successfully retreated endoscopically over a total follow-up period of 70 months [28].

Few studies and case series have evaluated FCSEMS for patients experiencing anastomotic biliary strictures after LDLT. In a small study examining the use of FCSEMS as salvage therapy following failure of standard approaches, patients with biliary anastomotic strictures after LDLT had a stricture resolution rate of 83%, with stent migration observed in 6%; however, the covered metal stent used in that study is not available in the United States [30]. Stent migration of FCSEMS and the resultant consequences would be of equal concern in patients having undergone LDLT compared to DDLT, and thus, FCSEMS should likely be reserved for refractory cases.

ERCP in patients with bilioenteric anastomosis is especially difficult, usually requiring deep enteroscopy to reach the bilioenteric anastomosis. The use of balloon enteroscopes to reach the anastomosis limits the types of accessories that can be used for the procedure owing the length of the enteroscope itself. Additionally, further difficulties arise due to the lack of an elevator and the small working channel. A few meta-analyses have examined the success rates of these procedures, with one showing an overall procedural success rate of 61.7% [31]. Ultimately, there is a significant learning curve for ERCP in altered anatomy, which can be successful in experienced hands [4, 27]. Bilioenteric anastomotic strictures can be less recalcitrant when compared to duct-duct anastomotic strictures, often requiring balloon dilation alone [32].

Case 1 Outcome

The patient underwent ERCP with cholangiography showing stenosis at the duct-to-duct anastomosis (Fig. 7.1a) *leading to the right anterior system. At the initial ERCP, this was dilated to 4 mm, and a 10 Fr plastic stent was successfully placed.*

An adult colonoscope was used to reach the hepaticojejunostomy with some difficulty, and limited cholangiography was performed, indicating stenosis at the hepaticojejunostomy. Given the severity of the stenosis, a guidewire could not be advanced into the right posterior system (Fig. 7.1b). *Percutaneous cholangiography was then performed by interventional radiology and was notable for dilated right posterior system leading to the stenosis at the hepaticojejunostomy* (Fig. 7.1c). *A percutaneous wire was able to traverse the hepaticojejunostomy and was coiled in the small bowel* (Fig. 7.1d). *The right posterior system was then able to be successfully accessed endoscopically using the rendezvous technique* (Fig. 7.1e). *The hepaticojejunostomy was balloon dilated* (Fig. 7.1f), *and a 10 Fr plastic stent was placed* (Fig. 7.1g).

The stenosis at the hepaticojejunostomy resolved quickly over subsequent ERCPs (Fig. 7.1h), *while the stenosis at the duct-to-duct anastomosis required further dilation and placement of multiple plastic stents. At 1 year, complete resolution of this stenosis was noted as well.*

Figure 7.1 Post living donor liver transplant biliary anastomotic strictures involving the duct-duct anastomosis and hepaticojejunostomy. Initial ERCP via the papilla showed stenosis at the duct-duct anastomosis in this patient who underwent LDLT (**a**, arrow), with associated upstream dilation of the right anterior system. A pediatric colonoscope was advanced to the hepaticojejunostomy, which was also noted to be stenosed, and a guidewire was unable to be passed into the right posterior system (**b**). A percutaneous cholangiogram was performed by interventional radiology (**c**), and a guidewire was able to traverse the stenosis at the hepaticojejunostomy and was coiled in the small bowel (**d**). Overall cholangiography findings of the right posterior system were notable for dilation of the bile ducts above the stenosis at the hepaticojejunostomy (**c**–**e**). Using the rendezvous technique, endoscopic access to the right posterior system was obtained (**e**). The stenosis at the hepaticojejunostomy was balloon dilated (**f**) and a 10 Fr plastic stent was successfully placed (**g**). This stenosis at the hepaticojejunostomy eventually resolved (**h**)

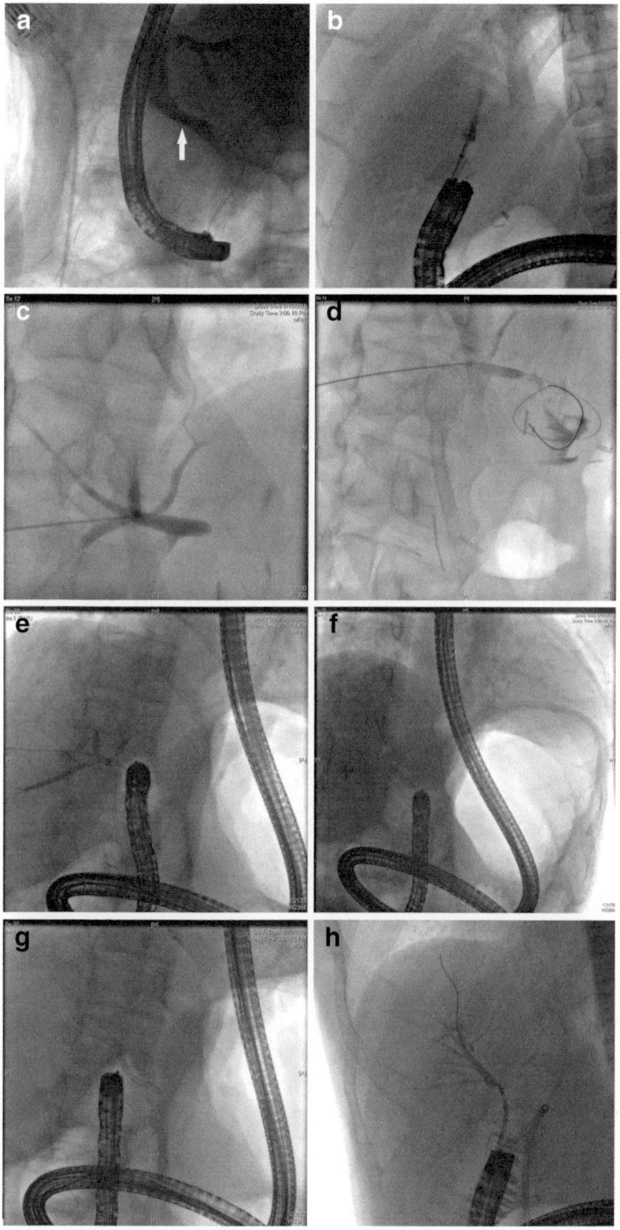
a
b
c
d
e
f
g
h

Case 2

A 62-year-old man with a history of chronic pancreatitis presented with symptoms of right upper quadrant and epigastric abdominal pain associated with nausea, pruritus, jaundice, and dark urine, worsening over the course of 1 week. He has also been experiencing intermittent fevers and chills. Initial lab tests on arrival were notable for marked elevation in transaminases and alkaline phosphatase, a total bilirubin of 7.0, and leukocytosis. Abdominal ultrasound is notable for marked dilation of the intrahepatic bile ducts. CT scan shows changes in the pancreatic parenchyma consistent with chronic pancreatitis and mild interstitial acute pancreatitis, with difficulty visualizing the extrahepatic bile duct.

Diagnosis and Assessment

The initial evaluation of a patient presenting with abdominal pain and physical findings concerning for possible biliary obstruction includes laboratory evaluation and imaging, which are paramount in establishing the diagnosis. With this patient's history of chronic pancreatitis, and without imaging evidence of a malignant mass, the etiology of biliary obstruction is most likely due to pancreatic fibrosis in the head of the pancreas, with resulting distal biliary stricture. Distal common bile duct stricture in the area of the head of the pancreas results from progressive fibrosis of the pancreatic parenchyma and develops in 3–46% of patients with chronic pancreatitis [10, 13, 33, 34].

Traditionally, bile duct strictures due to chronic pancreatitis do not need intervention unless there are signs and symptoms of biliary obstruction. These would include infectious symptoms due to cholangitis associated with elevations in transaminases and total bilirubin, and symptoms of biliary pain due to the formation of sludge and stones in a partially obstructed, dilated biliary system. While there is no evidence of distal pancreatic mass on CT scan, and the etiology is most likely stricture due to pancreatitis, it is still important to rule out a primary biliary malignancy with brushings for cytology. Placement of transpapillary parallel plastic stents is effective in 60–90% of cases [35]. As previously mentioned, balloon dilation with placement of increasing number of stents is performed sequentially every 3–4 months for up to 12 months. The stricture is considered resolved when the stricture waist has disappeared and contrast is able to freely drain from the biliary system [33].

Treatment and Management

On the spectrum of benign bile duct strictures, strictures due to chronic pancreatitis can be recalcitrant and respond least well to therapy with plastic stents [36]. In one observational study of 58 patients, the overall success rate at 12 months was only 38% [37]. The only predictor of success at 12 months was evidence of concomitant acute pancreatitis. This may indicate that the high recurrence rate of biliary strictures secondary to chronic pancreatitis may be due to the fibrotic, calcific nature of the disease.

As an alternative to plastic stents, fully covered self-expanding metal stents (FCSEMS) have been used in the treatment of benign biliary strictures. There are many potential advantages with FCSEMS, including easier deployment of a single stent compared to multiple plastic stents, larger post-deployment diameter, and less frequent and fewer endoscopic sessions. The FCSEMS can stay in place for 6 months before requiring removal, after which time there is a risk of stent occlusion and embedment due to the hyperplastic reaction of the biliary mucosa [33]. Disadvantages to FCSEMS include higher cost than plastic stents and potential difficulty with removal.

In a randomized trial comparing FCSEMS and plastic biliary stents in benign biliary strictures, FCSEMS were as effective as plastic stents and achieved resolution of strictures with fewer procedures (2.14 vs 3.24) [38]. In a systematic review and meta-analysis comparing FCSEMS and plastic biliary stents specifically in benign strictures due to chronic pancreatitis, FCSEMS showed higher clinical success at 12 months (77% vs 33%), lower incidence of late adverse events, and a lower number of ERCPs (1.5 vs 3.9). Despite the higher cost of FCSEMS when compared to plastic stents, there is evidence to show that the use of FCSEMS in benign biliary strictures due to chronic pancreatitis is cost-effective given the fewer number of ERCPs required [39].

Thus, while the use of simultaneous and increasing size/number of plastic stents in the treatment of benign biliary strictures is the generally preferred approach, when it comes to strictures due to chronic pancreatitis, we prefer the use of a fully covered self-expending metal stent.

Case 2 Outcome

The patient underwent ERCP, and a distal common bile duct stricture was confirmed (Fig. 7.2a). *Brushings of the stricture were performed, and the stricture was dilated to 6 mm with a biliary dilation balloon. A 10 Fr by 7 cm plastic stent was placed into the common bile duct* (Fig. 7.2b). *Cytology results from the brushings returned negative for malignancy. The patient's symptoms and lab findings improved significantly. He returned 3 months later for an ERCP, at which time the previously placed stent was removed, the stricture dilated to 8 mm, brushings repeated, and three parallel 10 Fr by 7 cm plastic stents were able to be placed. Cytology results again returned negative for malignancy, and the patient's stents were removed 3 months later, at which time the stricture was noted to have resolved.*

Four months after the removal of the biliary stents, the patient returned with similar symptoms to his original presentation (abdominal pain, itching, jaundice). Imaging confirmed a recurrent stricture. The patient underwent repeat ERCP, and the recurrent stricture was noted in the area of the head of the pancreas. At this time, a transpapillary 10 mm by 6 cm fully covered metal stent was successfully deployed (Fig. 7.2c).

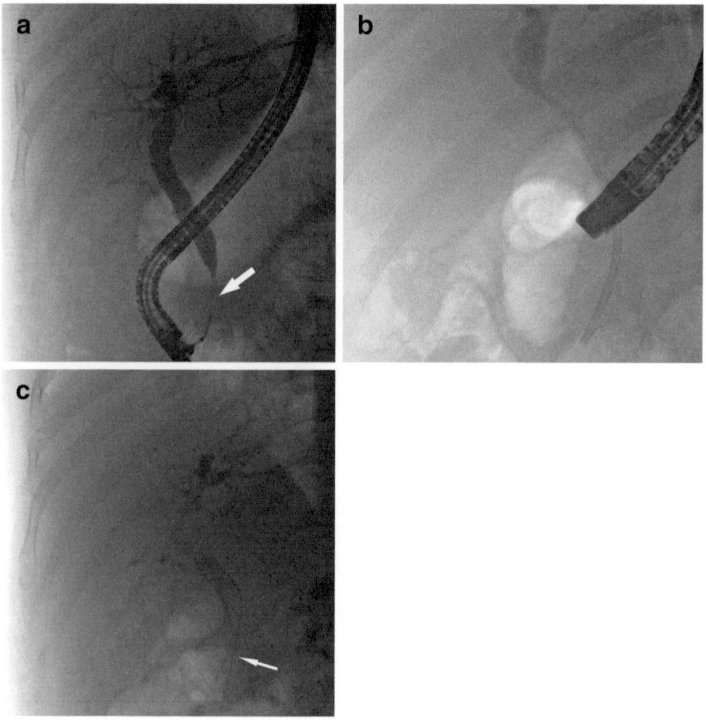

FIGURE 7.2 Biliary stricture due to chronic pancreatitis. Initial ERCP showed severe stricture of the common bile duct in the area of the head of the pancreas and associated upstream dilation of the main bile duct and intrahepatics (**a**, arrow). A transpapillary 10 Fr plastic stent was placed at the initial ERCP in order to traverse the stenosis (**b**). Eventually, the patient failed multiple plastic stents, and eventually, a transpapillary 10 mm by 6 cm fully covered self-expanding metal stent was placed to traverse the stricture (**c**). Note the waist in the body of the stent after initial placement in the area of the stenosis (arrow)

Bile Leaks

Introduction

Bile duct injury resulting in bile leak can occur following surgical procedures on the biliary system, including cholecystectomy, liver resection, and liver transplantation. The incidence of bile leak following cholecystectomy has varied and is estimated to occur in 0.4–1% of all cholecystectomies in the laparoscopic era, with some evidence to suggest a higher association with open cholecystectomies [40, 41]. The overall incidence of bile leaks following liver transplant is common, with one review of literature noting an incidence of 8.2%, and various studies showing a range of 2–25% [23, 42].

Case 3

A 34-year-old man with a history of cirrhosis due to alcohol use undergoes a living donor liver transplant and receives a donor right lobe. The transplant is initially uneventful, and the patient is discharged. A few days following discharge, the patient is seen urgently in transplant surgery clinic, where he is noted to have a distended/tender abdomen and bilious discharge from the incision site. He is admitted to the hospital and taken for a laparotomy, at which time a large amount of bile is washed out of the peritoneum, and leakage of bile is noted from the cut surface of the liver, which was repaired surgically. A Jackson-Pratt drain was left in place. Over the next 2 days, there was continuous drainage of bile from the JP drain, concerning for an ongoing bile leak.

Diagnosis and Assessment

Bile leaks are diagnosed clinically, often presenting as a biloma resulting in bile peritonitis or as persistent drainage of bile from a percutaneous drain in the right upper quadrant. Combined with a history of hepatobiliary surgical intervention, the presence of a collection of fluid on imaging, such as transabdominal ultrasonography or computed tomography, should raise significant suspicion for a bile leak. While US and CT scan are useful, these methods cannot reliably distinguish bile leaks from other postoperative fluid collections such as blood, serous fluid, or pus. In this way, MRCP, combined with hepatobiliary contrast-enhanced MR imaging, is useful in detecting biliary leak and differentiating it from other postoperative complications [43].

With respect to bile duct injuries following cholecystectomy, various classification systems have been proposed [44]. The Bismuth classification is based on the location of the injury in the biliary tract, specifically according to the distance from the biliary confluence [45]. However, this system does not include the wide spectrum of possible biliary injuries. The Strasberg classification consequently sought to expand the Bismuth classification and includes different types of injuries and leaks [46]. The most useful classification for endoscopists is likely the Amsterdam classification proposed by Bergman et al., where there are four types of postoperative bile duct injury: type A being a cystic duct or aberrant duct leak, type B being a major bile duct leak with or without concomitant stricture, type C being a bile duct stricture without a leak, and type D being a complete transection of the bile duct [47].

Bile leaks following hepatobiliary surgery such as liver resection and liver transplant are common and can be more complex when compared to cholecystectomy, occurring in up to 15% of all liver resections [48]. In a meta-analysis, the rate of biliary leakage after liver transplant was 8.2%, without significant difference between DDLT (7.8%) and LDLT (9.5%) [23]. Bile leaks following hepatobiliary surgery make up about 17% of all postsurgical bile leaks, with post-cholecystectomy leaks accounting for the rest [49].

Known risk factors for the development of bile leak following liver transplant include surgical technique, hepatic artery thrombosis, donors after cardiac death, prolonged warm and cold ischemia times, ABO blood group mismatch, and T-tube use [50].

Following liver transplant, leakage may develop at the anastomotic site, from the cystic duct remnant, from the cut surface of partial liver grafts in the case of LDLT, and following T-tube removal [25]. Anastomotic leaks or leaks resulting from anastomotic strictures are the most common type to occur in post-liver transplant patients, followed by complications due to the presence of a T-tube if a T-tube is placed at the time of surgery [51]. It should be mentioned that the current trend is toward no longer using T-tubes in the prevention of anastomotic strictures [52].

Treatment and Management

In early years prior to the development of minimally invasive endoscopic techniques, surgical repair or conversion to hepaticojejunostomy was primarily used, with resultant morbidity and mortality [48, 53–55]. However, in the era of therapeutic ERCP, the vast majority of bile leaks are able to be successfully treated endoscopically with a combination of sphincterotomy and placement of biliary stents, given that the continuity of the bile ducts is maintained, and the main ducts have not been completely transected. The goal of sphincterotomy and stent placement is twofold: to potentially bridge and cover the leak if possible, thereby allowing healing and/or to lead to preferential flow of bile through the papilla resulting in a reduced pressure gradient, thereby diminishing flow through the leak [53, 55].

As in post-cholecystectomy bile leaks, ERCP with sphincterotomy and stent placement is the minimally invasive treatment of choice in bile leaks following liver transplant. Overall, endoscopic therapy solves the problem in 85% of patients [13, 25, 56, 57]. However, when compared to bile leaks after cholecystectomy, the rates of success are somewhat lower in patients who undergo liver transplant or liver resection [58]. In one study, multiple ERCPs were successful in treating 95% of leaks following cholecystectomy, but only 86% of leaks following liver transplant or other hepatobiliary surgery [58].

Based on experience and literature, a general protocol for endoscopic therapy of bile leaks can be proposed [47, 48, 53–55, 58, 59]. Treatment should consist of cholangiography to localize and assess the severity of the leak, followed by sphincterotomy, and placement of a plastic biliary stent. The stent should cover or span the bile leak if possible (i.e., not in patients with a very peripheral leak or a terminal leak). Bilious output from the percutaneous drain should be monitored, and when complete resolution is suspected, repeat ERCP with stent removal and reassessment should be performed (typically 4–6 weeks following initial procedure). For persistent leaks (i.e., no improvement in bilious output within 2–3 days following initial ERCP), repeat ERCP with multiple plastic stents should be considered. For those who fail this treatment, ERCP with placement of a fully covered self-expanding metal stent (FCSEMS) can be attempted if the stent can be placed above the leak site [53, 59].

If endoscopic therapy has failed, then referral for surgery would be appropriate.

While some specific classification systems exist for bile leaks following cholecystectomy, a clinically useful method for the endoscopist to assess a postoperative bile leak would be a two-category system delineating low-grade (small) leaks and high-grade (large) leaks. Low-grade leaks would be classified as such if the leak is identified only after filling of the intrahepatic duct with contrast during cholangiography. High-grade leaks would be classified when there is substantial extravasation of contrast prior to filling of the intrahepatic bile duct at the time of cholangiography [48, 55, 60]. In one study, bile leak severity was the only independent factor associated with eventual success of endoscopic treatment following hepatobiliary surgery.

The use of FCSEMS in the treatment of posttransplant bile leaks has not been studied in detail. In one study examining the outcomes of FCSEMS in posttransplant bile leaks, there was a high rate of resultant common bile duct strictures, and removal was difficult in some cases, despite achieving resolution of bile leak [61]. Therefore, at this time, the use of FCSEMS is only recommended in select cases of refractory bile leaks, if at all [13, 25].

The success of endoscopic treatment for post-cholecystectomy bile duct leaks has been shown to be greater than 90% [53]. The success rate approaches 100% for Amsterdam type A bile duct injuries, which is the most common type of injury seen after a cholecystectomy [58, 62, 63]. For other types of leaks, the success rate is significantly lower. For patients with Amsterdam type B leak, the success rate has been reported to vary between 60% and 80%, and nearly all patients with a complete transection of a main bile duct (Amsterdam type D) typically require surgical repair [58, 62, 63].

Case 3 Outcome

The patient underwent ERCP 2 days following laparotomy. On cholangiography, there was immediate extravasation of contrast at the posttransplant biliary anastomosis. Additionally, it was noted that the leak also involved the branch leading to the right posterior ductal system. The intrahepatic ducts in the right posterior system and right anterior system eventually opacified with contrast (Fig. 7.3a). *With some difficulty, guidewires were able to be passed into both the right anterior and right posterior system* (Fig. 7.3b). *Two 8.5 Fr plastic stents were placed, both ending upstream above the location of the leak, with one in the right posterior system and one in the right anterior system* (Fig. 7.3c).

One day following the procedure, the patient's output of bile from the percutaneous drain was noted to be significantly reduced, and continued to improve the following day, at which time the patient was discharged.

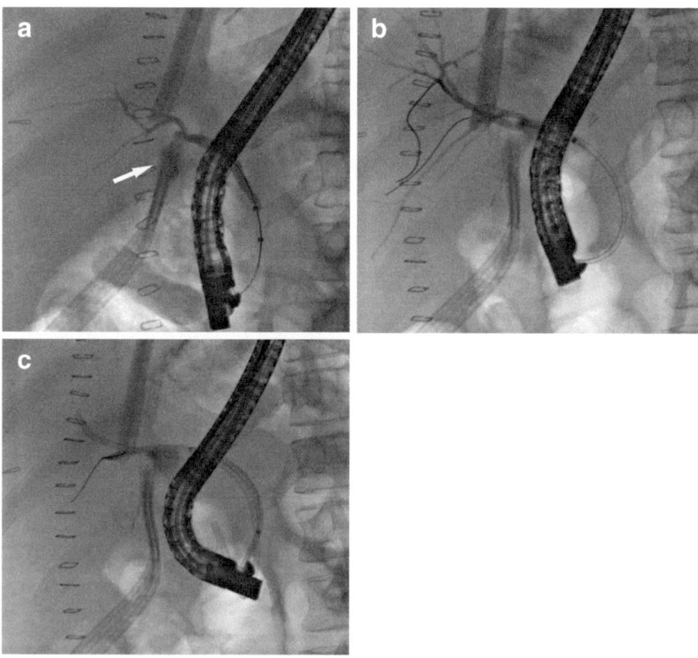

FIGURE 7.3 Bile leak at the anastomosis following living donor liver transplant. Initial ERCP showed immediate extravasation of contrast at the posttransplant biliary anastomosis, indicating a large bile leak involving the right posterior system (**a**, arrow). With significant difficulty due to the small, angulated ducts, two guidewires were placed into the biliary system, with one in the anterior system and one in the posterior system such that the bile leak was traversed (**b**). Two 8.5 Fr plastic stents were placed, both ending upstream above the location of the leak, with one in the right posterior system and one in the right anterior system (**c**)

Pearls and Pitfalls

- Endoscopic retrograde cholangiopancreatography (ERCP) is considered the first-line option for treatment of benign biliary strictures and has been shown to be safe and effective, with strong long-term results.
- A standard approach for the treatment of benign biliary strictures includes ERCP with sphincterotomy, balloon dilation of the stricture to the width of the bile duct, and placement of multiple plastic stents. ERCP is repeated with stent exchange every 3 months for up to 1 year until stricture resolution is achieved.
- Fully covered self-expanding metal stents (FCSEMS) are effective in treating benign biliary strictures, requiring a lower number of ERCPs; however, stent migration can be a significant concern.
- In patients having undergone living donor liver transplant (LDLT), the donor duct is typically smaller when compared to deceased donor liver transplant (DDLT), and the biliary system is often angulated, resulting in difficulty advancing a wire across the stenosis.
- FCSEMS are preferred in the treatment of bile duct strictures due to chronic pancreatitis because these strictures tend to be more recalcitrant and respond least well to therapy with plastic stents.
- The vast majority of bile leaks are able to be successfully treated endoscopically with a combination of sphincterotomy and placement of biliary stent, given that the continuity of the bile duct is maintained, and the main ducts have not been completely transected.
- The stent should cover or span the bile leak if possible (i.e., not in patients with a very peripheral leak or a terminal leak).
- Classifying bile leaks as low grade and high grade at the time of cholangiography can be helpful in determining treatment success.
- Anastomotic leaks or leaks resulting from anastomotic strictures are the most common type to occur in post-liver transplant patients.

- While multiple ERCPs may be beneficial in treating bile leaks following cholecystectomy, the success of subsequent ERCPs after failure of initial ERCP in bile leaks following hepatobiliary surgery and liver transplant is much lower.
- In both benign bile duct strictures and bile leaks following liver transplant, the use of FCSEMS should be reserved only for refractory cases.

References

1. Campos S, Silva N, Carvalho A. A new paradigm in gallstones diseases and marked elevation of transaminases: an observational study. Ann Hepatol. 2017;16:285–90.
2. Roche SP, Kobos R. Jaundice in the adult patient. Am Fam Physician. 2004;69:299–304.
3. Singh A, Gelrud A, Agarwal B. Biliary strictures: diagnostic considerations and approach. Gastroenterol Rep. 2015;3:22–31.
4. Hu B, Sun B, Cai Q, et al. Asia-Pacific consensus guidelines for endoscopic management of benign biliary strictures. Gastrointest Endosc. 2017;86:44–58.
5. Flum DR, Cheadle A, Prela C, et al. Bile duct injury during cholecystectomy and survival in medicare beneficiaries. JAMA. 2003;290:2168–73.
6. Welling TH, Heidt DG, Englesbe MJ, et al. Biliary complications following liver transplantation in the model for end-stage liver disease era: effect of donor, recipient, and technical factors. Liver Transpl Off Publ Am Assoc Study Liver Dis Int Liver Transplant Soc. 2008;14:73–80.
7. Hong SY, Hu X-G, Lee HY, et al. Long-term analysis of biliary complications after duct-to-duct biliary reconstruction in living donor liver transplantations. Liver Transpl Off Publ Am Assoc Study Liver Dis Int Liver Transplant Soc. 2018;24(8):1050–61.
8. Sundaram V, Jones DT, Shah NH, et al. Posttransplant biliary complications in the pre- and post-model for end-stage liver disease era. Liver Transpl Off Publ Am Assoc Study Liver Dis Int Liver Transplant Soc. 2011;17:428–35.

9. Abdallah AA, Krige JEJ, Bornman PC. Biliary tract obstruction in chronic pancreatitis. HPB. 2007;9:421–8.
10. Dumonceau J-M, Delhaye M, Tringali A, et al. Endoscopic treatment of chronic pancreatitis: European Society of Gastrointestinal Endoscopy (ESGE) clinical guideline. Endoscopy. 2012;44:784–800.
11. Costamagna G, Tringali A, Mutignani M, et al. Endotherapy of postoperative biliary strictures with multiple stents: results after more than 10 years of follow-up. Gastrointest Endosc. 2010;72:551–7.
12. Kuroda Y, Tsuyuguchi T, Sakai Y, et al. Long-term follow-up evaluation for more than 10 years after endoscopic treatment for postoperative bile duct strictures. Surg Endosc. 2010;24:834–40.
13. Dumonceau J-M, Tringali A, Blero D, et al. Biliary stenting: indications, choice of stents and results: European Society of Gastrointestinal Endoscopy (ESGE) clinical guideline. Endoscopy. 2012;44:277–98.
14. Lee DW, Jo HH, Abdullah J, et al. Endoscopic management of anastomotic strictures after liver transplantation. Clin Endosc. 2016;49:457–61.
15. Tabibian JH, Asham EH, Han S, et al. Endoscopic treatment of postorthotopic liver transplantation anastomotic biliary strictures with maximal stent therapy (with video). Gastrointest Endosc. 2010;71:505–12.
16. Kaffes A, Griffin S, Vaughan R, et al. A randomized trial of a fully covered self-expandable metallic stent versus plastic stents in anastomotic biliary strictures after liver transplantation. Therap Adv Gastroenterol. 2014;7:64–71.
17. Tal AO, Finkelmeier F, Filmann N, et al. Multiple plastic stents versus covered metal stent for treatment of anastomotic biliary strictures after liver transplantation: a prospective, randomized, multicenter trial. Gastrointest Endosc. 2017;86:1038–45.
18. Martins FP, De Paulo GA, Contini MLC, et al. Metal versus plastic stents for anastomotic biliary strictures after liver transplantation: a randomized controlled trial. Gastrointest Endosc. 2018;87:131.e1–131.e13.
19. Tarantino I, Traina M, Mocciaro F, et al. Fully covered metallic stents in biliary stenosis after orthotopic liver transplantation. Endoscopy. 2012;44:246–50.
20. Kim PTW, Testa G. Living donor liver transplantation in the USA. Hepatobiliary Surg Nutr. 2016;5:133–40.

21. Shah SA, Levy GA, Greig PD, et al. Reduced mortality with right-lobe living donor compared to deceased-donor liver transplantation when analyzed from the time of listing. Am J Transplant. 2007;7:998–1002.
22. Berg CL, Merion RM, Shearon TH, et al. Liver transplant recipient survival benefit with living donation in the model for endstage liver disease allocation era. Hepatol Baltim Md. 2011;54:1313–21.
23. Akamatsu N, Sugawara Y, Hashimoto D. Biliary reconstruction, its complications and management of biliary complications after adult liver transplantation: a systematic review of the incidence, risk factors and outcome. Transpl Int Off J Eur Soc Organ Transplant. 2011;24:379–92.
24. Liu CL, Fan ST, Lo CM, et al. Operative outcomes of adult-to-adult right lobe live donor liver transplantation: a comparative study with cadaveric whole-graft liver transplantation in a single center. Ann Surg. 2006;243:404–10.
25. Gómez CM, Dumonceau J-M, Marcolongo M, et al. Endoscopic management of biliary complications after adult living-donor versus deceased-donor liver transplantation. Transplantation. 2009;88:1280–5.
26. Samstein B, Smith AR, Freise CE, et al. Complications and their resolution in recipients of deceased and living donor liver transplants: findings from the A2ALL Cohort Study. Am J Transplant. 2016;16:594–602.
27. Tsujino T, Isayama H, Kogure H, et al. Endoscopic management of biliary strictures after living donor liver transplantation. Clin J Gastroenterol. 2017;10:297–311.
28. Hsieh T-H, Mekeel KL, Crowell MD, et al. Endoscopic treatment of anastomotic biliary strictures after living donor liver transplantation: outcomes after maximal stent therapy. Gastrointest Endosc. 2013;77:47–54.
29. Woo YS, Lee JK, Noh DH, et al. SpyGlass cholangioscopy-assisted guidewire placement for post-LDLT biliary strictures: a case series. Surg Endosc. 2016;30:3897–903.
30. Jang SI, Sung SY, Park H, et al. Salvage therapy using self-expandable metal stents for recalcitrant anastomotic strictures after living-donor liver transplantation. Therap Adv Gastroenterol. 2017;10:297–309.

31. Inamdar S, Slattery E, Sejpal DV, et al. Systematic review and meta-analysis of single-balloon enteroscopy-assisted ERCP in patients with surgically altered GI anatomy. Gastrointest Endosc. 2015;82:9–19.
32. Lee AY, Gregorius J, Kerlan RK, et al. Percutaneous transhepatic balloon dilation of biliary-enteric anastomotic strictures after surgical repair of iatrogenic bile duct injuries. PLoS One. 2012;7:e46478.
33. Familiari P, Boškoski I, Bove V, et al. ERCP for biliary strictures associated with chronic pancreatitis. Gastrointest Endosc Clin N Am. 2013;23:833–45.
34. Dumonceau J-M, Macias-Gomez C. Endoscopic management of complications of chronic pancreatitis. World J Gastroenterol. 2013;19:7308–15.
35. Elmunzer BJ. Endoscopic approaches to pancreatic disease. Curr Opin Gastroenterol. 2016;32(5):422–28.
36. Siiki A, Helminen M, Sand J, et al. Covered self-expanding metal stents may be preferable to plastic stents in the treatment of chronic pancreatitis-related biliary strictures: a systematic review comparing 2 methods of stent therapy in benign biliary strictures. J Clin Gastroenterol. 2014;48:635–43.
37. Cahen DL, van Berkel A-MM, Oskam D, et al. Long-term results of endoscopic drainage of common bile duct strictures in chronic pancreatitis. Eur J Gastroenterol Hepatol. 2005;17:103–8.
38. Coté GA, Slivka A, Tarnasky P, et al. Effect of covered metallic stents compared with plastic stents on benign biliary stricture resolution: a randomized clinical trial. JAMA. 2016;315:1250–7.
39. Behm BW, Brock A, Clarke BW, et al. Cost analysis of temporarily placed covered self expandable metallic stents versus plastic stents in biliary strictures related to Chronic pancreatitis. Gastrointest Endosc. 2007;65:AB211.
40. Veen EJ, Bik M, Janssen-Heijnen MLG, et al. Outcome measurement in laparoscopic cholecystectomy by using a prospective complication registry: results of an audit. Int J Qual Health Care J Int Soc Qual Health Care. 2008;20:144–51.
41. Karvonen J, Salminen P, Grönroos JM. Bile duct injuries during open and laparoscopic cholecystectomy in the laparoscopic era: alarming trends. Surg Endosc. 2011;25:2906–10.

42. Kochhar G, Parungao JM, Hanouneh IA, et al. Biliary complications following liver transplantation. World J Gastroenterol. 2013;19:2841–6.
43. Mungai F, Berti V, Colagrande S. Bile leak after elective laparoscopic cholecystectomy: role of MR imaging. J Radiol Case Rep. 2013;7:25–32.
44. Chun K. Recent classifications of the common bile duct injury. Korean J Hepatobiliary Pancreat Surg. 2014;18:69–72.
45. Bismuth H, Majno PE. Biliary strictures: classification based on the principles of surgical treatment. World J Surg. 2001;25:1241–4.
46. Strasberg SM, Hertl M, Soper NJ. An analysis of the problem of biliary injury during laparoscopic cholecystectomy. J Am Coll Surg. 1995;180:101–25.
47. Bergman JJ, van den Brink GR, Rauws EA, et al. Treatment of bile duct lesions after laparoscopic cholecystectomy. Gut. 1996;38:141–7.
48. Dechêne A, Jochum C, Fingas C, et al. Endoscopic management is the treatment of choice for bile leaks after liver resection. Gastrointest Endosc. 2014;80:626–633.e1.
49. Adler DG, Papachristou GI, Taylor LJ, et al. Clinical outcomes in patients with bile leaks treated via ERCP with regard to the timing of ERCP: a large multicenter study. Gastrointest Endosc. 2017;85:766–72.
50. Seehofer D, Eurich D, Veltzke-Schlieker W, et al. Biliary complications after liver transplantation: old problems and new challenges. Am J Transplant. 2013;13:253–65.
51. Sendino O, Fernández-Simon A, Law R, et al. Endoscopic management of bile leaks after liver transplantation: an analysis of two high-volume transplant centers. United Eur Gastroenterol J. 2018;6:89–96.
52. López-Andújar R, Orón EM, Carregnato AF, et al. T-tube or no T-tube in cadaveric orthotopic liver transplantation: the eternal dilemma: results of a prospective and randomized clinical trial. Ann Surg. 2013;258:21–9.
53. Canena J, Horta D, Coimbra J, et al. Outcomes of endoscopic management of primary and refractory postcholecystectomy biliary leaks in a multicentre review of 178 patients. BMC Gastroenterol. 2015;15:105.

54. Ahmad F, Saunders R, Lloyd G, et al. An algorithm for the management of bile leak following laparoscopic cholecystectomy. Ann R Coll Surg Engl. 2007;89:51–6.
55. Sandha GS, Bourke MJ, Haber GB, et al. Endoscopic therapy for bile leak based on a new classification: results in 207 patients. Gastrointest Endosc. 2004;60:567–74.
56. Rerknimitr R, Sherman S, Fogel EL, et al. Biliary tract complications after orthotopic liver transplantation with choledochocholedochostomy anastomosis: endoscopic findings and results of therapy. Gastrointest Endosc. 2002;55:224–31.
57. Solmi L, Cariani G, Leo P, et al. Results of endoscopic retrograde cholangiopancreatography in the treatment of biliary tract complications after orthotopic liver transplantation: our experience. Hepatogastroenterology. 2007;54:1004–8.
58. Tewani SK, Turner BG, Chuttani R, et al. Location of bile leak predicts the success of ERCP performed for postoperative bile leaks. Gastrointest Endosc. 2013;77:601–8.
59. Lee HW, Shah NH, Lee SK. An update on endoscopic management of post-liver transplant biliary complications. Clin Endosc. 2017;50:451–63.
60. Yabe S, Kato H, Mizukawa S, et al. Predictive factors for outcomes of patients undergoing endoscopic therapy for bile leak after hepatobiliary surgery. Dig Endosc Off J Jpn Gastroenterol Endosc Soc. 2017;29:353–61.
61. Phillips MS, Bonatti H, Sauer BG, et al. Elevated stricture rate following the use of fully covered self-expandable metal biliary stents for biliary leaks following liver transplantation. Endoscopy. 2011;43:512–7.
62. Rainio M, Lindström O, Udd M, et al. Endoscopic therapy of biliary injury after cholecystectomy. Dig Dis Sci. 2018;63:474–80.
63. Fathy O, Wahab MA, Hamdy E, et al. Post-cholecystectomy biliary injuries: one center experience. Hepatogastroenterology. 2011;58:719–24.

Chapter 8
Management of Concurrent Biliary and Duodenal Obstruction

Osama Altayar and Koushik Das

Case Presentations

Case 1

A 29-year-old man with history of ataxia-telangiectasia syndrome (*ATM* gene mutation) presented with 2 days of painless jaundice associated with nausea and vomiting. The patient was afebrile, hemodynamically stable, and physical exam revealed conjunctival telangiectasias and scleral icterus. Laboratory studies were remarkable for total bilirubin 11.7 mg/dL, direct bilirubin 9.7 mg/dL, and alkaline phosphatase 398 units/L. An abdominal ultrasound showed a distended gallbladder in addition to intrahepatic and extrahepatic biliary dilatation without identifiable filling defect. Magnetic resonance imaging with cholangiopancreatography (MRI/MRCP) demonstrated a 3.3 by 3.3 cm hypoenhancing mass in the distal duodenal bulb and descending duodenum resulting

O. Altayar · K. Das (✉)
Division of Gastroenterology, Washington University
School of Medicine, St. Louis, MO, USA
e-mail: k.das@wustl.edu

D. K. Mullady (ed.), *Dilemmas in ERCP*,
https://doi.org/10.1007/978-3-030-12741-1_8

in common bile duct (CBD) stricture and dilatation of the pancreatic duct without vascular invasion (Fig. 8.1).

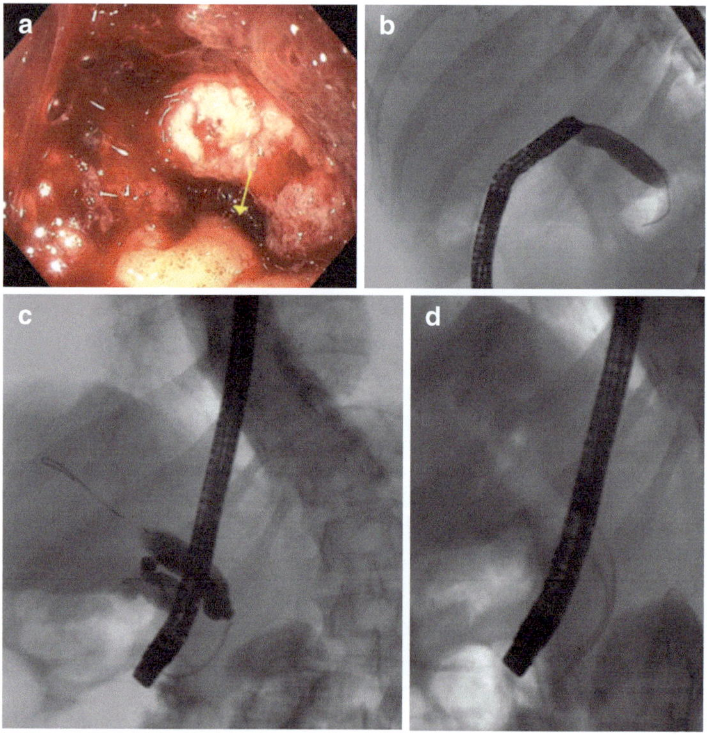

FIGURE 8.1 A 29-year-old man with history of ataxia-telangiectasia syndrome (ATM gene mutation) presented with a hypoenhancing mass in the distal duodenal bulb and descending duodenum resulting in common bile duct (CBD) stricture and dilatation of the pancreatic duct. Evaluation with upper endoscopy demonstrated a complete obstruction of the duodenal bulb due to a friable mass (**a**) that was successfully dilated under fluoroscopic guidance to 18 mm (**b**). Subsequently, passage of a duodenoscope was possible, and cholangiography demonstrated a severe, malignant-appearing distal bile duct stricture (**c**). An uncovered metallic biliary stent was successfully deployed (**d**, **e**), followed by the successful placement of an uncovered metallic duodenal stent (**f**, **g**) for palliation of the gastric outlet obstruction

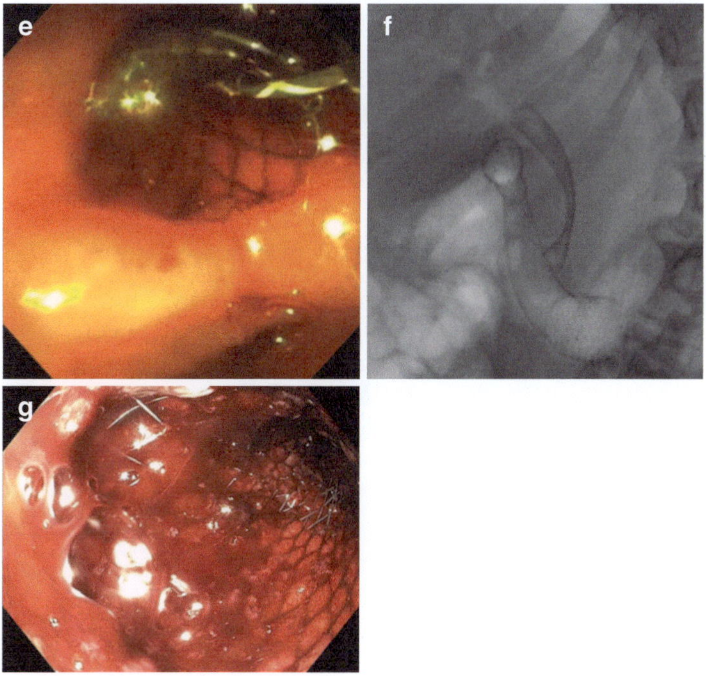

FIGURE 8.1 (continued)

Case 2

A 57-year-old woman presented with painless jaundice, and MRI/MRCP showed a porcelain gallbladder, Mirizzi's syndrome, and right adnexal cystic mass concerning for primary ovarian malignancy. Mirizzi's syndrome was palliated with ERCP, sphincterotomy, and plastic stent placement. Subsequent exploratory laparotomy, bilateral salpingo-oophorectomy, omentectomy, and subtotal cholecystectomy demonstrated metastatic gallbladder cancer with peritoneal and drop ovarian metastases. Postoperatively, the patient developed a left intrahepatic bile leak that was treated with stent placement. Over the next year, the patient was managed with plastic stent exchanges with a progressive, Bismuth IV severe hilar stricture involving the upper portion of the CBD in addition to the left main and right main hepatic ducts. Despite bilateral plastic stenting with fenestrated double pigtail plastic stents, she presented with cholangitis and gastric outlet obstruction (Fig. 8.2).

Case 3

A 59-year-old woman with a history of poorly differentiated duodenal cancer, managed with ERCP and plastic stent placement, underwent attempted Whipple procedure. Intraoperatively, she was found to have multiple liver metastases, so the Whipple operation was aborted. A gastrojejunostomy was performed to alleviate gastric outlet obstruction symptoms. However, postoperatively, the patient

FIGURE 8.2 A 57-year-old woman with a complex history of metastatic gallbladder cancer complicated by Bismuth IV hilar strictures previously managed with bilateral plastic stent placement now presents with septic shock and gastric outlet obstruction. The malignant gastric outlet obstruction was dilated to 18 mm under fluoroscopic guidance (**a**), and an Olympus JF slim duodenoscope was advanced to the major papilla. Limited cholangiography confirmed the persistence of a severe, complex hilar stricture (**b**). Subsequently uncovered metallic stents were placed in a Y-configuration for palliation of the hilar obstruction, and an uncovered duodenal stent was placed for the management of the gastric outlet obstruction (**c**, **d**). The patient returned several months later with recurrent cholangitis. After dilation of the previously place duodenal stent, the JF duodenoscope was advanced to the region of the major papilla (**e**). The uncovered metallic biliary stent was cannulated through the interstices of the duodenal stent with a guidewire, and the orifice was dilated to allow stent passage. Limited cholangiogram demonstrated persistence of a complex stricture of the left intrahepatic duct (**f**). Subsequently to 7 Fr plastic stents were successfully placed into the left intrahepatic duct with subsequent resolution of cholangitis (**g**)

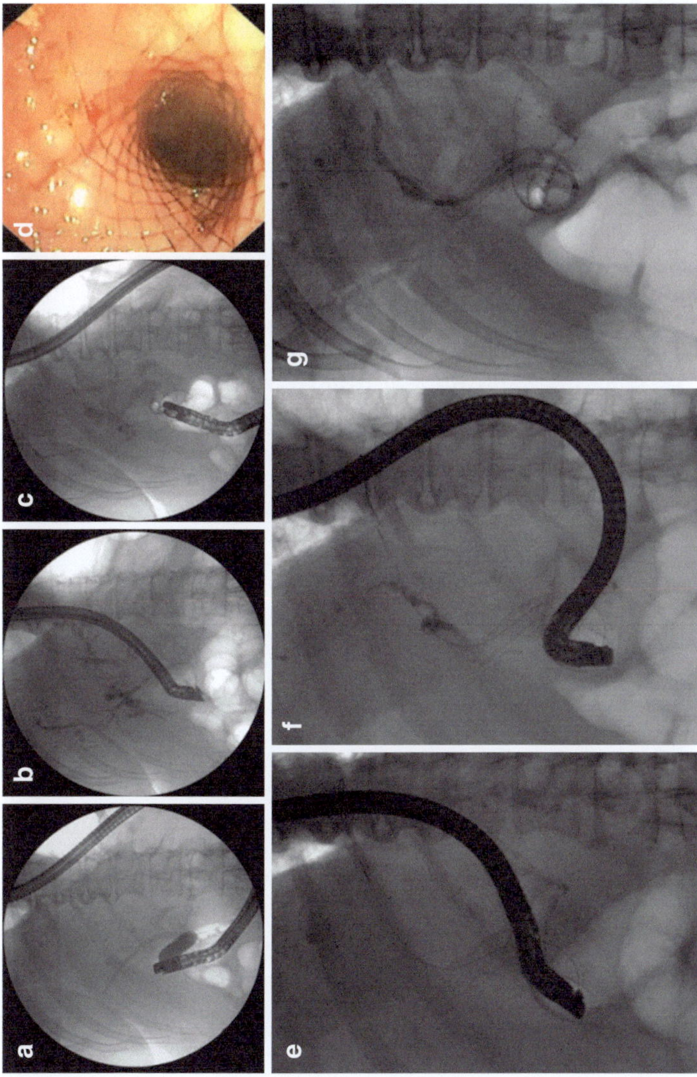
a
b
c
d
e
f
g

developed fever and obstructive jaundice with a total bilirubin 4.8 mg/dL and alkaline phosphatase 754 units/L (Fig. 8.3).

Assessment and Diagnosis

Concurrent biliary and duodenal obstruction (CBDO) occurs in both malignant and benign diseases. Among malignant etiologies, pancreatic adenocarcinoma is the most common, followed by ampullary cancer, gallbladder cancer, cholangiocarcinoma, gastric cancer, small bowel adenocarcinoma, intestinal and extraintestinal lymphoma, and metastatic diseases. Benign conditions, such as autoimmune pancreatitis, sclerosing mesenteritis, and Bouveret's syndrome, are much less common causes of CBDO [1].

Without therapy, the mean survival for patients presenting with malignant biliary obstruction is less than 200 days. Because most patients have advanced disease at the time of

Figure 8.3 A 59-year-old woman with a history of poorly differentiated duodenal cancer, managed with ERCP and plastic stent placement, underwent an aborted Whipple due to intraoperative identification of diffuse metastatic disease. A palliative surgical gastrojejunostomy was surgically created but the patient developed cholangitis and biliary obstruction postoperatively. Endoscopy demonstrated complete and untraversable obstruction at the level of the pylorus due to malignant infiltration (**a**). Subsequently the Olympus 1 T upper endoscope was able to be advanced retrograde through the gastrojejunostomy to the second portion of the duodenum (**b**, **c**). There was malignant infiltration of the duodenum distal to the papilla. Utilizing a sphincterotome with fluoroscopic guidance, a guidewire was able to be advanced adjacent to the previously placed plastic stent into the bile duct. Cholangiography confirmed a severe 2 cm distal biliary stricture with upstream dilation (**d**). Subsequently, an uncovered metallic biliary stent was deployed under fluoroscopic (**e**) and endoscopic (**f**) guidance, successfully (**g**)

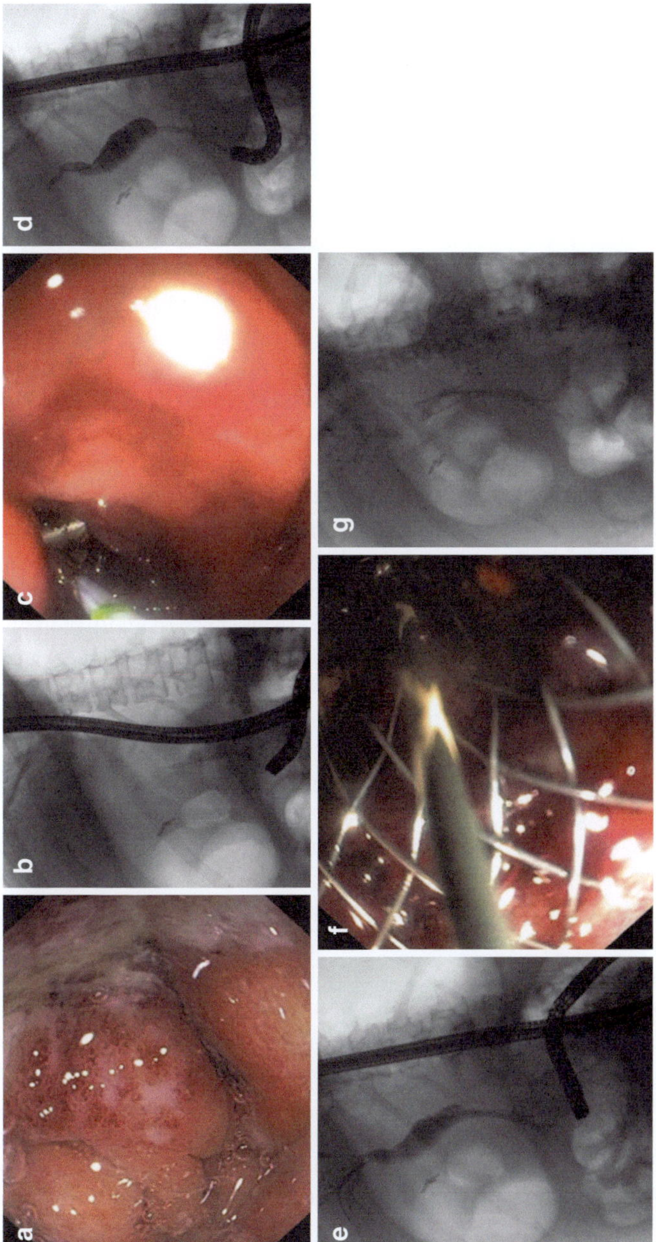
a
b
c
d
e
f
g

presentation, operative resection with curative intent is only possible in 10–15% of cases [2]. While there are not large series of patients with CBDO, published cohorts suggest that these patients have a worse prognosis, with as little as an 81-day median survival [3]. Given this prognosis, treatment must aim to palliate symptoms of duodenal obstruction, obstructive jaundice, and pain. While there is controversy about the best approach to palliative treatment, options include surgical approaches (biliary and gastric bypass with choledochojejunal and gastrojejunal anastomoses), percutaneous drainage options (percutaneous biliary drainage), and endoscopic approaches (endoscopic biliary and enteral stent placement).

Although the diagnosis of CBDO can be confirmed by endoscopic evaluation, clinical vigilance by incorporating clinical history, physical examination, and biochemical and radiographic findings can prevent unnecessary repeat procedures or delay in care. Patients usually present with symptoms of biliary obstruction including jaundice and pruritus with associated conjugated hyperbilirubinemia and imaging findings of biliary ductal dilatation. The difficulty usually arises in recognizing gastric outlet obstruction (GOO) before proceeding with endoscopic biliary decompression. Patients with GOO usually have nonspecific symptoms that could be explained by the primary disease, and it is important to have a low index of suspicion. Patients could present with nausea, vomiting, abdominal pain, early satiety, weight loss, dehydration, and undernutrition. Imaging might show large volume of gastric contents with or without a dilated stomach or duodenum. Oral and intravenous contrast are key due to their ability to establish the diagnosis, assess the stage of malignant diseases, evaluate the anatomy before procedures, and assess for possible contraindications and the extent and severity of luminal stenoses. The above findings in the right clinical settings should elicit the suspicion for CBDO in the pre-procedural setting.

Based on the timing of the development of the biliary obstruction compared to the development of the duodenal obstruction, patients with CBDO can be classified into three

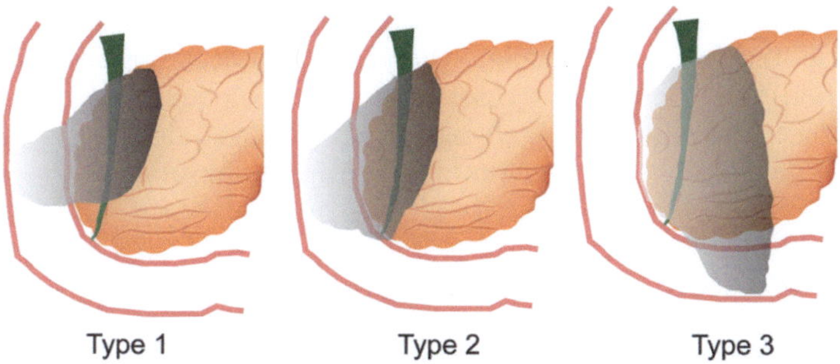

FIGURE 8.4 Anatomic subtypes of combined biliary and duodenal obstruction, as suggested by Mutignani et al. [3]

groups: (1) biliary obstruction followed by duodenal obstruction within weeks to months which is the most common scenario (as in the first and third cases above), (2) simultaneous biliary and duodenal obstruction (as in the second case above), or (3) duodenal obstruction followed by biliary obstruction (least common).

From an anatomic and prognostic standpoint, CBDO can be classified into three types based on the location of the duodenal obstruction in relation to the major papilla, as described by Mutignani et al. (Fig. 8.4) [3, 4]. Type 1 represents duodenal obstruction that occurs at the level of the duodenal bulb or upper genu of the pancreas without involvement of the major papilla as in the first case. Type 2 is duodenal obstruction at the level of the major papilla as in the second case. Type 3 is duodenal obstruction distal to the major papilla. Generally, combined endoscopic approaches are most readily achievable in type 3 and most challenging in type 2 when biliary cannulation is hampered by tumor involvement of the papilla.

The above classifications can affect the clinical approach, treatment strategy, and outcomes for a patient. For example, in the three cases discussed, while all presented with obstructive jaundice, in the first case, the diagnosis of GOO was delayed until the time of endoscopy. In the second case, the presence of ingrowth into the stents and worsening hilar mass on imaging were clues into the possible concurrent obstruction. While in the third case, the prior knowledge of the presence of the duodenal malignancy and GOO requiring surgical bypass were key in attempting a retrograde approach.

Treatment and Management

The management of benign etiologies of CBDO primarily focuses on the treatment of the underlying process in the cases of sclerosing mesenteritis or AIP or relief of the obstructing stone in the case of Bouveret's syndrome. We will focus here primarily on the management of malignant CBDO, which accounts for the vast majority of presentations in clinical practice.

In early stages, when the malignant disease can be resected, the role of endoscopy is to alleviate the symptoms and achieve biliary drainage while awaiting surgical resection. However, usually the presence of CBDO indicates at least locally advanced disease that is unresectable. Historically, unresectable disease was palliated surgically by performing double-bypass surgery, gastrojejunostomy with hepaticojejunostomy or choledochojejunostomy, at the time of the diagnostic laparotomy. With the advancement of radiographic and endoscopic technologies, surgical palliation is rarely done. From an endoscopic perspective, a common theme is to attempt to treat the biliary obstruction first. This is related to the increased difficulty of accessing the major papilla when it becomes jailed behind an enteric stent. In addition to traditional endoscopic approaches, endoscopic ultrasound-guided biliary access and lumen-apposing metal stents (LAMS) have advanced our ability to perform minimally invasive palliative procedures to alleviate the complications of malignant diseases including CBDO even in patients who are poor surgical candidates. Here we briefly discuss the management of isolated biliary and duodenal obstructions separately first, before discussing the different possible scenarios for CBDO based on the anatomical types described by Mutignani et al. [3].

Management of Malignant Biliary Obstruction

The current standard treatment for unresectable malignant biliary obstructions is transpapillary stenting. This can be achieved using plastic stents (PS) or self-expandable metal stents (SEMS). PS are safe and effective, are less expensive than SEMS, and can be easily replaced if occlusion occurs. SEMS were designed to extend the duration of patency utilizing a larger internal diameter and thereby reducing the frequency of re-intervention. SEMS are associated with lower complications rates, longer stent patency, and fewer re-interventions and lower costs after 1 year in comparison to PS, even in those patients with short survival times (<3 months) [5, 6]. Compared to uncovered SEMS (uSEMS), partially/fully covered SEMS (pc/fcSEMS) were developed to reduce the rate of tumor ingrowth; however there remain concerns of stent migration, sludge formation, stent-induced cholecystitis and pancreatitis, and tumor overgrowth [7]. The utility of covered SEMS is also limited to distal malignant biliary obstructions due to concerns for blocking the contralateral intrahepatic system or ipsilateral intrahepatic branches. A recent meta-analysis [8] and large single-center retrospective study [9] demonstrated no differences in the number of recurrent biliary obstructions or stent patency after 6 or 12 months, overall or median survival, median time to recurrent biliary obstruction, or rate of adverse events. Therefore, our practice is primarily to utilize fcSEMS upfront in palliation of clinically, highly suspicious malignant biliary strictures without an official tissue diagnosis when a patient is post-cholecystectomy [10] or in recanalization and preservation of an occluded indwelling uSEMS.

When the transpapillary approach fails, EUS-guided biliary drainage and percutaneous transhepatic biliary drainage (PTBD) with external or internal biliary drainage are both excellent options. The presence of ascites might limit such approaches due to the risk of infection, leakage, and migration of the drainage catheters.

Management of Malignant Duodenal Obstruction

The current treatment options for unresectable duodenal obstruction or GOO are endoscopic stenting with enteral SEMS, surgical gastrojejunostomy, or venting gastrostomy with or without the placement of a jejunal feeding extension. Regardless of the treatment strategy chosen, it is paramount that when a patient presents with suspected GOO, a nasogastric (NG) tube is placed to suction as soon as possible to reduce the risk of aspiration and facilitate endoscopic intervention as appropriate. We frequently allow 24 hours of drainage with an NG tube prior to attempting endoscopic intervention especially in patients with a distended stomach on imaging. The SUSTENT study demonstrated that enteral stents have no differences in survival or quality of life in comparison with surgical gastrojejunostomy, though surgical intervention was associated with fewer recurrent obstructive symptoms (28% vs 5%) occurring at a longer interval [11]. However, in aggregate, enteral stents are associated with faster resolution of GOO symptoms, shorter hospital stays, reduced cost, and no differences in survival for the management of intrinsic duodenal obstruction [12].

The use of LAMS for EUS-guided gastrojejunostomy is a new approach that may be considered in the hands of high-volume therapeutic endoscopists in patients who are poor surgical candidates and cannot undergo duodenal stenting [13]. In this technique, a small bowel loop is demarcated by placement of wire-guided balloon catheter, injection of contrast using a wire-guided nasobiliary tube or a peroral ultraslim endoscope, or a wire-guided double-balloon tube. Then, an echoendoscope is used to localize the demarcated small bowel loop, and a gastroenterostomy is formed by placement of a LAMS [14]. While the preliminary case series of this approach have been encouraging, further robust clinical experience is required before its routine use in clinical practice.

Management of Combined Biliary and Duodenal Obstruction (CBDO)

In type 1 CBDO (duodenal obstruction is proximal to the major papilla), the goal is to pass the duodenoscope through the stricture to the major papilla, if possible. The initial approach should employ gentle pressure to pass the duodenoscope or the utilization of a slim duodenoscope (i.e., JF) if available through the duodenal stricture. If that fails, a 15–16.5–18 mm TTS balloon dilator can be used to dilate the stricture under fluoroscopic guidance. Alternatively, a balloon-tipped catheter can be passed fluoroscopically to the third portion of the duodenum to anchor and pull the endoscope across the stricture. Once the major papilla is reached, biliary cannulation and SEMS placement are completed per usual fashion. Subsequent to placement of a biliary stent, a guidewire can be passed into the fourth portion of the duodenum, and an enteric stent can be placed under endoscopic and fluoroscopic guidance. The proximal end of the enteric stent should be positioned within the prepyloric area as type 1 duodenal obstruction tends to be in the duodenal bulb. Additionally, care should be taken to use a stent long enough to achieve a margin of 2 cm both proximal and distal to the margins of the duodenal stricture as SEMS tend to shorten by 25% during expansion. Ideally, if possible, the position of the biliary stent on fluoroscopy should be used as a guide to prevent deployment of the duodenal stent across the biliary stent, though this is often unavoidable. If the maneuvers above fail to allow the duodenoscope to traverse the duodenal stricture, the placement of the enteric stent under fluoroscopic guidance prior to achieving biliary drainage becomes necessary. The endoscopist should attempt to position the distal end of the enteric stent proximal to the papilla to facilitate later biliary cannulation, though this is often difficult to gauge on fluoroscopy alone. As biliary obstruction usually develops prior to the development of the duodenal stenosis, many patients have indwelling PS/SEMS in place which can help in localizing the papilla. Alternatively, it may be possible to advance a standard upper endoscope or ultrathin scope to the level of the papilla and mark this point either with a reference fluoroscopic image or with the placement of an endoscopic hemoclip. Once the duodenal stent is placed, the options are to either wait 1–3 days to allow the enteric stent to expand or to attempt to dilate the freshly deployed stent to 15 mm to allow scope passage in the same session.

Type 2 CBDO represents the most challenging anatomic type of CBDO, as the duodenal obstruction includes the level of the major papilla making biliary access very challenging. Identification of the papillary orifice is often difficult due to extensive tumor infiltration. Furthermore, maneuverability is usually limited, with little room to work between the head of the endoscope and medial/lateral walls of the strictured duodenum. In many cases, the biliary obstruction has developed prior to the duodenal obstruction, and thus patients present having an indwelling PS or occluded SEMS in place. Utilizing endoscopic and/or fluoroscopic cues can be critical in achieving biliary cannulation. If biliary access is gained, the patient can be treated in similar approach to type 1. If the stricture is not traversable, a duodenal stent can be placed across the duodenal stenosis first. However, the placement of this stent will invariably make identification of the major papilla more challenging. In some cases, after stent deployment, the papillary orifice may be identified or intuited based on the presence of bile streaking through the interstices of the duodenal stent, and biliary cannulation may be possible. If wire access can be established into the bile duct, ERCP can be performed through the interstices utilizing balloon dilation and/or argon plasma coagulation (APC) to create an opening in the metallic mesh sufficient to allow passage of the biliary stent. There has been some innovation in this area, with the creation of the Meditek BONASTENT M-Duodenal, which employs a central area of looser cross mesh that makes biliary cannulation potentially easier [15]. If biliary access cannot be achieved through a transpapillary approach after duodenal stent placement, then EUS-guided or percutaneous approaches can be utilized to gain biliary access.

EUS-guided cholangiography utilizes a curved linear echoendoscope to identify the intrahepatic bile ducts using a transgastric approach or the extrahepatic bile ducts using a transgastric or transduodenal approach. When accessing the biliary tree in this fashion, the options are either a rendezvous approach where EUS access is used to pass a wire antegrade to the papilla to facilitate transpapillary drainage or EUS-guided creation of a fistula (hepaticogastrostomy, choledochoduodenostomy, etc.). Under EUS guidance, the bile duct is identified and punctured using a 19-gauge access needle. After aspiration of bile and injection of contrast into the biliary tree to confirm appropriate access, a biliary wire is advanced into the biliary tree under fluoroscopic guidance. In the rendezvous approach, the wire is directed toward the papilla under fluoroscopic guidance. Once the wire is out of the papilla, the echoendoscope is withdrawn, and a duodenoscope is readvanced to the level of the papilla. Through the duodenoscope, the wire is retrieved and backloaded into the duodenoscope using snare or forceps. Over this wire, conventional transpapillary drainage and stent placement can then be performed with the distal end of the biliary stent deployed within the duodenal stent [16]. Alternatively, the EUS-placed wire emerging transpapillary can be used as a guide for traditional transpapillary cannulation if grasping the wire is challenging. We will typically utilize fcSEMS that traverse the point of EUS-guided access to minimize the risk of a leak. In a similar fashion, PTC can be used to perform rendezvous ERCP, in conjunction with interventional radiology. Alternatively, a hepaticogastrostomy (HGS) or choledochoduodenostomy (CDS) could be created with this approach. After the wire is advanced into the biliary tree via either transduodenal or transgastric puncture, verifying that there are no intervening structures or vasculature on EUS, dilation of the tract can be performed with a combination of push catheters and a 4 mm/6 mm balloon. Subsequently, a transmural fcSEMS or LAMS can be advanced in antegrade fashion and deployed to form a hepaticogastrostomy or choledochoduodenostomy [17, 18]. There are lower complication rates and leak rates associated with transpapillary drainage as opposed to the creation of fistulas. All of these techniques should be employed only in the hands of expertly trained therapeutic endoscopists at high-volume centers, with immediately available hepatobiliary surgery, and interventional radiology consultations given the potential for morbidity or even mortality should misdeployment or perforation occur. If this is not available or the case is not amenable, then percutaneous biliary access with the placement of a biliary stent across the papilla or external percutaneous drainage by an interventional radiologist is an excellent alternative.

In type 3 CBDO, as the duodenal obstruction is distal to the major papilla, endoscopic treatment is generally the most straightforward. These cases are the most uncommon and usually arise from pancreatic uncinate tumors. Although we still prefer achieving biliary drainage first to avoid unplanned jailing of the papilla, the order of which stent to place first is not as pivotal as in type 1 when the distance between the ampulla and the duodenal stricture is not close. It is important to keep in mind that the risk of duodenal reflux after biliary stenting is higher in patients with type 3 CBDO.

Outcomes of the Clinical Cases

Pre-procedural knowledge of the patient's anatomy and preparation for every type of CBDO, or combination therein, is crucial for real-time decision-making. It is also important to discuss and obtain appropriate consent from patients for possible dilation, placement of biliary and enteric stents when GOO is suspected, or even the specific performance of EUS-guided access procedures. As mentioned above, when a patient has suspected GOO, an NG tube must be placed, and the gastric contents should be suctioned for at least 24 hours before the procedure. In our practice, we perform all our procedures with fluoroscopy and with anesthesia support under general endotracheal intubation when GOO is suspected.

In the first case, the patient had type 1 CBDO with simultaneous biliary and duodenal obstruction. On initial attempt at ERCP, an Olympus TJF-160VF (13.2 mm outer diameter) and Olympus JF-140F (11.0 mm outer diameter) could not traverse a stricture at the distal duodenal bulb. The duodenoscope was exchanged for a straight-viewing Olympus GIF-H190 (9.2 mm outer diameter) gastroscope, and there was a large, infiltrating, obstructing mass in the distal portion of the duodenal bulb that was traversed with gentle pressure. The mass extended to 1.5 cm proximal of the ampulla. The stenosis was dilated using a 15–16.5–18 mm through the scope (TTS) balloon dilator to 18 mm. This made it possible for the Olympus TJF-160VF to traverse the stricture. Subsequently, biliary cannulation was achieved and cholangiography demonstrated a single severe stenosis in the distal CBD that was treated successfully with the placement of an uncovered self-expandable metallic stent (uSEMS). Finally, the duodenal stenosis was treated with the placement of a 22 mm × 9 cm enteral stent with the proximal end positioned within the prepyloric antrum and the distal end proximal to the biliary stent (Fig. 8.1). The patient's jaundice resolved, and he was able to advance his diet and receive outpatient neoadjuvant chemotherapy. Duodenal stent patency and biliary drainage were maintained for 6 months. His course was complicated by bleeding which was likely related to the combination of his ataxia-telangiectasia syndrome and the locally advanced tumor. The bleeding episodes were treated conservatively.

In the second case, the patient initially had a type 1 CBDO which was treated in a similar fashion to the first case, although the biliary obstruction was a hilar Bismuth IV lesion. She subsequently presented with a type 2 CBDO with tumor ingrowth through the stent interstices. In this case, ERCP was performed and demonstrated a severe duodenal bulb stenosis which was dilated with a 15–16.5–18 mm TTS balloon dilator to 18 mm under fluoroscopic guidance. She was noted to have occluded plastic stents which were removed, and a Bismuth IV stenosis was noted again. Due to the presence of malignant duodenal obstruction raising concern for possible inability to access the bile ducts should the plastic stent be replaced, the decision was made to place Y-configuration metallic biliary stents. Subsequently, a 10 mm × 8 cm uncovered metallic stent was placed into the left intrahepatic duct. A wire was advanced through the interstices of the first stent into the right anterior duct, and another 10 mm × 8 cm uncovered metallic stent was placed into the right main duct, extending beyond the papilla. Finally, the duodenal stenosis was managed with a 22 mm × 9 cm uncovered metallic stent with its proximal end in the prepyloric antrum. Two months later, the patient represented with fever, hypotension, bacteremia, and jaundice with total bilirubin 2.4 mg/dL and alkaline phosphatase 1002 units/L. She was found on contrast-enhanced computed tomography (CT) to have tumor ingrowth into the uncovered metallic stents and worsening infiltration of the soft tissue lesion into the hepatic hilum. Repeat ERCP was attempted through the duodenal stent and overlapping Y-configuration biliary stents. The duodenal stent was dilated with a 15–16.5–18 mm TTS balloon dilator to 18 mm under fluoroscopic guidance. The Olympus TJF-160VF duodenoscope was unable to traverse the stenosis, so it was exchanged for an Olympus JF-140F duodenoscope which was able to traverse the luminal stenosis. The biliary orifice was obscured by the overlaying duodenal stent. Utilizing fluoroscopic guidance, the bile duct was cannulated with a short-nosed traction sphincterotome through the interstices of the duodenal stent. The entire biliary tree contained multiple diffuse stenoses, likely due to secondary cholangiopathy from chronic cholangitis and obstruction. The interstices of the duodenal stent and distal CBD were dilated with an 8-mm balloon dilator. Finally, two double pigtail 7 Fr × 10 cm plastic biliary stents were placed 12 cm into the common bile duct extending into the left intrahepatic ducts (Fig. 8.2). Subsequently, the patient's fever, cholangitis, and jaundice rapidly resolved, and she was able to receive further palliative chemotherapy. Her course was complicated by recurrent cholangitis due to her hilar biliary strictures and cholangiopathy. She has been undergoing chemotherapy by her local oncologist and she had her plastic stents exchanged through the previously placed duodenal and biliary metal stents successfully for an episode of cholangitis 6 months later.

In the third case, the patient had biliary obstruction that was treated with PS initially and subsequently underwent palliative surgical gastrojejunostomy for a type 1 CBDO. She then developed biliary obstruction due to occlusion of the PS. In this case, upper GI endoscopy using Olympus GIF-1TQ160 endoscope demonstrated severe malignant infiltration and obstruction of the duodenum just beyond the level of the duodenal bulb that could not be traversed. Therefore, the afferent limb of the gastrojejunostomy was entered, and the scope was advanced retrograde with some difficulty to the area of the ampulla. There was malignant infiltration of the second portion of the duodenum noted retrograde, with a small portion of the previously placed plastic stent visible endoscopically. There appeared to be a necrotic cavity anatomically proximal to the level of the ampulla. Wire-guided biliary cannulation was achieved with a short-nosed sphincterotome utilizing fluoroscopic visualization to direct the sphincterotome tip in axis with the indwelling biliary stent. Cholangiogram demonstrated the indwelling plastic stent with a 2 cm distal CBD stricture with significant upstream ductal dilation to 18 mm. A 10 mm × 8 cm uSEMS was then successfully placed across the stricture with the distal end of the stent position beyond the ampullary mass in the distal duodenum. Bile and pus flowed through the stent (Fig. 8.3). Jaundice and leukocytosis rapidly resolved after the procedure, and it has been 9 months since without need for re-intervention. She continues to follow up with her oncologist for chemotherapy.

Reported Outcomes and Complications in Patients with CBDO

The evidence evaluating the role of the different endoscopic treatments for CBDO comes mainly from case series of malignant unresectable CBDO [19]. The largest published case series by Hamada et al. included 110 patients with a functional success rate of 95% including 90 patients who underwent ERCP, 10 who underwent EUS-guided CDS, and 10 who underwent EUS-guided HGS. In terms of the timing of the development of the duodenal obstruction, 61% of the patients developed the duodenal obstruction after the biliary obstruction with a median time of 2 months. In 12.7% of the patients, the duodenal obstruction preceded the biliary obstruction with a median time of 1 month. Survival was the longest in patients who developed simultaneous CBDO and patients who had type 2 CBDO. In terms of achieving biliary drainage, ERCP was successful in most patients who had type 1, type 3, or nonsimultaneous CBDO, while 30% of patients who had type 2 and 42% of the patients who had simultaneous CBDO required EUS-guided transmural drainage. In total, 33% of the patients developed recurrent biliary obstruction. Neither the sequence of the development nor the anatomical type of CBDO predicted the time to recurrent biliary obstruction. On the other hand, different treatment approaches had different rates of recurrence with 50% of EUS-guided CDS, 40% of EUS-guided HGS, and 31% of transpapillary drainage developing recurrent biliary obstruction. Regardless, all the patients underwent successful re-intervention for biliary drainage via ERCP, EUS-guided, and percutaneous approaches [20].

From a safety standpoint, ERCP had the lowest rate of adverse events at 8.9% followed by EUS-guided CDS (20%) and then EUS-guided HGS (50%). Adverse events associated with EUS-guided transmural drainage occurred early, within 30 days, in all the patients. Potential adverse events of the endoscopic interventions that attempt to alleviate CBDO include cholangitis, cholecystitis, pancreatitis, bleeding, perforation, stent migration, and bile leakage [20].

A recently conducted randomized controlled trial has shown no difference in efficacy or safety profile between ERCP or EUS-guided biliary drainage in patients with distal biliary obstruction due to pancreatic cancer [21]. However, one of the exclusion criteria was the presence of altered anatomy or inability to access the major papilla, which is a uniquely challenging scenario that might have led to higher rates of complications in line with prior CBDO case series [20]. Percutaneous drainage, in comparison to endoscopic intervention, has been associated with higher rate of adverse events and unscheduled re-interventions [22].

Pearls and Pitfalls

- Given the complexity, potential complications, and varied approaches to patients with CBDO, a multidisciplinary team that involves hepatobiliary surgery, oncology, interventional radiology, and interventional gastroenterology should evaluate and discuss each case individually prior to committing a patient to intervention.
- Understanding the anatomy and the different anatomical variations of CBDO is key in approaching the case efficiently. There should be a low index of suspicion for CBDO in patients who may not have classical, overt GOO symptoms, and contrast-enhanced cross-sectional imaging should be reviewed pre-procedure to help in procedure planning. Similarly, patients should be consented for both enteric and biliary stents when there is any suspicion for CBDO.
- Malignancy is the most common cause for unresectable CBDO. Such patients usually have poor performance status, and achieving both biliary drainage and duodenal stenting in one procedure may prevent periprocedural complications.
- It is important to set realistic expectations with the patients and their families that the intention of endoscopic intervention is palliation of symptoms and that the median survival remains modest.
- In general, when double stenting is performed, we recommend securing the biliary stent first when at

all possible before proceeding with enteric stent placement to maximize chances of transpapillary cannulation.

- Based on the results of observational studies, ERCP tends to be associated with the highest success rate, lowest risk of recurrent biliary obstruction, and best safety profile. Hence, we recommend exhausting attempts at biliary decompression via ERCP by a high-volume endoscopist prior to proceeding with EUS-guided or percutaneous approaches.
- EUS-guided biliary access should be performed in well-informed, selected patients, by endoscopists with sufficient experience and multidisciplinary support by interventional radiology and surgery. In particular, EUS-guided access should not be attempted in patients with biliary dilation <1 cm or those who have ascites.

References

1. Riff BP, DiMaio CJ. Endoscopic treatment of simultaneous malignant biliary and gastric outlet obstruction. In: Adler DG, editor. Advanced Pancreaticobiliary endoscopy. Cham: Springer International Publishing; 2016. p. 121–33.
2. Ryan DP, Hong TS, Bardeesy N. Pancreatic adenocarcinoma. N Engl J Med. 2014;371(11):1039–49.
3. Mutignani M, Tringali A, Shah SG, Perri V, Familiari P, Iacopini F, et al. Combined endoscopic stent insertion in malignant biliary and duodenal obstruction. Endoscopy. 2007;39(5):440–7.
4. Baron TH. Management of simultaneous biliary and duodenal obstruction: the endoscopic perspective. Gut Liver. 2010;4(Suppl 1):S50–6.
5. Almadi MA, Barkun A, Martel M. Plastic vs. self-expandable metal stents for palliation in malignant biliary obstruction: a series of meta-analyses. Am J Gastroenterol. 2017;112(2):260–73.

6. Walter D, van Boeckel PG, Groenen MJ, Weusten BL, Witteman BJ, Tan G, et al. Cost efficacy of metal stents for palliation of extrahepatic bile duct obstruction in a randomized controlled trial. Gastroenterology. 2015;149(1):130–8.
7. Tringali A, Hassan C, Rota M, Rossi M, Mutignani M, Aabakken L. Covered vs. uncovered self-expandable metal stents for malignant distal biliary strictures: a systematic review and meta-analysis. Endoscopy. 2018;50(6):631–41.
8. Almadi MA, Barkun AN, Martel M. No benefit of covered vs uncovered self-expandable metal stents in patients with malignant distal biliary obstruction: a meta-analysis. Clin Gastroenterol Hepatol. 2013;11(1):27–37e1.
9. Lee JH, Krishna SG, Singh A, Ladha HS, Slack RS, Ramireddy S, et al. Comparison of the utility of covered metal stents versus uncovered metal stents in the management of malignant biliary strictures in 749 patients. Gastrointest Endosc. 2013;78(2):312–24.
10. Siddiqui AA, Mehendiratta V, Loren D, Hong SK, Kowalski T. Fully covered self-expandable metal stents are effective and safe to treat distal malignant biliary strictures, irrespective of surgical resectability status. J Clin Gastroenterol. 2011;45(9):824–7.
11. Jeurnink SM, Steyerberg EW, van Hooft JE, van Eijck CH, Schwartz MP, Vleggaar FP, et al. Surgical gastrojejunostomy or endoscopic stent placement for the palliation of malignant gastric outlet obstruction (SUSTENT study): a multicenter randomized trial. Gastrointest Endosc. 2010;71(3):490–9.
12. Nagaraja V, Eslick GD, Cox MR. Endoscopic stenting versus operative gastrojejunostomy for malignant gastric outlet obstruction-a systematic review and meta-analysis of randomized and non-randomized trials. J Gastrointest Oncol. 2014;5(2):92–8.
13. Tyberg A, Perez-Miranda M, Sanchez-Ocana R, Penas I, de la Serna C, Shah J, et al. Endoscopic ultrasound-guided gastrojejunostomy with a lumen-apposing metal stent: a multicenter, international experience. Endosc Int Open. 2016;4(3):E276–81.
14. Itoi T, Baron TH, Khashab MA, Tsuchiya T, Irani S, Dhir V, et al. Technical review of endoscopic ultrasonography-guided gastroenterostomy in 2017. Dig Endosc. 2017;29(4):495–502.
15. Moon JH, Choi HJ, Ko BM, Koo HC, Hong SJ, Cheon YK, et al. Combined endoscopic stent-in-stent placement for malignant biliary and duodenal obstruction by using a new duodenal metal stent (with videos). Gastrointest Endosc. 2009;70(4):772–7.
16. Iwashita T, Yasuda I, Mukai T, Iwata K, Ando N, Doi S, et al. EUS-guided rendezvous for difficult biliary cannulation using

a standardized algorithm: a multicenter prospective pilot study (with videos). Gastrointest Endosc. 2016;83(2):394–400.
17. Iwashita T, Yasuda I, Doi S, Uemura S, Mabuchi M, Okuno M, et al. Endoscopic ultrasound-guided antegrade treatments for biliary disorders in patients with surgically altered anatomy. Dig Dis Sci. 2013;58(8):2417–22.
18. Itoi T, Isayama H, Sofuni A, Itokawa F, Kurihara T, Tsuchiya T, et al. Stent selection and tips on placement technique of EUS-guided biliary drainage: transduodenal and transgastric stenting. J Hepatobiliary Pancreat Sci. 2011;18(5):664–72.
19. Nakai Y, Hamada T, Isayama H, Itoi T, Koike K. Endoscopic management of combined malignant biliary and gastric outlet obstruction. Dig Endosc. 2017;29(1):16–25.
20. Hamada T, Nakai Y, Lau JY, Moon JH, Hayashi T, Yasuda I, et al. International study of endoscopic management of distal malignant biliary obstruction combined with duodenal obstruction. Scand J Gastroenterol. 2018;53(1):46–55.
21. Bang JY, Navaneethan U, Hasan M, Hawes R, Varadarajulu S. Stent placement by EUS or ERCP for primary biliary decompression in pancreatic cancer: a randomized trial (with videos). Gastrointest Endosc. 2018;88:9.
22. Lee TH, Choi JH, Park do H, Song TJ, Kim DU, Paik WH, et al. Similar efficacies of endoscopic ultrasound-guided transmural and percutaneous drainage for malignant distal biliary obstruction. Clin Gastroenterol Hepatol. 2016;14(7):1011–9 e3.

Chapter 9
ERCP in Recurrent Acute Pancreatitis

Jeffrey J. Easler

Abbreviations

CP	Chronic pancreatitis
ERCP	Endoscopic retrograde cholangiopancreatography
EUS	Endoscopic ultrasound
FNA	Fine needle aspiration
IRAP	Idiopathic recurrent pancreatitis
MRCP	Magnetic resonance cholangiopancreatography
PDv	Pancreas divisum

Case Presentations

Case 1

A 40-year-old male is referred for recurrent acute pancreatitis. He reports two episodes in the past 4 months of right

J. J. Easler (✉)
Division of Gastroenterology and Hepatology, Indiana University School of Medicine, Indianapolis, IN, USA
e-mail: jjeasler@iu.edu

D. K. Mullady (ed.), *Dilemmas in ERCP*,
https://doi.org/10.1007/978-3-030-12741-1_9

upper quadrant and epigastric abdominal pain, nausea, vomiting, and anorexia. He denies associated fevers or scleral icterus. He has a past medical history of hypertension, non-insulin-dependent diabetes, and morbid obesity (BMI 43). Hydrochlorothiazide was discontinued following his first attack of pancreatitis. He reports a remote history of binge drinking, but he denies alcohol intake in the context of recent attacks of pancreatitis. He reports tobacco use. He denies family history of pancreatitis, pancreatic cancer, or cystic fibrosis. In the clinic, he also reports daily postprandial abdominal pain. He has experienced a 10-pound weight loss.

Lipase levels with each attack of pancreatitis were 1131 and 1246 U/L (ULN 393 U/L). Liver function testing and calcium level were normal. Triglycerides were 161 mg/dL at the time of his first episode of pancreatitis.

Right upper quadrant ultrasound was performed. The study demonstrated a contracted gallbladder and was negative for gallbladder calculi or wall dilation. There was no evidence of intrahepatic or extrahepatic bile duct dilation. Contrast-enhanced CT scan of the abdomen and pelvis was performed with both episodes of pancreatitis and was negative for significant pathology. With both pancreatitis episodes he was managed conservatively with NPO status, IV fluids, and discharged on a liquid diet with instructions to advance to solids as an outpatient.

What is the next best diagnostic test?

Case 2

A 76-year-old male is referred with a diagnosis of IRAP. He has experienced three episodes of acute pancreatitis in the 12 months leading up to his referral. He denies scleral icterus or fevers. He denies current or prior alcohol abuse and does not smoke. Review of his medication list is unrevealing. He is status post cholecystectomy 5 years ago for recurrent right upper quadrant abdominal pain and low gallbladder ejection fraction on HIDA scan. No gallstones were seen on pathology. His medical history also is notable for coronary artery disease, non-insulin-dependent diabetes, dyslipidemia, hypertension, psoriasis, and chronic kidney disease. He has a BMI of 32.1. There is no family history of pancreatitis, pancreatic cancer, or cystic fibrosis. He is asymptomatic between episodes of pancreatitis.

Labs during attacks of pancreatitis reveal lipase levels between 315 and 11,159 U/L (ULN 78 U/L). His liver tests, calcium, and triglyceride levels are normal.

His workup includes a right upper quadrant ultrasound, which demonstrates a normal bile duct caliber.

Secretin-enhanced magnetic resonance cholangiopancreatography (s-MRCP) with contrast performed at the time of his last episode of pancreatitis demonstrated a 4 cm hypoenhancing peripancreatic lesion proximate to the tail of the pancreas. The lesion appears to have mass effect on the body/tail junction and has radiographic characteristics consistent with peripancreatic fat necrosis. The pancreatic duct is intact and demonstrates mild narrowing proximate to this lesion. There is no evidence of pancreas divisum (PDv). The common bile duct is normal.

An EUS one month following demonstrates interval decrease in the size of the peripancreatic fluid collection. The pancreatic parenchyma is otherwise unremarkable. The pancreatic duct measures 3.4 mm in the head and 0.6 mm in the body and is diminutive in the tail. The ampulla is normal. The bile duct is normal caliber without evidence of stones or sludge.

Further workup is performed which demonstrates an ANA of 1:80, IgG4 of 62 mg/dL, calcium level of 10 mg/dL, and CA19–9 of 16 units/mL, all within normal limits.

Pancreatitis four panel is negative for pathogenic variants in cystic fibrosis transmembrane regulator (CFTR), chymotrypsin C (CTRC), cationic trypsinogen (PRSS1), and serine protease inhibitor Kazal Type I (SPINK1) gene loci.

At the conclusion of the above workup, he returns to clinic 3 weeks after a subsequent attack of pancreatitis (lipase 1400 U/L). A contrast-enhanced CT scan demonstrated interstitial pancreatic in the region of the pancreatic head and near resolution of his peripancreatic fluid collection.

What is the next step in his care?

Case 3

A 43-year-old female is referred for recurrent acute pancreatitis. Her first episode occurred 13 years prior to presentation in clinic. She underwent cholecystectomy for suspicion of biliary pancreatitis at that time. She reports multiple, subsequent episodes of moderate to severe epigastric abdominal pain associated with nausea and anorexia lasting for 24–36 hours that were largely managed at home with a clear liquid diet. However, she presented recently twice to her local emergency room with severe, debilitating symptoms of abdominal pain, nausea, and vomiting. Biochemical testing revealed pancreatic enzyme elevations three times the upper limit of normal. Pancreatic enzyme levels between episodes were evaluated by her primary physician and are normal. She denies alcohol use. She is a prior smoker, having quit 11 years ago.

Workup from the referring center included normal calcium, IgG4, and triglyceride levels. She has a family history of pancreatic cancer in a paternal grandmother at age 40. An MRCP/MRI with contrast was also performed at the referring center demonstrated PDv anatomy. The dorsal pancreatic duct is approximately 2.5 mm in the head of the pancreas. There are no focal cystic or solid pancreatic lesions. No evidence of pancreatic side branches and/or pancreatic atrophy.

What is the next step in her care?

Case 4

A 59-year-old female was admitted for acute pancreatitis. She has a history of chronic lower back pain managed with opioid pain medications. However, over the past 9 months, she has experienced worsening, daily abdominal pain and thoracic-level back pain. In this setting her opioid pain medications have increased. She endorses a 15-pound weight loss over the past 2 months. Two outpatient CT scans of the abdomen and pelvis within the last 9 months were reportedly unremarkable. She has chronic constipation; however her pain does not change with defecation. She has a history of remote cholecystectomy for cholelithiasis. She has a history of remote, heavy alcohol abuse (10–12 servings of alcohol per day, abstinent for 15 years). She smokes one pack of cigarettes per day.

Labs in the emergency room demonstrated a lipase of 1661 (ULN 393), Alk Phos 159, ALT, and total bilirubin normal. A CT scan was performed in the emergency room upon presentation demonstrating a 2.4 cm low radiodensity lesion visualized in the uncinate portion of the pancreas with upstream pancreatic duct dilation to 5 mm. There are minimal interstitial and peripancreatic inflammatory changes.

She is managed with 3 cc/kg of lactate ringers for 36 hours. After 48 hours her nausea and anorexia improved, and she is tolerant of a clear liquid diet. However, she reports persistent abdominal pain.

What is the next step? When should this step be taken?

Diagnosis and Assessment of Recurrent Acute Pancreatitis

Understanding the Natural History of Recurrent Acute Pancreatitis and the Role of Endoscopic Therapy

Recurrent pancreatitis (RAP) is defined by multiple, self-limited episodes of typical abdominal pain syndrome associated with either pancreatic enzyme elevations three times the upper limit of normal and/or radiographic evidence of pancreatic inflammation [1]. Attacks generally are of a severity to require management in the emergency department or inpatient setting. Expert opinion defines RAP as a discrete syndrome from episodes of acute pancreatitis and/or flares of pain in the absence of comorbid chronic pancreatitis (CP) [2]. This distinction is important when considering the role of endoscopic therapy to prevent or manage RAP, as therapeutic strategies can differ significantly in the presence of CP and its local complications. Endoscopic therapies for patients with symptomatic CP are covered elsewhere in this book.

The risk for a recurrent attack of pancreatitis after an initial episode is 10–30% [3]. However patients with alcohol etiology and those without an identifiable etiology (idiopathic) are at greater risk for recurrence 24–30% [2, 4, 5]. Ongoing alcohol and tobacco use following a first attack of pancreatitis substantially increases risk for recurrence. This risk can be as high as 40–50% in patients that continue to drink and smoke in the setting of alcoholic and/or IRAP [4].

Counseling patients with RAP to abstain from alcohol and tobacco use cannot be over emphasized as a meaningful intervention. Data support alcohol and tobacco cessation interventions for RAP, as they correlate with favorable outcomes [1, 6, 7]. Intensive counseling for alcohol cessation has randomized controlled trial level data that supports it as an intervention that associates with remission of recurrent episodes of pancreatitis [6]. For this reason, endoscopic therapy should generally be avoided in patients with recurrent pancreatitis in the setting of ongoing alcohol abuse.

Initial Diagnostic Approach: Is It Biliary Pancreatitis?

A directed history and review of objective data with a focus on establishing an etiology are the first steps in the diagnostic algorithm for recurrent pancreatitis. Pancreatic enzyme levels, liver function tests, and abdominal imaging of the pancreas, biliary tree, and gallbladder are of particular interest. These baseline studies are of greatest value when collected during or within days of an attack of pancreatitis. This data is critical in identifying biliary disease as the etiology for recurrent pancreatitis. Biliary disease is implicated in 26–82% of attacks of acute pancreatitis. This figure varies significantly across populations of patients when stratifying by demographics and geographic regions [8–10]. With reference to biliary pancreatitis, elevated alanine aminotransferase (ALT) at the time of pancreatitis and imaging that confirms choledocholithiasis, choleithiasis, microlithiasis (stones <3 mm in size), or gallbladder sludge are specific for biliary pancreatitis [3, 11].

Why is it so important to identify biliary disease as an etiology for pancreatitis? Aside from being the most common nonalcoholic etiology for pancreatitis, there is a well-defined algorithm for deploying established, diagnostic studies and definitive therapies for biliary pancreatitis. For ERCP in particular, its role is defined by evidence-based predictors for retained common bile duct stone(s) at the time of presentation and is supported by published societal guidelines. If a single "very high" or several "high" predictors for choledocholithiasis are present at the time of biliary pancreatitis, an ERCP for stone extraction should be performed. If a single *high* predictor or *moderate* predictors are present, high-quality imaging of the extrahepatic bile duct should be performed and ERCP to follow if choledocholithiasis is confirmed [12] (Table 9.1). Meta-analysis-level data support the selective use of ERCP in the setting of biliary pancreatitis, with lower rates of mortality and local and systemic complications in subgroups of patients with cholangitis and/or biliary obstruction [13, 14].

Cholecystectomy is indicated in all patients that are surgical candidates with biliary pancreatitis to prevent subsequent episodes. This is preferably performed at index hospitalization or shortly thereafter in patients with mild, interstitial pancreatitis [1, 15]. Subsequent pancreatitis event rates in patients that fail to undergo cholecystectomy are as high as 13–15% at 1–2 years [16, 17].

In patients who do not undergo cholecystectomy, ERCP offers therapeutic benefit for prevention of recurrence. A recent comparative study also found that ERCP biliary sphincterotomy

Table 9.1 Predictors and suggested management strategy for possible choledocholithiasis in patients with biliary pancreatitis based on biochemical and imaging findings

Predictor	Type	Approach
Very strong	CBD stone visualized on imaging Clinical ascending cholangitis Bilirubin >4 mg/dL	ERCP if any present
Strong	Dilated CBD (>6 mm with gallbladder in situ) Bilirubin level (1.8–4 mg/dL)	ERCP if both present Advanced imaging[a] if single predictor
Moderate	Abnormal liver biochemical test(s) other than bilirubin Age > 55 years Clinical gallstone pancreatitis	Advanced imaging[a] if any present

Adopted from [12]
[a]IOC or intraoperative ultrasound at cholecystectomy, EUS, or MRCP

when deployed appropriately in biliary pancreatitis patients predicts a lower rate of readmission for subsequent pancreatitis in patients that fail to undergo cholecystectomy (HR 0.051 CI 0.047–0.55, $p < 0.0001$) [18].

Diagnostic Approach for "Idiopathic," Recurrent Pancreatitis

The etiology of recurrent pancreatitis remains uncertain in up to 30% of patients after obtaining a history, right upper quadrant ultrasound, and biochemical testing [2]. Patients can be designated as having IRAP only after alcoholic, biliary, and medication etiologies have been excluded. Note that medications implicated in pancreatitis have varying levels of evidence supporting their mechanism. Badalov et al. offer a thoughtful review weighting the levels of evidence for various medications implicated in acute pancreatitis [19].

A second-tier workup should be undertaken prior to deploying endoscopic therapies for IRAP. This includes an evaluation for structural pancreatic abnormalities, pancreatic neoplasia, metabolic, autoimmune (more often Type II), and genetic cofactors that either cause or associate with recurrent pancreatitis. This next tier evaluation can be tailored based on comorbid clinical conditions that are associated with each of the known etiologies for RAP (Table 9.2) [15].

Table 9.2 Selected etiologies of recurrent pancreatitis and associated clinical conditions, diagnostic findings

Category	Specific etiologies	Associated clinical conditions, diagnostic findings, and "pearls"
Biliary	Stones, microlithiasis (stones <3 mm), and sludge	Antecedent biliary colic Elevated transaminases, jaundice with pancreatitis Gallbladder pathology (stones, sludge) on ultrasound Bile duct dilation on imaging
Alcohol	Cofactor with tobacco abuse	Alcohol us >2/1 drinks daily or binge drinking: >5/3 drinks at drinking sessions for M/F
Implicated medications[a]	6-MP, azathioprine Carbimazole Codeine Hydrochlorothiazide Cytosine arabinoside Dapsone ACE inhibitors Furosemide Isoniazid Valproic acid Tetracycline Sulindac	Timing of pancreatitis follows initiation of medication Pancreatitis recurs with re-challenge Absence of competing etiology (e.g., alcohol)

(continued)

TABLE 9.2 (continued)

Category	Specific etiologies	Associated clinical conditions, diagnostic findings, and "pearls"
Metabolic	Hypertriglyceridemia	Metabolic syndrome Diabetes Concomitant or provoked by alcohol consumption
	Hypercalcemia	Hyperparathyroidism Sarcoidosis Paraneoplastic syndrome
Autoimmune	Type I (lymphoplasmacytic sclerosing pancreatitis)	Age > 60 Elevated IgG4, ANA IgG4 cells (>10/hpf) on tissue staining Biliary obstruction, strictures^{+} Pancreatic duct strictures without upstream dilation Focal pancreatic lesions^{+} or diffuse pancreatic enlargement
	Type II (idiopathic duct-centric pancreatitis)	Age < 60 $^{+}$(also often found in type II) More often RAP Coincident with inflammatory bowel disease Neutrophils infiltrating ductal cells, granulocyte epithelial lesion (GEL) on pathology
Congenital, structural	Pancreas divisum	Cofactor with tobacco, alcohol Cofactor with SPINK1, CFTR polymorphisms
	Todani type I/III choledochal cyst Anomalous pancreaticobiliary junction	Gallbladder and biliary malignancy (APBJ, type I cysts) Cystic dilation of biliary tree on imaging (type I/III cysts)

TABLE 9.2 (continued)

Category	Specific etiologies	Associated clinical conditions, diagnostic findings, and "pearls"
Genetic	PRSS1 SPINK1 CFTR CTRC	Onset childhood, young adult Cofactor with pancreas divisum
Neoplasia	Intraductal papillary mucinous neoplasm Pancreatic ductal adenocarcinoma Ampullary adenoma, adenocarcinoma	Pancreatitis onset, age > 55 Pancreatic duct dilation on imaging alone or with biliary dilation (double duct sign) Elevated CA19–9

[a]Truncated list of implicated medications

It is at this stage that high-quality imaging of the pancreas and biliary system plays a critical role in the diagnostic algorithm. Options for imaging include s-MRCP, EUS, and/or ERCP. Timing studies 3–4 weeks distant from an episode of pancreatitis is generally recommended, especially if occult neoplasia or congenital pancreatic duct abnormalities are a consideration. Ongoing inflammatory changes such as pancreatic edema, necrosis, and acute peripancreatic fluid collections can compromise the ability of imaging studies to delineate small, focal pancreatic lesions and image the pancreatic duct.

EUS is now considered a cornerstone of high-quality imaging to investigate IRAP. EUS is most effective for identifying occult biliary disease (biliary sludge, microlithiasis) when investigating IRAP with a sensitivity approaching 96% [3]. A recent meta-analysis confirmed EUS as the most sensitive imaging modality to identify occult biliary disease in the setting of pancreatitis [20]. The frequency with which occult biliary disease such as microlithiasis is implicated as a etiologic factor in IRAP varies (16–73%) and is reported across a heterogeneous group of studies [3]. EUS should strongly be considered for patients with a gallbladder in situ, antecedent biliary-type pain, LFT abnormalities juxtaposed to pancreatitis events, and/or pancreatitis events that follow cholecystectomy for cholelithiasis.

Acute pancreatitis is also a recognized clinical presentation in patients with ampullary or pancreaticobiliary neoplasia which is an etiologic factor in up to 5–7% of patients. EUS should be performed if neoplasia is suspected. EUS is sensitive for solid lesions smaller than 1–2 cm in diameter that involve the pancreas, extrahepatic bile duct, and ampulla. Fine needle aspiration (FNA) is able to further characterize neoplastic pancreatic lesions by providing a confirmatory tissue diagnosis. FNA also enhances the accuracy of EUS for the diagnosis of mucinous lesions of the main pancreatic duct and its side branches.

In which patients should we suspect neoplasia? A study of 218 patients presenting for EUS after acute pancreatitis described factors associated with pancreatic neoplasia as an etiology [21]. The study cohort was comprised of patients with a negative evaluation for gallstones and alcohol etiology. Adenocarcinoma was identified in 17% of patients, with 89% of the tumors found to be in the head of the pancreas. Intraductal papillary mucinous neoplasm (IPMN) was also found in an additional 3% of the cohort. Multivariable analysis identified age >50 (p = <0.008), weight loss >10 lbs (p = 0.003), smokers (p = <0.001), cholestasis (p = 0.035), pancreatic mass on imaging (p = 0.001), and pancreatic atrophy (p = 0.006) as independent predictors for malignancy in the setting of acute pancreatitis. EUS was found to be sensitive and specific for establishing the diagnosis in this cohort.

MRI/MRCP with contrast and s-MRCP has meta-analysis-level data suggesting that it is superior to EUS for identifying morphologic pancreatic abnormalities. Compared to diagnostic ERCP, s-MRCP risk profile is favorable as there is negligible risk for acute pancreatitis and the quality of imaging for the pancreatic duct is comparable [20].

Finally, the role of ERCP with or without manometry as a diagnostic modality for IRAP is diminishing. A study of ERCP with sphincter of Oddi manometry in 116 patients with IRAP identified a treatable cause in 37% patients. However, this included a mixture of anatomic abnormalities and biliary stones/sludge in addition to sphincter hypertension [22].

Arguably, with the exception of sphincter hypertension, MRCP and EUS are sensitive for these etiologies. The benefit of a noninvasive imaging first approach was elegantly demonstrated through a prospective study. Patients with IRAP underwent MRCP, EUS, and ERCP. Ultimately, the diagnostic yield for EUS and MRCP together was >60%. ERCP offered negligible interval diagnostic benefit [23]. Consequently, diagnostic ERCP for recurrent pancreatitis should be reserved for cases with a clear pre-procedure intention for sphincter of Oddi manometry. More importantly, ERCP for recurrent pancreatitis should be considered a therapeutic modality (e.g., sphincterotomy, stone extraction, stricture therapy) and be deployed to address an abnormality found on EUS and/or s-MRCP [24].

ERCP for the Management of Recurrent Acute Pancreatitis

ERCP in the setting of acute pancreatitis should be reserved for therapeutic intervention. It is only after completing components of second-tier workup and high-quality imaging that ERCP should be offered for RAP. ERCP endotherapy is either a directed therapy for RAP after discovery of occult biliary disease (e.g., CBD sludge), PDv, or in very select cases of neoplasia. ERCP with biliary sphincterotomy can be performed "empirically" in select patients with IRAP, but with limited data for its effectiveness. Empiric ventral pancreatic duct sphincterotomy should never be performed in IRAP.

The literature that reports the impact ERCP for the recurrent pancreatitis is predominantly comprised of retrospective studies and case series. Significant heterogeneity across studies in terms of patient selection, outcome measures (single AP recurrence, decline in episode, or progression to CP), length of follow-up, and therapeutic techniques (biliary, pancreatic, dual sphincterotomy, stent exchanges) makes it difficult to draw firm conclusions as to the impact of endoscopic therapy for RAP. As recurrent pancreatitis is an intermittent, episodic disease, long-term follow-up is required before meaningful conclusions can be drawn about the impact of endoscopic therapy.

Pancreas Divisum, Minor Papillotomy, and Dorsal Duct Stent Placement

Pancreas divisum (PDv) is a congenital, anatomic variant characterized by a failure of fusion of the main pancreatic between the dorsal and ventral anlage of the pancreas. In this setting, secretion from dorsal pancreatic anlage (which represents the majority of the functional pancreas) exclusively exits the minor papilla. As the most common anatomic variant of the pancreas, the frequency is 6–12% in autopsy series [25–27]. PDv is identified in 25% patients with recurrent acute pancreatitis and 33–43% in patients with IRAP and CP [26, 28]. It is most effectively identified using s-MRCP [20]. The mechanism for recurrent pancreatitis in PDv is believed to be from pancreatic secretions exiting through a diminutive pancreatic outlet (the minor papilla). This creates a functional pancreatic duct outlet obstruction, "dominant dorsal duct syndrome" [29]. However, studies have found that PDv is present at a significantly greater frequency in RAP patients with CFTR polymorphisms than in RAP patients without genetic polymorphisms. The mechanism for IRAP in the setting of PDv is now believed to be more complex than standalone, mechanical obstruction. It is now believed that PDv serves as compounding cofactor with other etiologies that further predispose patients to symptomatic pancreatitis [30, 31].

Endoscopic therapy focuses on alleviating obstruction at the level of the minor papilla through the technique of dorsal duct cannulation, minor papillotomy with or without stent insertion [29]. Literature on ERCP-minor papillotomy with or without dorsal duct stenting for recurrent acute pancreatitis identifies endoscopic therapy as an intervention that offers favorable results for preventing further attacks. A recent systematic review describes a quite favorable rate of "response" in RAP patients without CP at a median of 76% of patients across studies [27, 32–36].

However, the impact of therapeutic ERCP for RAP in PDv should be interpreted with caution. The literature is quite heterogeneous in terms of study design, follow-up, and the combination of dorsal duct therapeutic techniques. Importantly, the effectiveness of minor papillotomy alone is yet to be confirmed in randomized controlled trials. The only prospective, randomized, controlled trial reported results for serial dorsal duct stenting (5–7 Fr stents, total of 12 months decompression) without minor papillotomy. While the intervention group experienced fewer attacks of pancreatitis ($p = <0.05\%$), the median follow-up was also short (~2.5 years) following stent extraction [32]. Beyond the significant procedure burden of 12 months of serial stent exchanges, this approach is less often deployed by experts due to the high rates of stent-induced dorsal pancreatic duct changes in patients with PDv undergoing endotherapy (up to 50%) [27, 32].

ERCP with minor papilla cannulation and papillotomy is recognized as technically challenging by expert endoscopists and carries a significantly higher risk for early complications, namely, post-ERCP pancreatitis [29, 37, 38]. Interval stenosis of the minor papillotomy is an additional risk of papillotomy and occurs in 11–24% of patients [27, 33]. Consequently, follow-up endoscopic procedures are often required to further manage patients after minor papillotomy with or without stenting.

In spite of favorable data that supports endotherapy for PDv in the setting of RAP, this intervention remains an area of controversy given the risks and our evolving understanding of PDv as a cofactor in RAP. The risks and benefits of endoscopic therapy should be carefully discussed with a patient. The physician and patient should carefully weigh such factors as frequency of pancreatitis attacks, operator/center expertise, potential need for multiple procedures, presence of modifiable (alcohol, tobacco) and non-modifiable (CFTR, SPINK) cofactors for recurrent acute pancreatitis, and a patient's age and health status when considering endotherapy for RAP in the setting of PDv.

ERCP for Managing Congenital Abnormalities of Pancreaticobiliary Tree

Congenital pancreaticobiliary malformations are readily diagnosed on MRI/MRCP and represent a minority of patients with RAP [39]. Todani Type III choledochal cysts ("choledochocele") are congenital cystic abnormalities of the common bile duct within the ampulla of Vater. The papilla will display a focally cystic, protuberant appearance on cross-sectional imaging and when viewed endoscopically from within the duodenum. Pancreatitis is the most common presentation of choledochoceles (38–70%) presumably caused by a combination of mechanical outflow obstruction, increased pancreatic duct pressures, formation of biliary stones, and/or reflux of bile into the pancreatic duct. Endoscopic biliary sphincterotomy is considered therapeutic and is a reasonable alternative to resection as the potential for malignancy is low relative to other types of choledochal cysts [40]. Anomalous pancreaticobiliary junction occurs in 0.2% of populations of European descent but is more common in Asian populations and is associated with choledochal cysts (40–70%). These patients can present with pancreatitis by similar mechanisms as choledochocele. ERCP with biliary sphincterotomy may also benefit these patients in preventing further episodes of pancreatitis [41]. However, due to a much greater risk for malignancy, surgical referral for cholecystectomy with or without resection of the extrahepatic bile duct in the presence of choledochal cyst is also recommended in surgical candidates.

Idiopathic Recurrent Pancreatitis, Sphincter of Oddi Manometry, and Sphincterotomy

Sphincter of Oddi dysfunction (SOD) is found in 30–78% of RAP patients [24]. Literature suggests endoscopic sphincterotomy for sphincter "spasm," when identified, may eliminate recurrent pancreatitis in 50–75% of patients with SOD [42–44].

The impact of sphincterotomy on IRAP is best described in the form two, conflicting retrospective studies. A study by Wehrmann et al. reported outcomes in 37 patients with IRAP managed with biliary, pancreatic, or dual duct endoscopic sphincterotomy. The relapse rate was also 50% in the cohort. In patients with recurrent attacks, a lower frequency of episodes was observed after intervention after more than 10 years of follow-up. This study is hindered by lack of a comparison group managed without ERCP [45]. Das et al. reported retrospective comparative data for IRAP patients from the North American Pancreatitis Study (NAPS) cohort. In this study IRAP patients were stratified and analyzed based on a management strategy of either "medical therapy" or sphincterotomy. Rates of recurrent pancreatitis between groups managed with medical therapy versus sphincterotomy were similar ($p = 0.63$). Rates of pancreatitis were observed to decline across both groups with follow-up. However, while a comparative study, there were some notable limitations to this study design. Length of follow-up to potentially capture events was nearly twice as long for patients managed with sphincterotomy (11.8 vs 6.8 years, $p = 0.003$). Also, baseline disease activity appeared to differ between groups, with the number of preceding attacks of pancreatitis found to be greater in the sphincterotomy group (3 vs 2, $p = 0.039$) and the rate to progression to CP was also higher in the sphincterotomy group (27% vs 18%, $p = 0.46$). These two studies offer long-term follow-up data on the impact of sphincterotomy on not only any recurrence of pancreatitis but also episode density which is perhaps the most important metric for therapy in IRAP. Their conflicting findings highlight the limitations in studying the effectiveness of sphincterotomy for IRAP retrospectively. The potential for unmeasured confounders related to differences in upfront selection of patients for sphincterotomy and variability in the subsequent duration of monitoring for events will consistently hinder studies with retrospective designs [46].

The only published prospective, randomized controlled trial dedicated to evaluating endotherapy for IRAP patients allocated patients to therapeutic approaches based on the presence of pancreatic SOD (PSOD) at manometry [24]. The primary outcome was a single, recurrent attack of pancreatitis after intervention. The median length of follow-up for this cohort was quite substantial at 78 months (IQR, 35–108 months). PSOD patients were randomized to biliary or biliary with pancreatic sphincterotomy. Recurrence of acute pancreatitis after intervention was similar between groups managed with either of the sphincterotomy approaches (48 vs 47%, $p = 1.0$). Patients without PSOD were randomized to sham or biliary sphincterotomy and recurrence rates of acute pancreatitis also found to be similar (11 vs 27%, $p = 0.60$). The impact of sphincterotomy on the frequency of pancreatitis (episode density) was not analyzed in this study, nor was the study powered to assess the impact of sphincterotomy vs sham. PSOD was associated with a risk of subsequent episodes of AP after intervention. Overall, this study concluded that a dual sphincterotomy approach (pancreatic and biliary) for patients with PSOD offers little interval advantage over a biliary sphincterotomy alone.

Conflicting data exists on the impact of sphincterotomy therapy on the natural history of IRAP. While it appears that IRAP recurs in approximately 50% of patients managed with a sphincterotomy, it is unclear if this can be attributed to the intervention or the natural history of the disease with observation. Based on the only randomized, controlled trial, if sphincterotomy is selected to manage a patient with IRAP, biliary sphincterotomy alone may be the most appropriate technique. The role of sphincter of Oddi manometry to identify SOD in IRAP is even more perplexing. Based on Cote et al., SOD may identify an aggressive phenotype. However, given that SOD is quite prevalent (50–75%) in RAP patients and does not predict response to therapy, many experts deploy an approach of empiric sphincterotomy without manometry.

Further, randomized studies with long-term follow-up that compare sphincterotomy to medical therapy/observation are required. These studies should assess the impact of sphincterotomy on not only recurrence but also the episode density of pancreatitis after intervention/enrollment. At this time, it is reasonable to offer biliary sphincterotomy to IRAP patients with an aggressive RAP phenotype. Pancreatic sphincterotomy in this context should be avoided based on a randomized prospective study, a high restenosis rate (20–30%), and consequent potential for repeat procedures to manage restenosis as a late, iatrogenic complication [3, 47]. Sphincterotomy for IRAP should be offered after a careful discussion of the risks (post-ERCP pancreatitis, interval sphincter stenosis), benefits, and alternatives (empiric cholecystectomy, observation).

ERCP for Management of Pancreatitis in the Setting of Pancreaticobiliary Neoplasia

Adenoma is the most common form of neoplasia of the ampulla. Pancreatitis is an infrequent presentation for these patients, occurring in 5% at presentation [48]. Endoscopic therapy in the form papillectomy with or without pancreatic sphincterotomy has technical success rates (defined by complete tumor resection at 3–6-month follow-up) of 46–92%. However, rates of post-procedure complications are high (8–42%), with post-ERCP pancreatitis the most frequent [48, 49]. While papillectomy effectively removes the obstructing lesion implicated in pancreatitis attacks, data regarding the success of this technique for realizing durable resolution of pancreatitis episodes remains poorly characterized and is largely unmeasured across studies. However, given obstruction is the most likely mechanism for RAP in these patients, is reasonable to offer endoscopic papillectomy to ampullary adenoma patients afflicted with RAP and expect resolution of pancreatitis with resection of the lesion.

Acute pancreatitis complicates 7–67% of patients with IPMN referred to tertiary centers for management. Reported rates of pancreatitis are higher in patients referred for resection, as this is a guideline level indication for surgery. Studies are conflicted as to whether differences in rates of pancreatitis exist across morphologic subtypes (e.g., side branch, mixed and main pancreatic duct lesions) [50, 51]. The mechanism for recurrent pancreatitis is suspected to be intermittent pancreatic duct obstruction from the passage of mucin excreted from neoplastic epithelium. ERCP endoscopic therapy is a potential alternative for patients that are not candidates for or refuse resection [52]. Specifically, pancreatic sphincterotomy may prevent recurrent episodes of pancreatitis based on small case series. The largest case series ($n = 16$) evaluating this approach reported complete resolution of pancreatitis in 69% of patients (mean follow-up 24.9 months). A median numbers 3.5 episodes (+/– 2.3) were observed before sphincterotomy which decreased to 0.56 (+/–1.03) after sphincterotomy ($p = < 0.0001$). Further, comparative studies are needed to evaluate this technique as a viable alternative to resection for IPMN complicated by RAP.

Case Outcomes

Case 1: Occult Biliary Pancreatitis (Fig. 9.1)

EUS was performed as an outpatient. Hyperechoic, mobile material was visualized in the gallbladder consistent with layer sludge. Mobile hyperechoic material was also visualized in the bile duct, which measured up to 7 mm in diameter. The pancreatic duct was normal in caliber, measuring up to 1.5 mm in the head of the pancreas. The pancreatic duct could be followed from the ventral to dorsal anlage, excluding PDv. The EUS was followed by an ERCP. Dark bile with particulate sludge was visualized endoscopically exiting the bile duct prior to cannulation. Biliary cannulation, biliary sphincterotomy, and balloon sweep clearing the bile duct of sludge were performed. The patient was referred for laparoscopic cholecystectomy. He has since advanced to a solid diet and is now 3 months without a recurrent pancreatitis event.

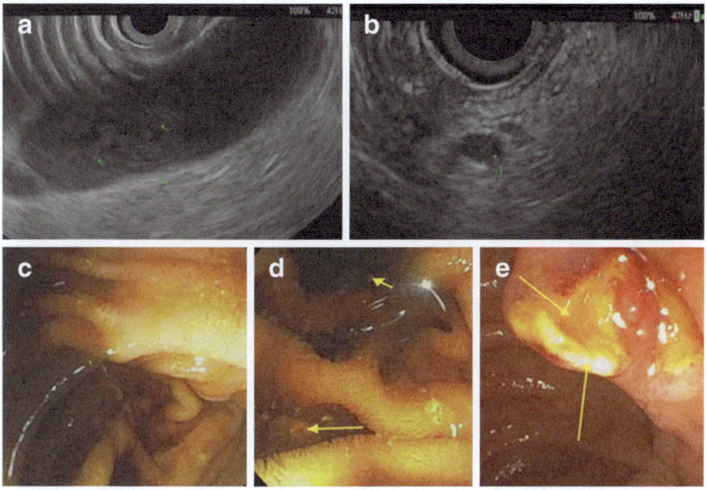

FIGUER 9.1 (**a**) EUS imaging demonstrating gallbladder sludge (green arrows), (**b**) EUS imaging from the duodenal bulb demonstrating bile duct sludge (green arrows). (**c**/**d**) Duodenoscope images of the region of the ampulla demonstrating dark bile with particulate sludge. (**e**) Ampulla following sphincterotomy

This patient-reported biliary colic, was with a gallbladder in situ, and possessed risk factors for biliary disease (morbid obesity, diabetes). CT scan has limited sensitivity for gallstone disease and cholelithiasis (sensitivity <65%). Right upper quadrant ultrasound is sensitive for gallstones (>95%). In this case the gallbladder was contracted at the time of the sonogram, which diminishes the sensitivity for small stones and layering sludge. ALT alone has limitations in its negative predictive value even when normal at the time of pancreatitis. EUS was performed as the suspicion for biliary disease remained high in spite of his negative diagnostic studies. ERCP followed given the presence of bile duct sludge. Cholecystectomy followed for definitive prophylaxis from further RAP events.

Case 2: Sphincterotomy for IRAP

Given an extensive workup that was unrevealing for an etiology, absence of CP, and multiple episodes of pancreatitis within a 12-month span, we offered endoscopic therapy. A temporary pancreatic stent was placed, and a biliary sphincterotomy was performed. He is now more than 12 months without recurrent pancreatitis, which based on his pre-intervention disease activity suggests a favorable response. Further follow-up will be required to gauge the overall impact.

Case 3: Minor Papillotomy for PDv (Fig. 9.2)

After a careful discussion of the risks, benefits, and alternatives, therapeutic ERCP was performed. Cannulation of the minor papilla was successful. Pancreatogram was consistent with PDv and without features of CP. A minor papillotomy was performed with a sphincterotome, and a 3 Fr by 8 cm prophylactic pancreatic stent was placed. Rectal indomethacin was administered. Following the procedure, she experienced new epigastric abdominal pain and nausea. She was administered IV fluids at 3 cc/kg/hour and admitted for suspiscion of post-ERCP pancreatitis, confirmed by biochemical testing the following day (Lipase 1848 U/L, ULN 59). She was admitted for 48 hours and ultimately discharged on a solid diet. Follow-up KUB at 15 days from ERCP confirmed spontaneous migration of her pancreatic stent.

She has been without an episode of recurrent pancreatitis for the past 3.5 years.

Case 4: Pancreatic Ductal Adenocarcinoma (Fig. 9.3)

Given the finding of suspicious pancreatic mass (discrete, low radiodensity, upstream pancreatic duct dilation) visualized on cross-sectional imaging in the setting of a concerning clinical scenario for cancer (antecedent pain, weight loss), the deci-

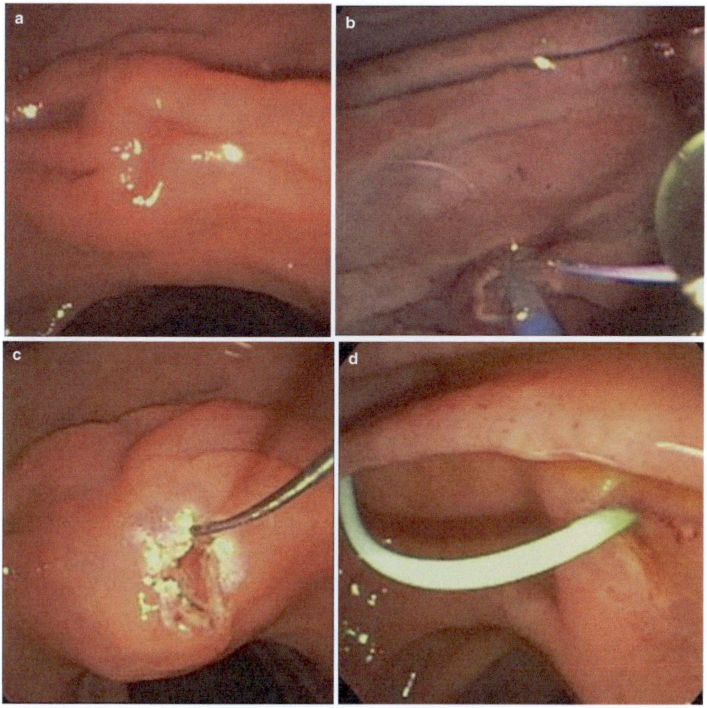

FIGURE 9.2 (**a**) Minor papilla, second portion of the duodenum. (**b**) Cannulation and minor papillotomy performed utilizing a sphincterotome. (**c**) Endoscopic view of the minor papillotomy, 0.018 inch guidewire positioned across the minor papilla in the dorsal pancreatic duct. (**d**) Prophylactic dorsal pancreatic duct stent placed

sion was made to perform an EUS. The decision was made to perform the EUS procedure prior to discharge, as we believe that the lesion would be readily identified for sampling. Specifically, the lesion as visualized on cross-sectional imaging and pancreatic inflammatory changes were minimal. EUS demonstrated a hypoechoic mass in the uncinate portion of the pancreas. FNA on-site cytopathology was suspicious for adenocarcinoma, with confirmatory final pathology. The lesion demonstrated abutment of the superior mesenteric

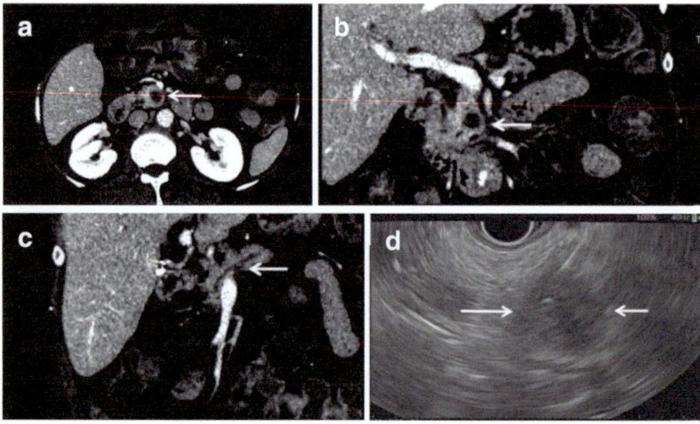

Figure 9.3 (**a/b**) Low radiodensity mass in the uncinate of the pancreas (arrows) visualized on cross section and coronal CT scan images. (**c**) Upstream pancreatic duct dilation on coronal CT scan images. (**d**) EUS images with a linear echoendoscope of the uncinate pancreas from second portion of the duodenal, mass visualized (arrows)

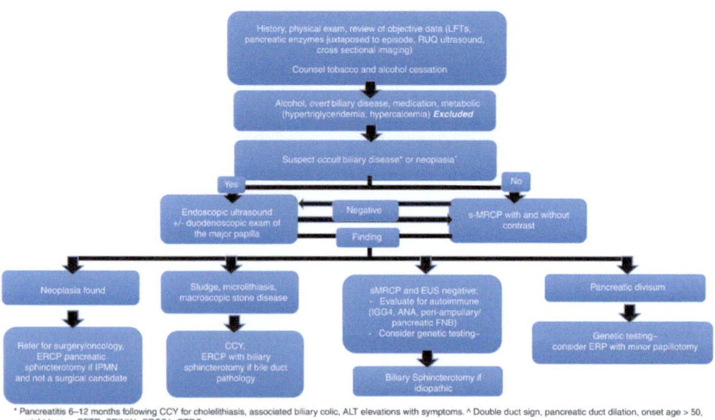

Figure 9.4 Diagnostic and therapeutic algorithm for recurrent acute pancreatitis

vein. The visualized left lobe of the liver was negative for focal lesions. The bile duct was normal. She was referred to oncology and pancreaticobiliary surgery. EUS-celiac plexus neurolysis was later performed due to persistent, severe abdominal pain. She was able to advance to a solid diet prior to discharge.

Pearls and Pitfalls (Fig. 9.4)

- ERCP for recurrent pancreatitis should be avoided in patients with alcoholic pancreatitis and in patients with non-biliary pancreatitis that are abusing alcohol.
- Smoking cessation should be emphasized for patients with RAP.
- Overt and occult biliary disease are among the most common identifiable etiologies for recurrent acute pancreatitis, and as ERCP endotherapy or surgery may be definitive interventions, biliary disease is a central, early consideration during the diagnostic workup.
- In patients with IRAP, significant inflammatory changes and that do not have a discrete mass on cross-sectional imaging, advanced imaging should be delayed 3–4 weeks, especially if structural abnormalities or occult neoplasia is a consideration.
- EUS is often the advanced imaging study of choice for RAP patients, especially if biliary disease or neoplasia is suspected.
- S-MRCP is the advanced imaging study of choice for RAP patients with suspected pancreatic ductal pathology.
- Diagnostic ERCP should be avoided in patients with IRAP.
- Therapeutic minor papillotomy may offer benefit for patients with recurrent pancreatitis in the setting of pancreas divisum.

- Sphincter of Oddi manometry and sphincterotomy for IRAP remains an area of controversy. Based on available data sphincterotomy, with or without manometry may be performed for IRAP after an extensive workup and careful discussion of the risks, benefits, and alternatives.
- Biliary sphincterotomy without pancreatic sphincterotomy is the best approach for ERCP endotherapy in IRAP based on available data.

References (Suggested Readings *)

1. Crockett SD, Wani S, Gardner TB, Falck-Ytter Y, Barkun AN. American Gastroenterological Association Institute clinical guidelines C. American Gastroenterological Association Institute guideline on initial management of acute pancreatitis. Gastroenterology. 2018;154:1096–101.
2. Das R, Yadav D, Papachristou GI. Endoscopic treatment of recurrent acute pancreatitis and smoldering acute pancreatitis. Gastrointest Endosc Clin N Am. 2015;25:737–48.
3. Guda NM, Muddana V, Whitcomb DC, et al. Recurrent acute pancreatitis: international state-of-the-science conference with recommendations. Pancreas. 2018;47:653–66.*
4. Ahmed Ali U, Issa Y, Hagenaars JC, et al. Risk of recurrent pancreatitis and progression to chronic pancreatitis after a first episode of acute pancreatitis. Clin Gastroenterol Hepatol. 2016;14:738–46.
5. Lankisch PG, Breuer N, Bruns A, Weber-Dany B, Lowenfels AB, Maisonneuve P. Natural history of acute pancreatitis: a long-term population-based study. Am J Gastroenterol. 2009;104:2797–805; quiz 806.*
6. Nordback I, Pelli H, Lappalainen-Lehto R, Jarvinen S, Raty S, Sand J. The recurrence of acute alcohol-associated pancreatitis can be reduced: a randomized controlled trial. Gastroenterology. 2009;136:848–55.
7. Sadr-Azodi O, Andren-Sandberg A, Orsini N, Wolk A. Cigarette smoking, smoking cessation and acute pancreatitis: a prospective population-based study. Gut. 2012;61:262–7.
8. Zheng Y, Zhou Z, Li H, et al. A multicenter study on etiology of acute pancreatitis in Beijing during 5 years. Pancreas. 2015;44:409–14.

9. Garg SK, Sarvepalli S, Campbell JP, et al. Incidence, admission rates, and predictors, and economic burden of adult emergency visits for acute pancreatitis: data from the National Emergency Department Sample, 2006 to 2012. J Clin Gastroenterol. 2018:1.
10. Papachristou GI, Machicado JD, Stevens T, et al. Acute pancreatitis patient registry to examine novel therapies in clinical experience (APPRENTICE): an international, multicenter consortium for the study of acute pancreatitis. Ann Gastroenterol. 2017;30:106–13.
11. Fogel EL, Sherman S. ERCP for gallstone pancreatitis. N Engl J Med. 2014;370:1956.
12. Committee ASoP, Maple JT, Ben-Menachem T, et al. The role of endoscopy in the evaluation of suspected choledocholithiasis. Gastrointest Endosc. 2010;71:1–9.*
13. Tse F, Yuan Y. Early routine endoscopic retrograde cholangiopancreatography strategy versus early conservative management strategy in acute gallstone pancreatitis. Cochrane Database Syst Rev. 2012;5:CD009779.
14. Petrov MS, van Santvoort HC, Besselink MG, van der Heijden GJ, van Erpecum KJ, Gooszen HG. Early endoscopic retrograde cholangiopancreatography versus conservative management in acute biliary pancreatitis without cholangitis: a meta-analysis of randomized trials. Ann Surg. 2008;247:250–7.
15. Tenner S, Baillie J, DeWitt J, Vege SS. American College of G. American College of Gastroenterology guideline: management of acute pancreatitis. Am J Gastroenterol. 2013;108:1400–15; 16.
16. Kamal A, Akhuemonkhan E, Akshintala VS, Singh VK, Kalloo AN, Hutfless SM. Effectiveness of guideline-recommended cholecystectomy to prevent recurrent pancreatitis. Am J Gastroenterol. 2017;112:503–10.
17. Kim SB, Kim TN, Chung HH, Kim KH. Small gallstone size and delayed cholecystectomy increase the risk of recurrent Pancreatobiliary complications after resolved acute biliary pancreatitis. Dig Dis Sci. 2017;62:777–83.
18. Qayed E, Shah R, Haddad YK. Endoscopic retrograde cholangiopancreatography decreases all-cause and pancreatitis readmissions in patients with acute gallstone pancreatitis who do not undergo cholecystectomy: a Nationwide 5-year analysis. Pancreas. 2018;47:425–35.
19. Badalov N, Baradarian R, Iswara K, Li J, Steinberg W, Tenner S. Drug-induced acute pancreatitis: an evidence-based review. Clin Gastroenterol Hepatol. 2007;5:648–61; quiz 4.*

20. Wan J, Ouyang Y, Yu C, Yang X, Xia L, Lu N. Comparison of EUS with MRCP in idiopathic acute pancreatitis: a systematic review and meta-analysis. Gastrointest Endosc. 2018;87:1180–8 e9.*
21. Tummala P, Tariq SH, Chibnall JT, Agarwal B. Clinical predictors of pancreatic carcinoma causing acute pancreatitis. Pancreas. 2013;42:108–13.
22. Venu RP, Geenen JE, Hogan W, Stone J, Johnson GK, Soergel K. Idiopathic recurrent pancreatitis. An approach to diagnosis and treatment. Dig Dis Sci. 1989;34:56–60.
23. Mariani A, Arcidiacono PG, Curioni S, Giussani A, Testoni PA. Diagnostic yield of ERCP and secretin-enhanced MRCP and EUS in patients with acute recurrent pancreatitis of unknown aetiology. Dig Liver Dis. 2009;41:753–8.
24. Cote GA, Imperiale TF, Schmidt SE, et al. Similar efficacies of biliary, with or without pancreatic, sphincterotomy in treatment of idiopathic recurrent acute pancreatitis. Gastroenterology. 2012;143:1502–9 e1.*
25. Stimec B, Bulajic M, Korneti V, Milosavljevic T, Krstic R, Ugljesic M. Ductal morphometry of ventral pancreas in pancreas divisum. Comparison between clinical and anatomical results. Ital J Gastroenterol. 1996;28:76–80.
26. Cotton PB. Congenital anomaly of pancreas divisum as cause of obstructive pain and pancreatitis. Gut. 1980;21:105–14.
27. Heyries L, Barthet M, Delvasto C, Zamora C, Bernard JP, Sahel J. Long-term results of endoscopic management of pancreas divisum with recurrent acute pancreatitis. Gastrointest Endosc. 2002;55:376–81.
28. Gonoi W, Akai H, Hagiwara K, et al. Pancreas divisum as a predisposing factor for chronic and recurrent idiopathic pancreatitis: initial in vivo survey. Gut. 2011;60:1103–8.
29. Fogel EL, Toth TG, Lehman GA, DiMagno MJ, DiMagno EP. Does endoscopic therapy favorably affect the outcome of patients who have recurrent acute pancreatitis and pancreas divisum? Pancreas. 2007;34:21–45.
30. Bertin C, Pelletier AL, Vullierme MP, et al. Pancreas divisum is not a cause of pancreatitis by itself but acts as a partner of genetic mutations. Am J Gastroenterol. 2012;107:311–7.
31. Garg PK, Khajuria R, Kabra M, Shastri SS. Association of SPINK1 gene mutation and CFTR gene polymorphisms in patients with pancreas divisum presenting with idiopathic pancreatitis. J Clin Gastroenterol. 2009;43:848–52.

32. Lans JI, Geenen JE, Johanson JF, Hogan WJ. Endoscopic therapy in patients with pancreas divisum and acute pancreatitis: a prospective, randomized, controlled clinical trial. Gastrointest Endosc. 1992;38:430–4.
33. Lehman GA, Sherman S, Nisi R, Hawes RH. Pancreas divisum: results of minor papilla sphincterotomy. Gastrointest Endosc. 1993;39:1–8.
34. Satterfield ST, McCarthy JH, Geenen JE, et al. Clinical experience in 82 patients with pancreas divisum: preliminary results of manometry and endoscopic therapy. Pancreas. 1988;3:248–53.
35. Liao Z, Gao R, Wang W, et al. A systematic review on endoscopic detection rate, endotherapy, and surgery for pancreas divisum. Endoscopy. 2009;41:439–44.
36. Kanth R, Samji NS, Inaganti A, et al. Endotherapy in symptomatic pancreas divisum: a systematic review. Pancreatology. 2014;14:244–50.*
37. DiMagno MJ, Wamsteker EJ. Pancreas divisum. Curr Gastroenterol Rep. 2011;13:150–6.
38. Moffatt DC, Cote GA, Avula H, et al. Risk factors for ERCP-related complications in patients with pancreas divisum: a retrospective study. Gastrointest Endosc. 2011;73:963–70.
39. Takuma K, Kamisawa T, Hara S, et al. Etiology of recurrent acute pancreatitis, with special emphasis on pancreaticobiliary malformation. Adv Med Sci. 2012;57:244–50.
40. Law R, Topazian M. Diagnosis and treatment of choledochoceles. Clin Gastroenterol Hepatol. 2014;12:196–203.
41. Samavedy R, Sherman S, Lehman GA. Endoscopic therapy in anomalous pancreatobiliary duct junction. Gastrointest Endosc. 1999;50:623–7.
42. Testoni PA, Caporuscio S, Bagnolo F, Lella F. Idiopathic recurrent pancreatitis: long-term results after ERCP, endoscopic sphincterotomy, or ursodeoxycholic acid treatment. Am J Gastroenterol. 2000;95:1702–7.
43. Jacob L, Geenen JE, Catalano MF, Geenen DJ. Prevention of pancreatitis in patients with idiopathic recurrent pancreatitis: a prospective nonblinded randomized study using endoscopic stents. Endoscopy. 2001;33:559–62.
44. Kaw M, Brodmerkel GJ Jr. ERCP, biliary crystal analysis, and sphincter of Oddi manometry in idiopathic recurrent pancreatitis. Gastrointest Endosc. 2002;55:157–62.
45. Wehrmann T. Long-term results (>/= 10 years) of endoscopic therapy for sphincter of Oddi dysfunction in patients with acute recurrent pancreatitis. Endoscopy. 2011;43:202–7.

46. Das R, Clarke B, Tang G, et al. Endoscopic sphincterotomy (ES) may not alter the natural history of idiopathic recurrent acute pancreatitis (IRAP). Pancreatology. 2016;16:770.*
47. Dufault DL, Elmunzer BJ, Cotton PB, Williams A, Cote GA. Adverse events and Reinterventions following pancreatic endoscopic Sphincterotomy. Pancreas. 2018;47:880–3.
48. Irani S, Arai A, Ayub K, et al. Papillectomy for ampullary neoplasm: results of a single referral center over a 10-year period. Gastrointest Endosc. 2009;70:923–32.
49. Ardengh JC, Kemp R, Lima-Filho ER, Dos Santos JS. Endoscopic papillectomy: the limits of the indication, technique and results. World J Gastrointest Endosc. 2015;7:987–94.
50. Jang JW, Kim MH, Jeong SU, et al. Clinical characteristics of intraductal papillary mucinous neoplasm manifesting as acute pancreatitis or acute recurrent pancreatitis. J Gastroenterol Hepatol. 2013;28:731–8.
51. Venkatesh PG, Navaneethan U, Vege SS. Intraductal papillary mucinous neoplasm and acute pancreatitis. J Clin Gastroenterol. 2011;45:755–8.
52. Tanaka M, Fernandez-del Castillo C, Adsay V, et al. International consensus guidelines 2012 for the management of IPMN and MCN of the pancreas. Pancreatology. 2012;12:183–97.

Chapter 10
Minor Papilla Cannulation

Dhairya Mehta and Zachary L. Smith

Case Presentation

A 44-year-old male with history of alcoholism and recurrent attacks of acute pancreatitis was evaluated for acute-onset epigastric abdominal pain radiating to the back and nausea for 3 days. Laboratory tests showed an elevated serum lipase at 152 U/L (reference range 9–82 U/L) and elevated total bilirubin at 2.9 mg/dl (reference range 0.0–1.2 mg/dl). CAT scan of the abdomen showed a 6 cm by 5 cm by 7 cm cystic lesion in the pancreatic head most likely representing a pseudocyst in the setting of recurrent pancreatitis. There was adjacent mass effect on the lower common bile duct (CBD) resulting in mild upstream extrahepatic and intrahepatic biliary dilatation.

D. Mehta
University Hospitals Cleveland Medical Center, Gastroenterology and Liver Disease, Cleveland, OH, USA

Z. L. Smith (✉)
Division of Gastroenterology and Liver Disease, University Hospitals Digestive Health Institute, Case Western Reserve University School of Medicine, Cleveland, OH, USA
e-mail: zachary.smith2@uhhospitals.org

D. K. Mullady (ed.), *Dilemmas in ERCP*,
https://doi.org/10.1007/978-3-030-12741-1_10

Pancreatic duct (PD) was noted to have mild diffuse dilation, likely from the mass effect of the aforementioned pseudocyst. An endoscopic ultrasound examination revealed a 5 cm by 6 cm hypoechoic and homogenous cyst in the pancreatic head causing mild extrinsic compression in the prepyloric region of the stomach, as well as the duodenal bulb. EUS-guided cystenterostomy was not technically feasible due to the lack of a safe needle tract for fistula creation. Subsequently, an ERCP was performed to evaluate for CBD and PD strictures. Ventral PD cannulation was achieved through the major papilla. After contrast injection, only a short portion of the ventral PD toward the ampulla was opacified, followed by acinarization of the ventral PD in pancreatic head suggesting pancreas divisum. Major papilla sphincterotomy was performed and one 5 Fr by 3 cm plastic stent was placed in the ventral PD for post-ERCP pancreatitis prophylaxis. Subsequently, the dorsal PD was cannulated via the minor papilla using a tapered tip cannula. Contrast injection through the dorsal PD resulted in duct opacification up to the tail with no communication with the ventral PD, confirming the diagnosis of complete pancreas divisum. A 10 mm stricture was identified in the head and genu of the pancreas with upstream PD dilation. Contrast was seen extravasating into the pseudocyst from the upstream body of the pancreas. A dorsal sphincterotomy was performed, and one 7 Fr by 9 cm plastic stent was placed, 8 cm into the dorsal PD. The patient experienced relief from his symptoms and was discharged the following day.

This case highlights the importance a priori recognition of pancreatic ductal anatomy, successful minor papilla cannulation, and the ability to deliver therapeutic interventions through the minor papilla into the dorsal pancreatic duct.

Pancreatic Anatomy

The normal adult pancreas originates from the fusion of the ventral pancreatic bud with the dorsal pancreatic bud. The ventral pancreatic bud forms the uncinate process and the main pancreatic duct (PD) in the head (duct of Wirsung), while the dorsal pancreatic bud forms the rest of the head, neck, body, and tail of the pancreas as well as the rest of the main PD and the accessory PD (duct of Santorini). As the embryonic pancreas develops, the ventral PD forms a communication with the dorsal PD to form the main PD. The portion of the dorsal PD toward the ampulla (downstream to the communication with the ventral PD) either regresses or opens into the duodenum via the minor papilla. Normally, all or almost all of the pancreatic secretions are drained through the main PD via the major papilla (Fig. 10.1).

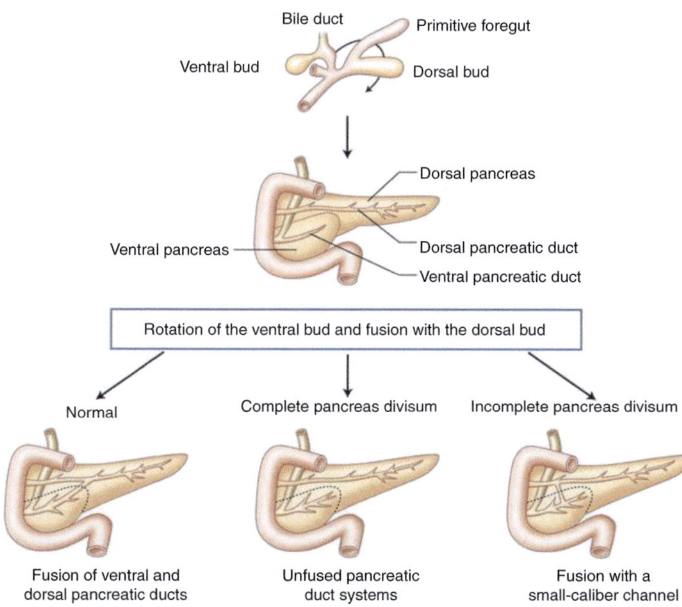

FIGURE 10.1 Formation of the normal pancreas and pancreas divisum during embryological development. The schematic illustration above represents the embryological formation of the normal pancreas and abnormalities in this process that lead to the development of pancreas divisum. (Reproduced with permission from Springer Nature. Luther and Casey [11])

In complete pancreas divisum, the ventral PD fails to communicate with the dorsal PD. Thus the bulk of the pancreatic secretions are drained through the accessory PD via the minor papilla, while the ventral PD drains only a small portion of the head and the uncinate process (Fig. 10.2). In incomplete pancreas divisum, a rudimentary communication exists between the dorsal and ventral ducts; however the majority of drainage occurs via the dorsal PD at the minor papilla. The term pseudo-divisum (or functional divisum) is used when the pancreas has normal ductal anatomy, but most of the pancreatic secretions are still drained through the patent accessory duct via the minor papilla. This most commonly occurs when a stone or a stricture blocks the downstream part of the main PD toward the ampulla (embryonic ventral PD) redirecting the pancreatic secretions to flow through the accessory duct via the minor papilla. Therefore, in symptomatic pancreas divisum or pseudo-divisum patients, cannulation of the minor papilla may be necessary to provide appropriate endotherapeutic interventions (Fig. 10.3).

The Role of Pancreatic Endotherapy

Therapeutic maneuvers within the PD (so-called pancreatic endotherapy) have evolved over the last two decades. Due to its minimally invasive nature and the relatively lower risk of procedure-related morbidity when compared to surgical drainage, pancreatic endotherapy has become the preferred initial management for symptomatic chronic pancreatitis associated with ductal obstruction, as well as other indications. The role of ERCP in chronic pancreatitis is discussed in more detail in Chap. 11 and therefore here will only be discussed superficially. While chronic pancreatitis associated with stones and strictures remains the most common indication for pancreatic endotherapy, other conditions such as recurrent acute pancreatitis (RAP) possibly due to pancreas divisum and the management of duct leaks, disruptions, and peripancreatic fluid collections are also common indications.

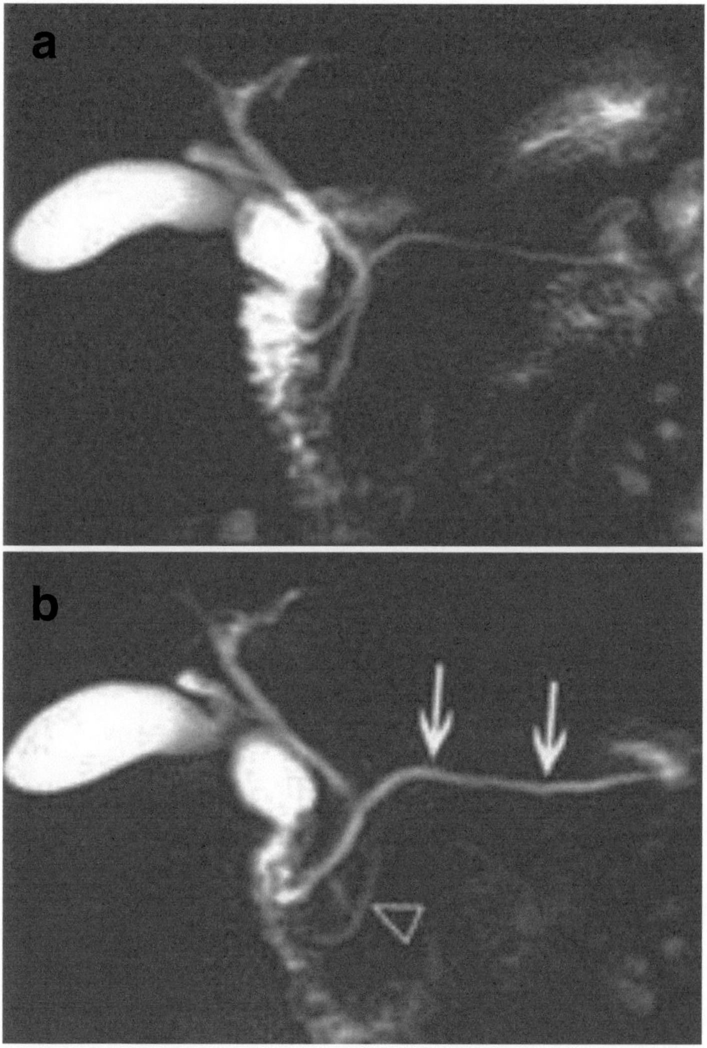

FIGURE 10.2 MRCP of pancreas divisum. MRCP images (**a**, **b**) show the main pancreatic duct (image (**b**), white arrows) crossing the common bile duct (image (**b**), black arrow head) and draining via the minor papilla. (Image courtesy of Raj Paspulati, MD, Department of Radiology, University Hospitals Cleveland Medical Center, Cleveland, Ohio, USA)

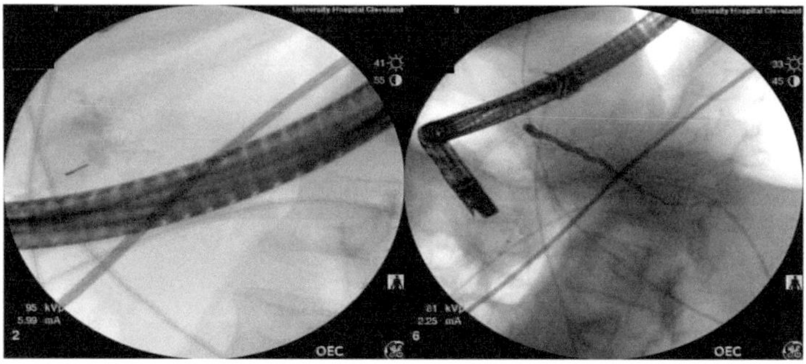

FIGURE 10.3 Fluoroscopic pancreatogram findings in a patient with complete pancreas divisum: (**a**) Acinarization of a ventral pancreatic duct (VPD) via the major papilla, (**b**) complete opacification of the main pancreatic duct via the minor papilla. A stent was placed in the acinarized VPD (arrow) via the major papilla

Other less common indications which have been reported include therapy for santoriniceles, resection of adenomatous polyps around the minor papilla, and transpapillary drainage of a dorsal duct intraductal papillary mucinous neoplasm (IPMN). While the majority of pancreatic endotherapy is performed by cannulation of the ventral PD at the major papilla, there are certain instances where cannulation of the minor papilla is required.

Indications and Planning for Minor Papilla Cannulation

Cannulation of the PD via the minor papilla is performed most commonly in two circumstances: the first is to aid in endotherapy in the setting of pancreas divisum, and the second is when the main PD cannot be accessed due to a failed cannulation or when deep-wire access and cannulation via the ventral PD is not achievable. The latter scenario most commonly occurs in the setting of ductal stones or strictures in the ventral PD. Sometimes, ventral PD distortion, such as an ansa loop, can prevent advancement of the guidewire beyond the head of the pancreas when cannulated through the major papilla. In such cases, cannulation of the accessory PD via the minor papilla may facilitate deep advancement of the guidewire and delivery of successful endotherapy.

Successful endoscopic retrograde pancreatography (ERP) through the minor papilla necessitates a patent accessory duct that communicates with the main PD upstream. Accessory duct patency estimates have ranged from 12% to 82%, depending on the method used (e.g., CT scan, MRCP, autopsy series) [1]. Therefore, knowledge of the PD anatomy, ahead of the planned ERP, by magnetic resonance cholangiopancreatography (MRCP) or endoscopic ultrasound (EUS) is extremely helpful before undertaking this technically challenging procedure. Having a good understanding of the underlying ductal anatomy before attempting endotherapy via the minor papilla may result in an increase in technical success while mitigating the risk of adverse events.

Identification and Duodenoscope Position

The minor papilla is typically located on the medial wall of the descending duodenum, at the 1 o'clock position, proximal to the major papilla. Because of its location, just beyond the superior duodenal angle, it is typically best viewed with the duodenoscope in the "long" position (i.e., with a loop in the greater curvature of the stomach). In contrast to the major papilla, viewing the minor papilla in the "short" position (i.e., after reduction of the loop in the greater curvature) often results in duodenoscope positional instability. Because of the difficult nature of minor papilla cannulation, duodenoscope stability is paramount, and we prefer to attempt minor papilla cannulation with the duodenoscope in the long position. As viewed endoscopically, the minor papilla can vary widely in its appearance. While it is often rather obvious, it can also be subtle and very difficult to locate (Fig. 10.4). In the event of a subtle minor papilla which is difficult to visualize, several adjunctive techniques have been described to aid in its detection. Intravenous (IV) secretin has been studied in a small

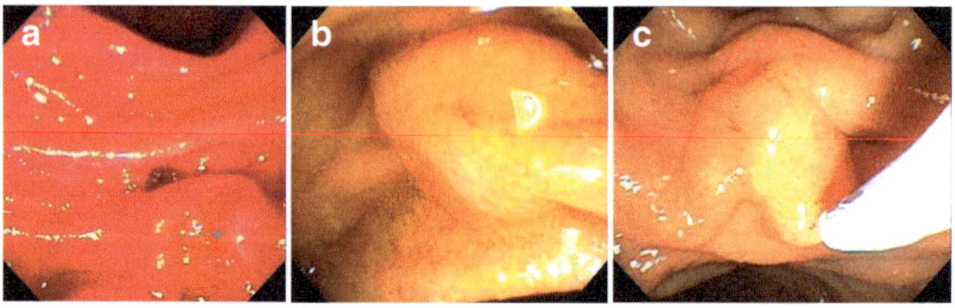

FIGURE 10.4 Varying appearances of minor papillae. (**a**) Small white flat spot (blue arrow), (**b**) moderately sized, protuberant, (**c**) larger minor papilla with visible intraduodenal ductal segment

randomized controlled trial in patients with a prior failed minor papilla cannulation. The use of IV secretin resulted in an improvement in minor papilla cannulation from 7.7% in the placebo group to 81.3% in the secretin group [2]. Dyes used in chromoendoscopy such as methylene blue and indigo carmine, with and without the concomitant use of IV secretin, have also been used to spray over the region of the minor papilla to help in its identification. Endoscopic ultrasound-guided injection of methylene blue into the dorsal PD has also been described [3]. With the current widespread shortage of indigo carmine and the expense of IV secretin, we prefer to spray a dilute methylene blue solution (1–2 mLs with 8–9 mLs of saline) in cases where the minor papilla is difficult to locate. This typically results in the minor papilla having a whitish appearance against a blue mucosal background (Fig. 10.5).

Cannulation Devices and Guidewires

Once the minor papilla is identified, preparations are made for cannulation. Due to the smaller size of the papillary orifice, techniques often differ when compared to cannulating the ventral PD or bile duct at the major papilla. Most standard sphincterotomes used for biliary cannulation have a distal tip outer diameter (OD) ranging from 4 to 5 Fr. The size

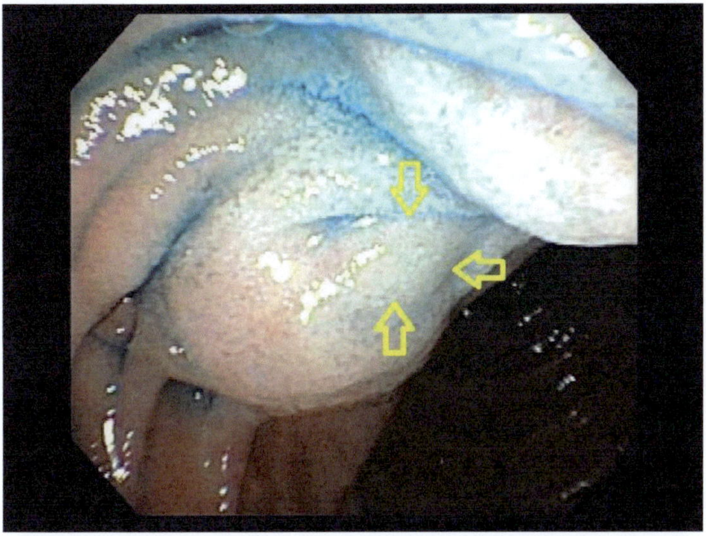

FIGURE 10.5 Use of methylene blue sprayed over duodenal mucosa in region of minor papilla to help identify orifice (arrows)

of these cannulating devices however may be too large when attempting to cannulate the minor papilla. Therefore, in planned minor papilla cannulation, it may be preferable to utilize a cannula or sphincterotome with a smaller OD ranging from 3 to 4 Fr. Older generation ERCP cannulas with small tapered tips are typically single-lumen devices meaning that the guidewire must be removed in order to inject contrast through the device. Several newer double-lumen models now exist (Tables 10.1a, 10.1b and 10.1c). Additionally, several sphincterotomes with smaller tapered distal tips are available for use. The distal OD of these tapered sphincterotomes is typically around 4 Fr, and they come with the advantages of having multiple lumen capabilities (i.e., allowing simultaneous wire access as well as contrast injection) and a sphincterotomy cutting wire.

As with cannulating devices, minor papilla cannulation also commonly requires the use of smaller diameter guidewires. Guidewires with diameters of 0.018, 0.020, 0.021, and 0.025

Table 10.1a Sphincterotomes

Company model	Distal tip outer diameter (F)	Cut wire length (mm)	Compatible guidewire	Working length (cm)	Comments
Boston Scientific					
Dreamtome	4.4, 4.9	20, 30	0.035		Preloaded with guidewire
Hydratome	4.4, 4.9	20, 30	0.035		Preloaded with guidewire
Jagtome	3.9, 4.4, 4.9	20, 30	0.025, 0.035		Preloaded with guidewire
Autotome	3.9, 4.4, 4.9	20, 30	0.025, 0.035		
TRUEtome	3.9, 4.4, 4.9	20, 30	0.025, 0.035		Over-the-wire guidewire
Ultratome	5.5	20, 30	0.035		Short nose tip
Ultratome XL	5.5	20, 30	0.035	200	Short nose tip20 mm tip length available

Stonetome	5.5	20, 30	0.035	200	With balloon (11.5 mm) above or below the cut wire
Needle Knife	5.5		0.035		Needle-knife tip
Microknife XL	5.5, 7.0		0.035	200	Needle-knife tip
Cook Medical					
Cannulotome	5.0	20, 25, 30	0.035	200	
DASH	5.5, 6.0, 6.5		0.021, 0.025, 0.035	196	Preloaded with guidewire
Fusion OMNI	5.5, 7.0		0.021, 0.035	200	Preloaded with guidewire
Minitome	4.0		0.021	200	
Ultrataper	4.0		0.021	200	
Tritome	5.0	20, 25, 30	0.035	200	
Fusion Needle Knife			0.035	200, 320	Needle-knife tip
Billroth II	5.0			200	

(continued)

Table 10.1a (continued)

Company model	Distal tip outer diameter (F)	Cut wire length (mm)	Compatible guidewire	Working length (cm)	Comments
Fusion IDE-Tome			0.035	200	
Conmed					
Trupass	4.3	20, 30	0.035	190	Short nose tip
Apollo 3AC	4.5	20, 30	0.035		5 mm tip length
Apollo 3	5	20, 30	0.035		8, 20 mm tip length
Olympus					
CleverCut	3.9, 4.4	20, 25, 30	0.025, 0.035	195	CleverCut® coating Preloaded with guidewire 2 or 3 lumen modelsVariable tip length – 3, 7, 15, 30 mm

TABLE 10.1B ERCP Cannulas

Company model	Distal tip outer diameter (F)	Shape of distal tip	Working length (cm)	Compatible guidewire	Comments
Boston Scientific					
ERCP cannula		Standard, tapered, ball tip	210	0.035	Straight tip
Tandem XL	5.5	Tapered	200	0.035	Straight tip
Contour	5.0	Standard, tapered, ultratapered, 5-4-3, ball tip	210	0.018, 0.025, 0.035	Angled tip
Flouro tip	5.0	Standard, tapered, ultratapered	210	0.025, 0.035	Angled tip
Cook Medical					
ERCP	3.5, 5.5	Standard, taper	200	0.021, 0.035	
Fusion	6.0, 7.0	DomeTip	200	0.035	
Glo-Tip	3.0, 3.5, 4.0, 4.5, 5.5	Standard, angled, tapered, ultratapered	200, 320	0.018, 0.021, 0.035	

(continued)

TABLE 10.1B (continued)

Company model	Distal tip outer diameter (F)	Shape of distal tip	Working length (cm)	Compatible guidewire	Comments
Haber RAMP	6.0	tapered	200	0.035	Accepts 3 guidewires
Huibregtse-Katon	5.5	Ball tip	200		
Cramer	5.5	1 mm/23 gauge blunt needle tip	200	N/A	
Conmed					
Conmed ERCP cannula	4.5	Standard	190	0.035	Straight and angled-tip models available
Olympus					
Soft sheath	2.5, 3.0, 3.5, 4.0, 6.0	Standard, tapered, split, ball tip	195	0.025, 0.035	
Stiff sheath	2.5, 3.5, 4.0, 4.5	Standard, tapered, split	195	0.025, 0.035	

Table 10.1c Guidewires

Company model	Maximum outer diameter (inch)	Working length (cm)	Shape of distal tip	Comments
Boston Scientific				
Dreamwire	0.035	260, 450	Straight, angled	Stiff model available
Hydra Jagwire	0.035	260, 450	Straight, angled	Stiff model available
Jagwire	0.025, 0.035, 0.038	260, 450	Straight, angled	Stiff model available;trip tip available
Navipro	0.018, 0.025, 0.035	260	Straight, angled	Stiff model available
Cook Medical				
Acrobat 2	0.025, 0.035	205, 260, 450	Straight, angled	25 mm hydrophilic coating model available
Delta	0.025, 0.035	260	Straight, angled	Full length hydrophilic coating
Fusion LoopTip	0.035	205, 260, 450		
Roadrunner	0.018	260, 480		

(continued)

TABLE 10.1C (continued)

Company model	Maximum outer diameter (inch)	Working length (cm)	Shape of distal tip	Comments
Standard	0.035	480		
Tracer Hybrid	0.035	480	Straight, angled	15 and 25 mm hydrophilic coating models
Tracer Metro	0.021, 0.025, 0.035	260, 480, 600	Straight, angled	
Conmed				
Conmed ERCP guidewire	0.025, 0.035	260, 450	Straight, angled	Stiff model available;torquable angled tip
Olympus				
VisiGlide	0.025, 0.029	270, 450	Straight, angled	

inches are most commonly used when cannulating the minor papilla. It is vital to understand the specifications of the cannulating device being used before selecting the preferred guidewire as several of the smaller tapered cannulas and sphincterotome models will not accommodate wires larger than 0.021 or 0.025 inches (Table 10.1a, 10.1b and 10.1c). Guidewires used in pancreatic endotherapy can have a straight or angled hydrophilic tip. Straight-tip wires may carry an advantage in cannulation because of their reliable trajectory; however angled-tip wires can provide added maneuverability in small diameter and tortuous ducts and can promote alpha loop formation.

Minor Papilla Cannulation Technique

Preparation

For planned minor papilla cannulation, we typically begin with a tapered sphincterotome with a 3.9 Fr distal OD loaded with a straight-tip 0.021 or 0.025 inch hydrophilic wire. However, we have additional accessories ready in the event that cannulation is not successful. These include a 0.018 inch guidewire, a 3 Fr tapered cannula, a needle-knife papillotome, and a 5.5 Fr catheter designed with a 1 mm/23 gauge blunt needle (Cramer cannula, Cook Endoscopy).

Wire-Guided Cannulation

We prefer the wire-guided cannulation (WGC) technique, exposing the wire a few millimeters out of the tip of the sphincterotome. The wire engages the papilla, and with gentle probing, cannulation can be achieved. This technique allows for the wire, the smallest part of the collective armamentarium being used, to engage the small orifice first resulting in less trauma and mucosal edema. Once the wire has entered the dorsal PD, a limited contrast injection often helps delineate the ductal anatomy enough to advance the wire safely upstream toward the body and tail. Doing so will result in a safer navigation, reducing the chance of accidental wire perforation of a PD side branch. Judicious use of contrast in the PD is imperative. Care should be taken to inject as little contrast as possible in order perform the task at hand as over-injection of contrast, even in patients with chronic pancreatitis, increases the risk of post-ERCP pancreatitis. After wire position is secured within the PD, a 3–6 mm minor papillotomy is performed, and the necessary endotherapy is undertaken.

Alternative Techniques if WGC Fails

In the event that cannulation in the above manner is not successful, we often will make further attempts with a 0.018 inch guidewire with either the sphincterotome or a smaller 3 Fr tapered cannula. If this fails, final attempts are made with a 5.5 Fr catheter designed with a 1 mm/23 gauge blunt needle tip to engage the minor papilla and delineate the dorsal PD with contrast. Due to the small gauge of the needle tip, this catheter does not accommodate ERCP guidewires. We make a concerted effort to attempt early freehand papillotomy prior as repeated cannulation attempts can cause significant mucosal trauma and edema to the minor papilla. Mucosal edema may obscure the normal landmarks, thereby potentially making a freehand papillotomy less safe. After freehand papillotomy, WGC is reattempted in the above manner. If cannulation remains unsuccessful, we do not perform endoscopic ultrasound (EUS)-guided intraductal methylene blue injection or rendezvous in the same session as these procedures require a more detailed discussion and informed consent process prior to proceeding.

Minor Papillotomy

Endoscopic minor papillotomy is useful in most circumstances where minor papilla cannulation is indicated. In all cases, minor papillotomy facilitates the advancement of accessories such as extraction balloons and stents, as well as making cannulation during any subsequent ERCP easier. Minor papillotomy can be performed by various methods. The method preferred by most endoscopists uses a pull-type sphincterotome. After deep-wire cannulation is achieved, the sphincterotome is advanced over the wire and into the dorsal PD. With the duodenoscope in the long position, a papillotomy directed toward the 12 o'clock position is performed. The length of papillotomy is tailored toward the size and position of the circular fold of the minor papilla but typically ranges from 3 to 5 mm in size. In the event that the sphincterotome is not able to traverse the minor papilla, one can consider using a tapered catheter dilator and reattempting to advance the sphincterotome thereafter. In the event the sphincterotome is still not able to intubate the papilla, papillotomy with a needle knife can be performed. This can be done over the guidewire or over a small diameter PD stent.

When other cannulation methods have failed, a freehand access minor papillotomy with a needle knife can aid in successful cannulation. With the needle engaging the papillary orifice and the papilla en face, cutting is again directed toward the 12 o'clock position (Fig. 10.6). For access papillotomy, smaller cuts of 2–3 mm are often enough to facilitate successful cannulation while minimizing the risks of adverse events such as duodenal perforation. Regardless of the method chosen, we recommend placing a PD stent after minor papillotomy to reduce the incidence of post-ERCP pancreatitis and papillary restenosis.

With regard to generator settings, we do not utilize a pure-cut mode so as to avoid an uncontrolled zipper cut at the smaller minor papilla. Whether using a sphincterotome, or a needle knife, we utilize the same generator settings for minor papillotomy. When using an ERBE generator (ICC200, VIO 200S or 300D, ERBE USA, Marietta, GA), we perform minor papillotomy with the following settings: ENDO CUT I, Effect 2, cutting duration 3, and cutting interval 3. We also utilize Olympus generators (ESG 100, Olympus of America, Inc. Center Valley, PA) and in these circumstances use the pulse cut mode at 120 W.

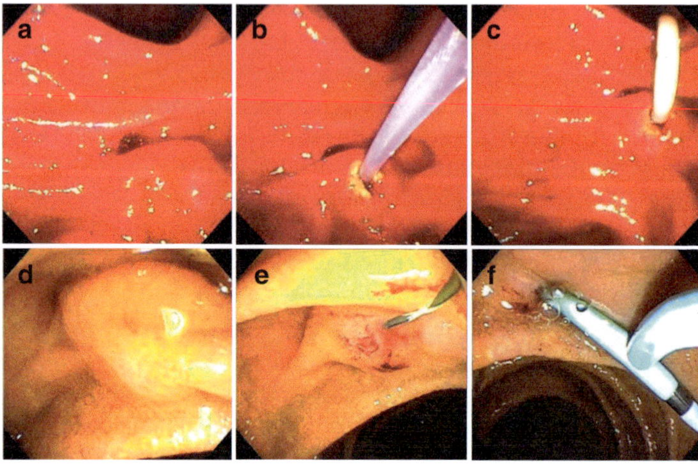

FIGURE 10.6 Minor papilla cannulation and papillotomy techniques: The top row demonstrates a small minor papilla (**a**) is accessed using a freehand needle-knife papillotomy technique (**b**), and a pancreatic duct stent is placed (**c**). The bottom row demonstrates a more obvious minor papilla (**a**) accessed atraumatically via wire-guided cannulation (**b**). After papillotomy with a standard traction sphincterotome, a pancreatic duct stent is placed (**f**)

At the completion of the procedure, if a minor transpapillary stent was not otherwise placed for therapeutic purposes, we place a short 3–5 Fr PD stent and obtain an abdominal X-ray in 4 weeks to assess for spontaneous migration. Stents that have not migrated are removed endoscopically if no further intervention is planned within the PD.

Endotherapies Through the Minor Papilla

Chronic Pancreatitis

The endoscopic therapy of chronic pancreatitis is discussed in detail elsewhere in Chap. 12. Published literature suggests that skilled endoscopists are able to perform all endoscopic therapeutic interventions through the minor papilla that have traditionally been performed via the major papilla [4–6]. These interventions include minor papillotomy, accessory or main PD stricture dilation, PD stent placement and PD stone extraction, mechanical lithotripsy and less commonly, and pancreatoscopy with or without electrohydraulic lithotripsy. PD stone clearance takes a median of two to three ERPs per patient, and the success rate ranges from 74% to 91% [4, 8, 9]. Extracorporeal shock wave lithotripsy (ESWL) is commonly applied beforehand to break larger stones into smaller fragments. Successful PD stricture resolution with balloon dilation followed by sequential stent upsizing ranges from 52% to 91% and also requires multiple procedures [4, 5, 8, 9]. In patients with chronic pancreatitis and ventral PD obstruction, minor papilla endotherapy has been associated with a reduction in pain by >50% ranging from 58 to 96% (average around 75%) and a reduction in narcotic medication requirement by >50% around 43% [4, 5, 9].

Symptomatic Pancreas Divisum

Pancreas divisum is the most common congenital anomaly of the pancreatic ductal system occurring with a prevalence of roughly 7%. The vast majority of people with pancreas divisum remain asymptomatic during their lifetime. A small subset of patients, however, develop complications including RAP, chronic pancreatitis, chronic abdominal pain, and cystic dilation of the dorsal PD, known as a santorinicele. The efficacy of endotherapy for symptomatic pancreas divisum varies based on clinical manifestation. Reported clinical outcomes include resolution of improvement in the number of RAP episodes (62–81%) [7], improvement in patient-reported pain (31–90%) [7], and a decrease in emergency room visits and hospital admissions (43–89%) [7]. Minor papilla endotherapy appears to be more successful in the subpopulation of patients with RAP (77%) compared to patients with chronic pancreatitis (52%) or "pancreatitis-type pain" (47%) [7].

Moreover, the therapeutic effect of endotherapy tends to fade with longer periods of follow-up. These results have also been shown in a recently published systematic review evaluating 22 studies [10]. Subsequent pancreatic surgery, for minor papilla endotherapy failure, or persistent symptom control, has been reported to be necessary in 22.5–46% [4, 7].

Adverse Events

Reported short-term adverse event rates vary widely in the literature from 0% to 26%, depending on the technique used to cannulate the minor papilla and the population of the study [5, 7]. Post-ERCP pancreatitis is the most common reported adverse event with a pooled incidence of 10% [7]. This higher than usual pancreatitis rate should be interpreted with caution, as minor papilla endotherapy is performed on medically complex and sick patients who already commonly have recurrent acute or chronic pancreatitis and are often opioid dependent. To further emphasize the point, 7–21% of patients report worsening abdominal pain and an increase in narcotic use even after technically successful endotherapy [4, 5]. Increasing number of cannulation attempts is associated with a higher risk of post-ERCP pancreatitis [5]. Post-papillotomy bleeding and infections have been reported in 1–4% patients [4–6]. Procedure-related perforations and deaths are rare.

Pearls and Pitfalls

- Minor papilla cannulation is useful in select cases including pancreas divisum or obstruction of the ventral PD at the major papilla.
- The minor papilla is located at the 1 o'clock position proximally in relation to the major papilla and is best viewed and accessed with the duodenoscope in the "long" position. Adjunctive measures such as methy-

lene blue spray can aid in the detection of a subtle minor papilla.
- Smaller access devices and wires are often needed for successful minor papilla cannulation.
- Whether performed by freehand needle knife, or with a sphincterotome, minor papillotomy necessitates the subsequent placement of a PD stent at the conclusion of the procedure.
- The main adverse event associated with minor papilla cannulation is post-ERCP pancreatitis, which may occur at a slightly higher rate when compared to ventral PD cannulation at the major papilla. The other adverse event profiles are similar when compared to ventral PD cannulation at the major papilla.

References

1. Gabbrielli A, Pandolfi M, Mutignani M, et al. Efficacy of main pancreatic duct endoscopic drainage in patients with chronic pancreatitis, continuous pain, and dilated duct. Gastrointest Endosc. 2005;61:576–81.
2. Devereaux BM, Fein S, Purich E, et al. A new synthetic porcine secretin for facilitation of cannulation of the dorsal pancreatic duct at ERCP in patients with pancreas divisum: a multicenter, randomized, double-blind comparative study. Gastrointest Endosc. 2003;57(6):643–7.
3. Dewitt J, Mchenry L, Fogel E, et al. EUS-guided methylene blue pancreatography for minor papilla localization after unsuccessful ERCP. Gastrointest Endosc. 2004;59(1):133–6.
4. Brown NG, Howell DA, Brauer BC, et al. Minor papilla endotherapy in patients with ventral duct obstruction: identification and management. Gastrointest Endosc. 2017;85(2):365–70.
5. Wang W, Gong B, Jiang WS, et al. Endoscopic treatment for pancreatic diseases: needle-knife-guided cannulation via the minor papilla. World J Gastroenterol. 2015;21(19):5950–60.
6. Fujimori N, Igarashi H, Asou A, et al. Endoscopic approach through the minor papilla for the management of pancreatic diseases. World J Gastrointest Endosc. 2013;5(3):81–8.

7. Michailidis L, Aslam B, Grigorian A, et al. The efficacy of endoscopic therapy for pancreas divisum: a meta-analysis. Ann Gastroenterol. 2017;30(5):550–8.
8. Song MH, Kim MH, Lee SK, et al. Endoscopic minor papilla interventions in patients without pancreas divisum. Gastrointest Endosc. 2004;59(7):901–5.
9. Brauer BC, Chen YK, Ringold DA, et al. Peroral pancreatoscopy via the minor papilla for diagnosis and therapy of pancreatic diseases. Gastrointest Endosc. 2013;78(3):545–9.
10. Kanth R, Samji NS, Inaganti A, et al. Endotherapy in symptomatic pancreas divisum: a systematic review. Pancreatology. 2014;14(4):244–50.
11. Luther J, Casey BW. Pancreas divisum and minor papilla interventions. In: Adler D, editor. Advanced pancreaticobiliary endoscopy. Cham: Springer; 2016.

Chapter 11
ERCP in Chronic Pancreatitis

Antonio R. Cheesman and Christopher J. DiMaio

Case Presentation

A 65-year-old male with alcohol- and tobacco-related chronic calcific pancreatitis with recurrent acute on chronic pancreatitis flares presented for further evaluation and management of abdominal pain. Initial magnetic resonance cholangiopancreatography (MRCP) revealed a severely atrophic pancreas with diffuse main pancreatic duct (MPD) dilatation up to 11 mm; multiple intraductal stones, including a 17 mm one at the head of pancreas (HOP); and scattered parenchymal calcifications (Figs. 11.1 and 11.2).

Given these findings and the presence of pancreatic-type pain, the decision was made to attempt MPD decompression by ERCP. The first ERCP proved technically challenging requiring multiple combinations of accessories for MPD access, ultimately revealing a severe 3-cm-long MPD stricture at the HOP with upstream dilation and multiple proximal filling defects (6–15 mm). The stricture was dilated, and a single 5 Fr pigtail plastic stent was placed (Fig. 11.3).

A. R. Cheesman · C. J. DiMaio (✉)
Division of Gastroenterology, Icahn School of Medicine at Mount Sinai, New York, NY, USA
e-mail: christopher.dimaio@mountsinai.org

D. K. Mullady (ed.), *Dilemmas in ERCP*,
https://doi.org/10.1007/978-3-030-12741-1_11

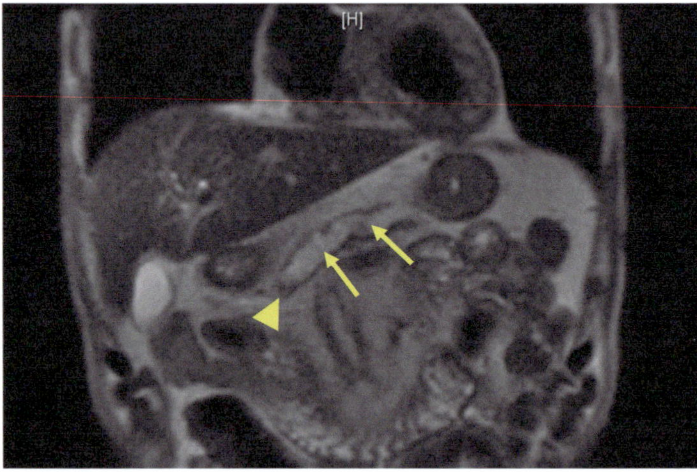

FIGURE 11.1 Coronal MRI/MRCP image demonstrating a markedly dilated main pancreatic duct (arrows) with stricture in the pancreatic duct in the head (arrowhead)

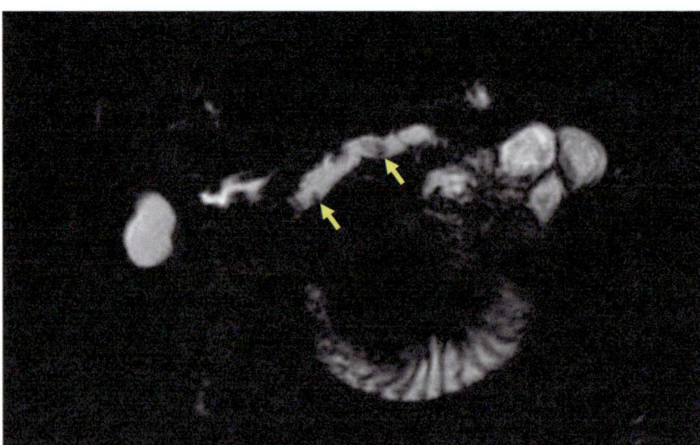

FIGURE 11.2 MRCP image demonstrating dilated main pancreatic duct and scattered intraductal stones (arrows)

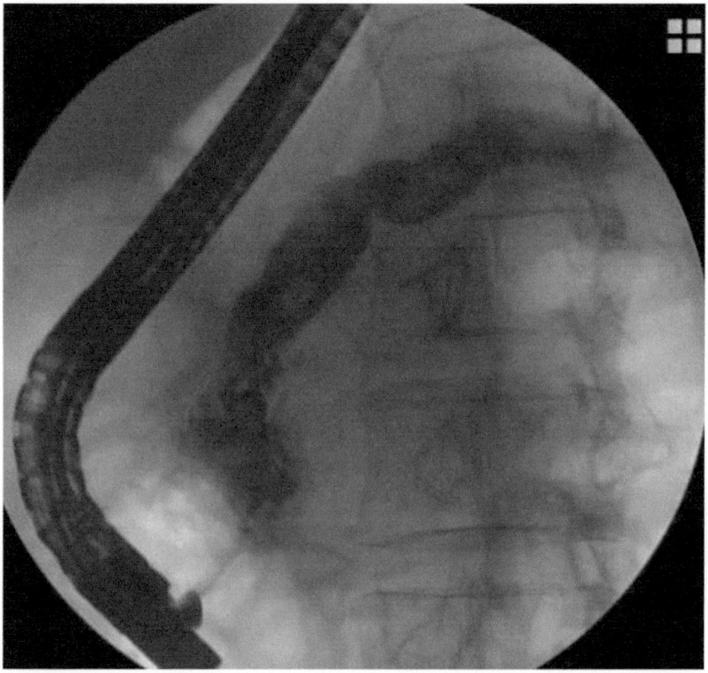

FIGURE 11.3 Pancreatogram demonstrating marked dilation of the pancreatic duct upstream from a severe stricture in the pancreatic head and multiple filling defects consistent with intraductal stones

Repeat ERCP 1 month later was performed. The pancreatic stent was removed and repeat stricture dilation performed; however attempts at stone removal by balloon sweep and basket use were unsuccessful. A new single 7 Fr pigtail plastic stent was placed with limited improvement in pain after 4 weeks. Given high-grade stricture persistence with proximal non-drainable MPD dilation on pancreatography and multiple filling defects, the decision was made to place an 80 × 60 mm fully covered self-expanding metal stent (FC-SEMS) to the MPD (Fig. 11.4).

The patient progressed well with improved pain control. At a follow-up ERCP session, MPD access was performed

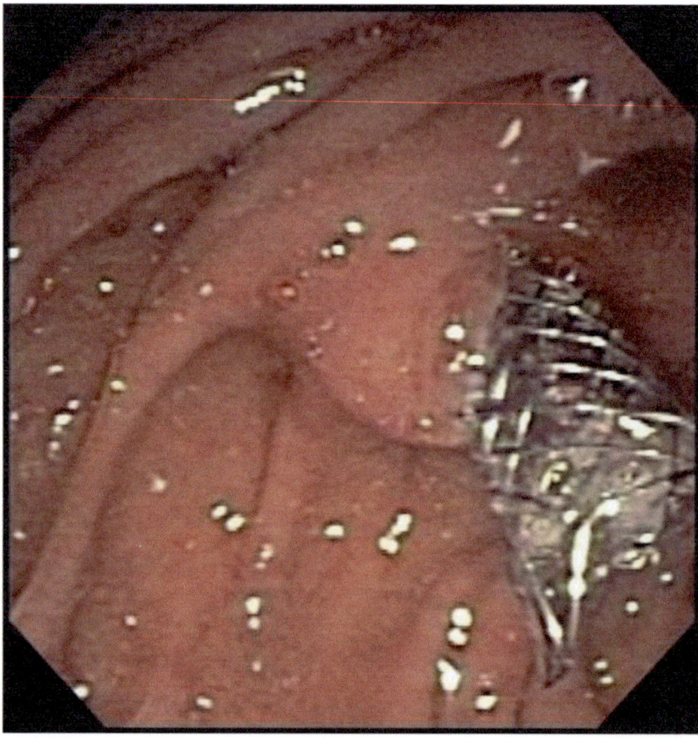

FIGURE 11.4 Intraduodenal portion of fully covered metallic biliary stent which was placed into the main pancreatic duct due to the persistence and severity of the pancreatic duct stricture despite previous dilation and plastic stenting

through the indwelling metal stent with balloon sweeps for direct stone extraction. Pancreatoscopy confirmed no proximal strictures or residual stones, so the stent was removed revealing now a large 20 mm stone impacted at the ventral pancreatic duct. Through-the-scope electrohydraulic lithotripsy (EHL) proved unsuccessful given the location of the stone, just superior to the ampulla, so a new 10 Fr straight plastic stent was placed (Fig. 11.5).

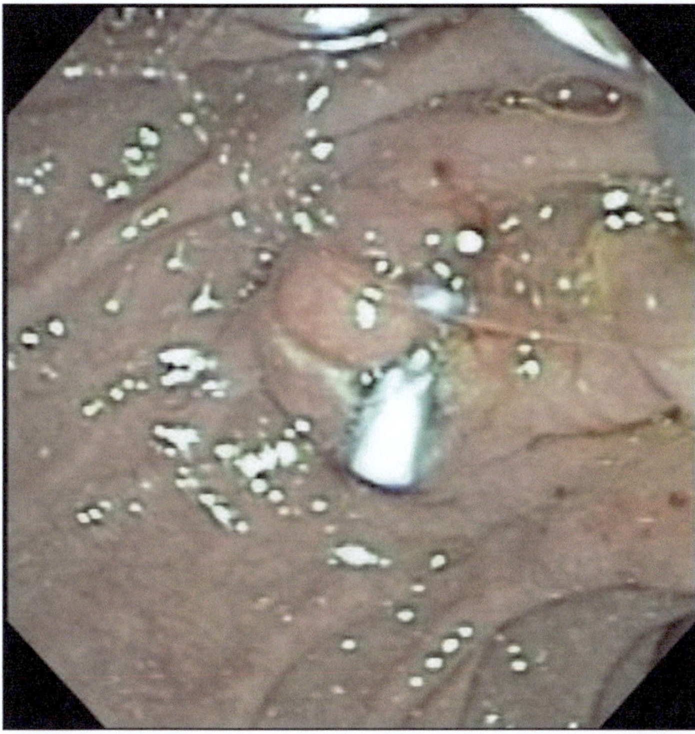

FIGURE 11.5 Following removal of the fully covered metallic stent, the large stone in the pancreatic head could not be fragmented via EHL, so a plastic pancreatic duct stent was placed

Extracorporeal shock wave lithotripsy (ESWL) was then performed successfully. Follow-up ERCP however revealed proximal stent migration into the MPD which failed multiple attempts at removal. Repeat pancreatoscopy showed stent impaction adjacent to a large residual stone (Fig. 11.6). This was successfully treated by EHL, though repeat attempts at stent removal proved unsuccessful. The decision was made to leave the plastic stent in place. The patient continued to prog-

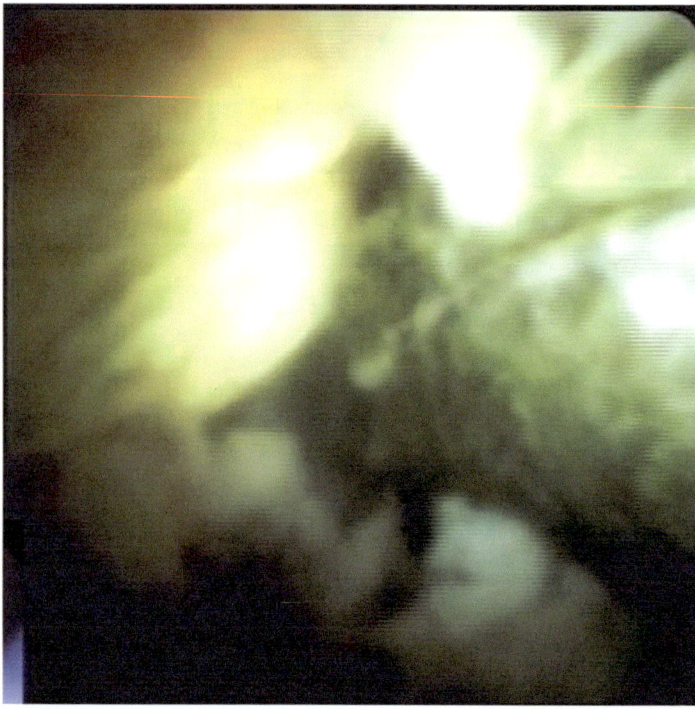

Figure 11.6 At follow-up ERCP following the removal of the fully covered metallic stent and a session of ESWL, the previously placed plastic pancreatic duct stent had migrated proximally into the pancreatic duct with persistence of the large pancreatic duct stone, both seen here on pancreatoscopy

ress well with absence of pain and no further interventions after 3 years of follow-up (Fig. 11.7).

Diagnosis/Assessment

The patient previously described presented with recurrent acute pancreatitis exacerbations superimposed on underlying chronic debilitating pain. As such, evaluation for treatable targets and potential new local complications was warranted.

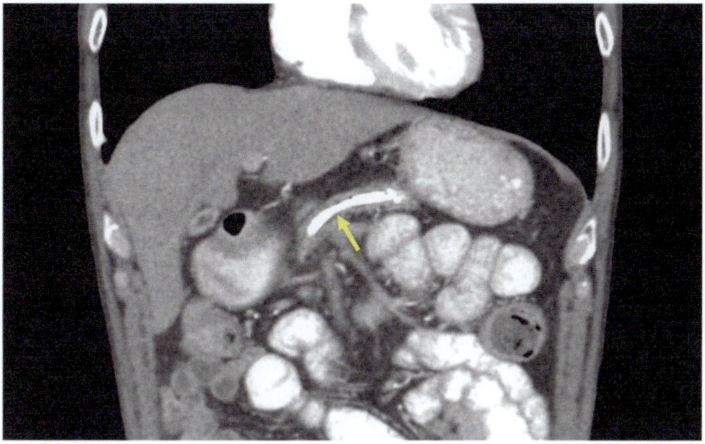

Figure 11.7 Coronal CT image with entirely intraductal pancreatic duct stent (arrow)

The importance of complete alcohol and tobacco abstinence was extensively discussed with the patient, and this cannot be emphasized enough, as its impact on disease progression is very well established. In addition, the response to endoscopic therapy and subsequent decisions in management may be more difficult to assess in the absence of alcohol and tobacco cessation.

Despite careful evaluation of MRCP results prior to therapeutic planning, dilation and stenting were performed across a HOP stricture which ultimately proved to be a large impacted stone at the distal MPD; highlighting that strictures, intraductal stones, and parenchymal calcifications may be difficult to differentiate. There should be a low threshold for EUS evaluation, and one must have appropriate understanding of the patient's CP morphology to select appropriate treatment and be prepared for unexpected findings requiring changes in endoscopic management or referral for surgical evaluation.

Finally, it is crucial to set expectations and review potential complications. As discussed later, a significant proportion of patients do not attain long-term benefit from endoscopic therapy, and selected cases may ultimately require surgery with variable results. Next, we will discuss the existing literature on the assessment of pain, pancreatic stones, and strictures in patients with CP.

Chronic Pancreatitis Pain

Pain is one of the most common and disabling features of CP, presenting in approximately 85% of patients during the disease course [4, 5]. Whether spontaneous resolution of pain occurs ("burnout") is controversial but has been reported in up to 53% of patients after a median of 10 years from diagnosis [6]. Classically two types of pain are described, "Ammann type A," which refers to short-lasting pain episodes separated by long pain-free intervals, and "Ammann type B," which presents with severe continuous non-resolving pain with or without recurrent pain exacerbations, which in turn may represent new local complications of CP.

Pain itself is multifactorial and may result from active inflammation and tissue ischemia, altered nociception (pain threshold, nerve damage, peripheral and central sensitization), local complications (pancreatic duct obstruction, inflammatory masses, pseudocysts, and pancreatic cancer), remote complications (common bile duct obstruction, duodenal obstruction, and small intestinal bacterial overgrowth), and opioid-induced complications (constipation and narcotic bowel syndrome) [4].

When evaluating and managing pain in CP, one must always consider and treat secondary causes of pain. As such, imaging including computed tomography (CT), MRCP, and in selected cases endoscopic ultrasound (EUS) are important to evaluate for strictures, stones, inflammatory masses, and malignancy, which may result in common bile duct (CBD) or MPD obstruction leading to increased intraductal and parenchymal pressure, pancreatic ischemia, and acute inflammation with recurrent acute pancreatitis or chronic pain [2].

Pancreatic Duct Stones

Pancreatic stones result from crystallization and deposition of calcium carbonate due to significant reduction in bicarbonate, citrate, and pancreatic stone protein in the setting of CP. Usually, pancreatic duct stones tend to be hard and sharp; however, occasionally proteins may precipitate forming plugs and stones with softer consistency. MPD strictures reduce flow and lead to stasis, thus facilitating intraductal stone formation [7].

Pancreatic stones can be single or multiple and may be difficult to differentiate from intraparenchymal calcifications on CT particularly when using intravenous (IV) contrast; in addition, as previously noted MPD strictures and stones often coexist. As such, MRCP and/or EUS should always be performed prior to therapeutic attempts. Proximal MPD dilation on MRCP or EUS confirms presence of an obstructive component.

Pancreatic Duct Strictures

Pancreatic strictures can result from acute or chronic pancreatitis, autoimmune pancreatitis, trauma, endoscopic or surgical interventions, and malignancy. Strictures may be single or multiple and are classified as dominant when there is associated ≥6 mm upstream MPD dilatation or contrast outflow obstruction alongside a 6 Fr catheter inserted into the MPD [8]. Refractory strictures are persistent symptomatic dominant strictures despite 1 year of appropriate stent therapy (10 Fr) [9]. In addition, MPD narrowing may result from extrinsic compression by masses or large parenchymal and side-branch stones.

Similar to the evaluation of pancreatic stones, MRCP and/or EUS should be considered. In addition, depending on the level of suspicion, EUS and pancreatoscopy may be required for tissue acquisition to rule out underlying malignancy.

Treatment/Management

The patient previously described presented with multiple challenges for endoscopic management, including difficult MPD access due to a large impacted stone at the HOP initially presumed to be a stricture, and further presence of multiple stones proximally throughout the MPD.

Appropriate identification of the large impacted HOP stone could have led to earlier attempts at ESWL and/or pancreatoscopy-guided intraductal lithotripsy prior to dilation and stenting efforts. While direct balloon-assisted stone extraction failed, and plastic stent placement to the MPD provided limited benefit, placement of a FC-SEMS led to pain relief and facilitated spontaneous passage of upstream MPD stones.

In a recent population-based cohort study of patients with CP and a median follow-up of 10 years, 23% underwent endoscopic therapy, while 11% required surgery [10]. This more closely reflects the general population prevalence, while other studies quoting higher numbers primarily include pancreatic referral centers. For those patients in which invasive procedures are required, however, typically multiple interventions are performed over several years.

Chronic Pancreatitis Pain

In general, nonoperative strategies for managing pain are used before considering more invasive therapies. However, endoscopic therapy, ESWL, and surgery should be considered early in the management of specific structural pathologies, and this should be carefully pursued before patients become opiate dependent [2]. It has been suggested, at least from the surgical literature, that early intervention where the operative indication is pain is associated with improved outcomes including postoperative pain-free status and decreased opiate requirements for patients treated within an optimal cutoff of 26.5 months since CP diagnosis [11].

Endoscopic therapy may restore luminal patency with variable success by removing or bypassing obstructing stones, dilating or stenting strictures, and sealing MPD disruptions. It must be noted however that the amendment of structural abnormalities may not always translate in clinical improvement. Centrally mediated pain and other secondary causes of pain including gastroparesis, small intestinal bacterial overgrowth, and narcotic bowel syndrome can play a role [4].

Pancreatic sphincterotomy is routinely performed in all cases to facilitate therapeutic access to the MPD and stone elimination [12–19]. Biliary sphincterotomy may also be added in selected cases where there is associated cholestasis, CBD obstruction, or cholangitis [8, 20].

As previously mentioned, there is limited to no role for endoscopic management of asymptomatic stones or strictures in CP patients, other than ruling out underlying malignancy in appropriate cases [9]. There is only limited evidence regarding the use of endoscopic therapy in asymptomatic patients to prevent development of exocrine or endocrine pancreatic dysfunction, and a large multicenter study in patients with painful CP in the setting of MPD obstruction due to strictures and/or stones showed no benefit [21].

Pancreatic Duct Stones

Pancreatic stones can be managed by ESWL with or without endoscopic removal, retrograde MPD access and direct removal, or through-the-scope lithotripsy.

Standard endoscopic retrograde pancreatoscopy techniques with sphincterotomy and direct stone removal can be attained by means of extraction balloons, retrieval baskets, and forceps. However in general this is not recommended for stones >5 mm in size, stones impacted proximal to MPD strictures, or those proximal to the pancreatic head given low technical success rates (9–17%) [22, 23] and high risk for complications [8]. In particular there is a risk of basket impaction with the stone behind a stricture.

ESWL achieves successful stone fragmentation in up to 90% of patients [24, 25]. Effective fragmentation has been previously defined as breakdown of stones into fragments of 3 mm or smaller [25, 26]. This in turn leads to spontaneous stone elimination in 70–88% of cases [26, 27]. Similar to outcomes of ERCP-guided stone removal, patients with MPD in the pancreatic head have the best outcomes with ESWL [28]. ESWL alone may provide long-term pain relief in up to 70–96% of patients [26, 27, 29–32]. The use of ESWL however is often limited by local expertise and availability.

In a small randomized controlled trial of ESWL alone vs. ESWL combined with endoscopic removal for management of painful obstructing chronic pancreatitis, there were no differences in post-procedural MPD diameter or pain relapse (ESWL 38% vs. combined therapy 45%) after 2-year follow-up. The cost however was three times higher for those in the combined therapy group [28].

In a large meta-analysis of ESWL with or without adjunct endoscopic stone removal, complete ductal clearance was attained in 70.7%, pain resolution was reported in 52.7%, and pain improvement in another 33.4%, while narcotic use decreased in 79.7% of patients [33].

Based on the available literature, the United European Guidelines recommend ESWL of obstructing stones $\geq$5 mm with immediate endoscopic extraction unless there is considerable local experience with ESWL use for pancreatic stones.

Common contraindications to ESWL include coagulopathy, interposing organ structures, pregnancy, and presence of pacemakers or defibrillators.

Finally, peroral pancreatoscopy with through-the-scope intraductal lithotripsy can be achieved by EHL or laser lithotripsy (LL).

A single center study [23] including 33 patients treated with EHL and 6 patients treated with LL noted complete stone clearance in 70% of patients, with an adverse event rate of 10%. In a multicenter retrospective study [34] of 28 patients with MPD stones who had otherwise failed ERCP (79%), ESWL (32%), and EHL (18%), LL achieved complete ductal clearance in 79% after a median of 1 session, with only mild adverse events reported (29%). A recent review [35] on the topic also noted a tendency for higher stone clearance rates by use of LL compared to EHL. Subsequently, the largest study to date by Brewer Gutierrez et al. [36] on 103 pts. with CP and MPD stones demonstrated higher success rates for LL (100%) vs. EHL (81%), with similar rates of adverse events (8–9%), in patients that had otherwise failed ESWL in 12% and ERCP extraction in 87% of cases.

One of the potential advantages to take into consideration during therapeutic planning is that direct peroral intraductal lithotripsy may provide an opportunity to address concurrent MPD strictures and complete treatment at index ERCP. There is however limited literature on their relative efficacy and safety compared to ESWL, and for the time being the decision to pursue these techniques as opposed to ESWL should be based on local expertise.

The United European Guidelines recommend ESWL of stones ≥5 mm obstructing the MPD with immediate endoscopic extraction unless there is considerable ESWL experience [9].

Pancreatic Duct Strictures

Pancreatic strictures can be managed by dilation and stenting.

Isolated MPD stricture dilation without stenting has a limited role given its short-lasting effect. The typical initial approach is single plastic stent placement; however MPD stricture resolution in this scenario is still only approximately 60% after the initial procedure [8]. Larger diameter plastic stents (10 vs. ≤8.5 Fr) are typically preferred based on studies showing improved outcomes with lower hospitalization rates [37].

Given limited stricture resolution after a single intervention, repeat procedures are usually required. Both scheduled and "on-demand" stent exchanges have been explored. On-demand exchanges are performed for interval symptom onset which may relate to stent occlusion that aims to reduce the number of ERCP sessions [38].

Studies looking at scheduled stent exchanges at less than 6-month intervals have shown worse outcomes [39]. On the other hand, a large study of repeated "on-demand" single plastic stent placement with or without ESWL, (median overall stent dwell time of 23 months) showed 62% of patients achieved adequate pain control without need for re-intervention during a median follow-up time of 27 months. For those who relapsed, 80% of cases occurred during the first year after stent removal [17].

The expert recommendation is for scheduled stent exchanges – these are typically performed every 6–12 months – with additional on-demand interventions as needed [8, 9]. Stent removal without replacement can be considered if there is adequate contrast outflow after upstream ductal filling and easy passage of a 6 Fr catheter beyond the stricture [8, 9].

Multiple simultaneous plastic stents may also be employed; this is typically reserved for refractory strictures. In a study of patients that failed single plastic stent placement, resolution was achieved in 84% of cases without additional complications after a median follow-up of 38 months (maximal stents allowed by stricture, median 3, individual size 8.5–11.5 Fr) [40].

Uncovered self-expanding metal stents (UC-SEMS) should not be used. There is limited data for the use of FC-SEMS. Prior reports noted high migration (40%) and stricture recurrence rates [41, 42]. More recently, a small study looking at outcomes of 6 mm diameter FC-SEMS used in benign CP-related MPD strictures, on plastic stent refractory patients, showed pain and radiological improvement in over 80% of cases, with a median post-stent removal follow-up of 47.3 months, after a median stent dwell time of 7.5 months during which there were no migration events [43].

Adverse events from MPD stent placement include acute pancreatitis, duct injury or long-term stent-related duct changes, stent migration and occlusion, bleeding, and infections with abscess formation.

The United European Guidelines recommend the use of single 10 Fr plastic stents with scheduled exchanges – these are typically performed every 6–12 months – with additional on-demand interventions as needed and consideration of multiple simultaneous plastic stents vs. a 3–6-month trial of FC-SEMS for refractory strictures. Surgical drainage procedures should also be considered for refractory and multifocal strictures [9].

Difficult MPD access may result from impassable stones and/or strictures in the proximal MPD or presence of an altered postsurgical anatomy, in which case the trans-papillary approach may not be feasible. In this scenario EUS-guided MPD access can be pursued. Large performance studies on ERCP have shown canalization failure rates of up to 10% [44, 45], while this may be higher in those with CP for the reasons pointed out before.

Indications for EUS-guided MPD access include inaccessible major and minor papilla or pancreaticoenterostomy site by ERCP in patients with ductal disruption/fistula or symptomatic MPD obstruction with associated dilation [46, 47].

Contraindications include non-dilated MPD, multifocal MPD strictures, long distance from gastrointestinal (GI) tract wall or intervening organs/vessel through puncture route, thrombocytopenia, and coagulopathy [46, 47].

EUS-guided MPD access may be achieved by antegrade, with or without rendezvous technique, or by a retrograde approach. In the trans-enteric antegrade technique without rendezvous, MPD stenting is conducted by transluminal stent placement through the GI tract (typically the stomach or duodenum) into the MPD toward and across the papilla, while in the rendezvous variant, a guidewire is advanced in antegrade fashion across the papilla or anastomotic site, followed by retrograde stent insertion into the MPD. The other less commonly used retrograde stenting approach involves transluminal stenting through the GI tract toward the pancreatic tail. In general, the rendezvous approach should be favored whenever the papilla is accessible.

The combined technical success rate on small retrospective series of various forms of EUS-guided MPD access is

79% [47], while a recent large multicenter study of EUS-guided pancreatic duct drainage in 80 patients showed it to be as high as 89% [48]. The overall adverse event rate is 18–21% according to various reports [47, 49]. Most common complications include acute pancreatitis, MPD disruption and leakage, hematomas, bleeding, pancreatic abscess formation, and GI perforation.

Outcomes are closely related to technical expertise; EUS-guided MPD access is technically demanding and should be performed by endoscopists adequately trained in this procedure. The general recommendation is for EUS-guided rendezvous approach to MPD access after failed ERCP whenever the papilla is accessible to endoscopic examination.

Outcomes

The patient previously described progressed well on the long-term follow-up with adequate pain control and no need for further interventions after successful HOP stone fragmentation by consecutive therapy with ESWL and EHL. The plastic stent however was left in place at the MPD after multiple failed attempts at removal in the setting of proximal migration. The relative contribution of the indwelling plastic stent to the patient's indolent clinical course however is difficult to interpret and may be related to "pancreatic burn out." Finally, it must be noted that consideration for surgical MPD drainage would have also been a reasonable option if the patient had remained considerably symptomatic.

Critical appraisal of the outcomes of endoscopic therapy is reviewed, with brief discussion on the indications and comparative outcomes of surgical management in CP.

A large multicenter study [21] with over 1000 patients on endoscopic therapy for painful CP with MPD obstruction due to strictures (47%), stones (18%), or their combination (32%) revealed long-term clinical success rates, defined as improvement or resolution of pain, to be as low as 65% after a median of 4 ERCP sessions with pancreatic sphincterotomy, stenting, and use of ESWL at the endoscopist's discretion. This was driven largely by adjustments after intention to treat analysis due to the large number of patients requiring surgery (24%) during the mean 4.9 years of follow-up time. There were however no significant differences in outcomes based on index presentation (strictures, stones, or their combination).

Another large meta-analysis [3], including 11 studies and over 1500 patients, on the efficacy of endoscopic therapy for the treatment of painful CP using a similar approach revealed immediate pain relief in up to 88% of patients, but this was reduced to only 67% after the first month and decreased further during a mean of 47 months of follow-up. The adverse event rate was 7.8% after each individual endoscopic intervention. Stents (4–11.5 Fr) were selected according to MPD stricture characteristics, and both on-demand and fixed stent exchange schedules were used at the endoscopist's discretion.

While endotherapy is a viable first-line therapeutic modality for painful obstructing CP, an individualized treatment plan should be developed after detailed pancreatic ductal anatomy evaluation, and early surgical consultation should be sought in cases of complex morphology with pancreatic ductal pathology in the body or tail, multifocal strictures or stones, refractory strictures, and inflammatory masses.

Studies looking at early vs. delayed multimodality surgical intervention for painful CP, where the operative indication was exclusively pain, have shown an optimal cutoff of 26.5 months since the diagnosis of CP for long-term pain control and opioid independence [11].

Otherwise, two small studies comparing endoscopic therapy vs. multimodality surgical intervention for painful obstructive CP have demonstrated superior pain control outcomes on long-term follow-up after surgery (37 vs. 14% and 75 vs. 32%) [50, 51], leading to a Cochrane Review favoring surgical management where applicable [52]. It must be noted however that the endoscopic techniques used in the two studies included may not reflect the current standard of care.

The United European Guidelines recommend that surgical evaluation be considered for the management of inflammatory masses, multifocal strictures and/or stones affecting the pancreatic body or tail, or refractory strictures. However endoscopic therapy may still be attempted initially, with referral for surgical consideration if there is no clinical response after 6–8 weeks [9].

Table 11.1 Endoscopic therapies for chronic pancreatitis

Pancreatic sphincterotomy
Pancreatic duct stone extraction
Direct endoscopic extraction with or without extracorporeal shock wave lithotripsy
Intraductal electrohydraulic or laser lithotripsy
Pancreatic duct stricture dilation and stenting
Pancreatic duct leak stenting
Biliary sphincterotomy
Common bile duct stricture dilation and stenting
Drainage of pancreatic pseudocysts

Pearls and Pitfalls

- When considering endoscopic therapy in patient with chronic pancreatitis (Table 11.1), patient selection is key to successful clinical outcomes. The main indication to pursue ERCP and endoscopic decompression is for the relief of chronic pancreatitis-associated pain or recurrent acute pancreatitis attributed to pancreatic duct obstruction.
- Endocrine insufficiency, exocrine insufficiency, and weight loss are not strong indications to pursue pancreatic decompression as a significant clinical response is not expected to occur in the majority of cases.

- Chronic pancreatitis patients suffering from pain but without evidence of pancreatic duct stone, stricture, or dilation should not be offered endoscopic decompression.
- Patients with obstructing disease (stones and/or strictures) localized to the head/neck/proximal body and those in whom intervention is initiated during early course of pain onset tend to have the best response to endoscopic decompression.
- Tobacco and alcohol cessation should be strongly emphasized to all patients with chronic pancreatitis, as cessation may lead to significant relief of pain, and continued use will result in accelerated disease progression and may reduce the therapeutic response to endoscopic interventions.
- The process of pain development and progression in chronic pancreatitis is complex, typically starting at the local level (i.e., pancreatic inflammation, obstruction, ischemia) and evolving to a more centrally mediated process as the disease course progresses. As such, the inclusion of pain management specialists should be sought out sooner rather than later.
- In patients who are not responsive to therapeutic endoscopy, alternative sources of discomfort should be sought out, including chronic pancreatitis-associated biliary obstruction, luminal obstruction, pancreatic duct disruption/leak, pancreatic exocrine insufficiency, GI dysmotility, small bowel bacterial overgrowth, and occult malignancy.
- Surgical intervention should not be considered a failure on the part of the endoscopist. Surgery has a major role in the management of chronic pancreatitis, and data suggests that it may be the more preferable approach in select patients.
- Patients with chronic pancreatitis are at increased risk for the development of pancreatic adenocarcinoma. Thus, any significant change in pain pattern, weight loss, or clinical course should prompt an evaluation for pancreatic cancer.

References

1. Tillou JD, Tatum JA, Jolissaint JS, Strand DS, Wang AY, Zaydfudim V, et al. Operative management of chronic pancreatitis: a review. Am J Surg. 2017;214(2):347–57.
2. Kleeff J, Whitcomb DC, Shimosegawa T, Esposito I, Lerch MM, Gress T, et al. Chronic pancreatitis. Nat Rev Dis Primers. 2017;3:17060.
3. Jafri M, Sachdev A, Sadiq J, Lee D, Taur T, Goodman A, et al. Efficacy of endotherapy in the treatment of pain associated with chronic pancreatitis: a systematic review and meta-analysis. JOP. 2017;18(2):125–32.
4. Drewes AM, Bouwense SAW, Campbell CM, Ceyhan GO, Delhaye M, Demir IE, et al. Guidelines for the understanding and management of pain in chronic pancreatitis. Pancreatology. 2017;17(5):720–31.
5. Gachago C, Draganov PV. Pain management in chronic pancreatitis. World J Gastroenterol. 2008;14(20):3137–48.
6. Lankisch PG. Natural course of chronic pancreatitis. Pancreatology. 2001;1(1):3–14.
7. Tandan M, Talukdar R, Reddy DN. Management of pancreatic calculi: an update. Gut Liver. 2016;10(6):873–80.
8. Dumonceau JM, Delhaye M, Tringali A, Dominguez-Munoz JE, Poley JW, Arvanitaki M, et al. Endoscopic treatment of chronic pancreatitis: European Society of Gastrointestinal Endoscopy (ESGE) Clinical Guideline. Endoscopy. 2012;44(8):784–800.
9. Löhr JM, Dominguez-Munoz E, Rosendahl J, Besselink M, Mayerle J, Lerch MM, et al. United European Gastroenterology evidence-based guidelines for the diagnosis and therapy of chronic pancreatitis (HaPanEU). United European Gastroenterol J. 2017;5(2):153–99.
10. Machicado JD, Chari ST, Timmons L, Tang G, Yadav D. A population-based evaluation of the natural history of chronic pancreatitis. Pancreatology. 2018;18(1):39–45.
11. Yang CJ, Bliss LA, Freedman SD, Sheth S, Vollmer CM, Ng SC, et al. Surgery for chronic pancreatitis: the role of early surgery in pain management. Pancreas. 2015;44(5):819–23.
12. Farnbacher MJ, Mühldorfer S, Wehler M, Fischer B, Hahn EG, Schneider HT. Interventional endoscopic therapy in chronic pancreatitis including temporary stenting: a definitive treatment? Scand J Gastroenterol. 2006;41(1):111–7.

13. Cremer M, Devière J, Delhaye M, Baize M, Vandermeeren A. Stenting in severe chronic pancreatitis: results of medium-term follow-up in seventy-six patients. Endoscopy. 1991;23(3):171–6.
14. Ponchon T, Bory RM, Hedelius F, Roubein LD, Paliard P, Napoleon B, et al. Endoscopic stenting for pain relief in chronic pancreatitis: results of a standardized protocol. Gastrointest Endosc. 1995;42(5):452–6.
15. Smits ME, Badiga SM, Rauws EA, Tytgat GN, Huibregtse K. Long-term results of pancreatic stents in chronic pancreatitis. Gastrointest Endosc. 1995;42(5):461–7.
16. Vitale GC, Cothron K, Vitale EA, Rangnekar N, Zavaleta CM, Larson GM, et al. Role of pancreatic duct stenting in the treatment of chronic pancreatitis. Surg Endosc. 2004;18(10):1431–4.
17. Eleftherladis N, Dinu F, Delhaye M, Le Moine O, Baize M, Vandermeeren A, et al. Long-term outcome after pancreatic stenting in severe chronic pancreatitis. Endoscopy. 2005;37(3):223–30.
18. Ishihara T, Yamaguchi T, Seza K, Tadenuma H, Saisho H. Efficacy of s-type stents for the treatment of the main pancreatic duct stricture in patients with chronic pancreatitis. Scand J Gastroenterol. 2006;41(6):744–50.
19. Weber A, Schneider J, Neu B, Meining A, Born P, Schmid RM, et al. Endoscopic stent therapy for patients with chronic pancreatitis: results from a prospective follow-up study. Pancreas. 2007;34(3):287–94.
20. Kim MH, Myung SJ, Kim YS, Kim HJ, Seo DW, Nam SW, et al. Routine biliary sphincterotomy may not be indispensable for endoscopic pancreatic sphincterotomy. Endoscopy. 1998;30(8):697–701.
21. Rösch T, Daniel S, Scholz M, Huibregtse K, Smits M, Schneider T, et al. Endoscopic treatment of chronic pancreatitis: a multicenter study of 1000 patients with long-term follow-up. Endoscopy. 2002;34(10):765–71.
22. Farnbacher MJ, Schoen C, Rabenstein T, Benninger J, Hahn EG, Schneider HT. Pancreatic duct stones in chronic pancreatitis: criteria for treatment intensity and success. Gastrointest Endosc. 2002;56(4):501–6.
23. Attwell AR, Brauer BC, Chen YK, Yen RD, Fukami N, Shah RJ. Endoscopic retrograde cholangiopancreatography with per oral pancreatoscopy for calcific chronic pancreatitis using endoscope and catheter-based pancreatoscopes: a 10-year single-center experience. Pancreas. 2014;43(2):268–74.

24. Nguyen-Tang T, Dumonceau JM. Endoscopic treatment in chronic pancreatitis, timing, duration and type of intervention. Best Pract Res Clin Gastroenterol. 2010;24(3):281–98.
25. Tandan M, Reddy DN, Santosh D, Vinod K, Ramchandani M, Rajesh G, et al. Extracorporeal shock wave lithotripsy and endotherapy for pancreatic calculi-a large single center experience. Indian J Gastroenterol. 2010;29(4):143–8.
26. Ohara H, Hoshino M, Hayakawa T, Kamiya Y, Miyaji M, Takeuchi T, et al. Single application extracorporeal shock wave lithotripsy is the first choice for patients with pancreatic duct stones. Am J Gastroenterol. 1996;91(7):1388–94.
27. Inui K, Tazuma S, Yamaguchi T, Ohara H, Tsuji T, Miyagawa H, et al. Treatment of pancreatic stones with extracorporeal shock wave lithotripsy: results of a multicenter survey. Pancreas. 2005;30(1):26–30.
28. Dumonceau JM, Costamagna G, Tringali A, Vahedi K, Delhaye M, Hittelet A, et al. Treatment for painful calcified chronic pancreatitis: extracorporeal shock wave lithotripsy versus endoscopic treatment: a randomised controlled trial. Gut. 2007;56(4):545–52.
29. Tandan M, Reddy DN, Talukdar R, Vinod K, Santosh D, Lakhtakia S, et al. Long-term clinical outcomes of extracorporeal shockwave lithotripsy in painful chronic calcific pancreatitis. Gastrointest Endosc. 2013;78(5):726–33.
30. Tadenuma H, Ishihara T, Yamaguchi T, Tsuchiya S, Kobayashi A, Nakamura K, et al. Long-term results of extracorporeal shockwave lithotripsy and endoscopic therapy for pancreatic stones. Clin Gastroenterol Hepatol. 2005;3(11):1128–35.
31. Delhaye M, Vandermeeren A, Baize M, Cremer M. Extracorporeal shock-wave lithotripsy of pancreatic calculi. Gastroenterology. 1992;102(2):610–20.
32. Seven G, Schreiner MA, Ross AS, Lin OS, Gluck M, Gan SI, et al. Long-term outcomes associated with pancreatic extracorporeal shock wave lithotripsy for chronic calcific pancreatitis. Gastrointest Endosc. 2012;75(5):997–1004.e1.
33. Moole H, Jaeger A, Bechtold ML, Forcione D, Taneja D, Puli SR. Success of extracorporeal shock wave lithotripsy in chronic calcific pancreatitis management: a meta-analysis and systematic review. Pancreas. 2016;45(5):651–8.
34. Attwell AR, Patel S, Kahaleh M, Raijman IL, Yen R, Shah RJ. ERCP with per-oral pancreatoscopy-guided laser lithotripsy for calcific chronic pancreatitis: a multicenter U.S. experience. Gastrointest Endosc. 2015;82(2):311–8.

35. Beyna T, Neuhaus H, Gerges C. Endoscopic treatment of pancreatic duct stones under direct vision: revolution or resignation? Systematic review. Dig Endosc. 2018;30(1):29–37.
36. Brewer Gutierrez O, Raijman I, Shah R, Elmunzer J, Webster G, Pleskow D, et al. International multicenter study on digital single operator pancreatoscopy for the management of pancreatic stones. DDW Gastrointest Endoscop. 2018:AB68–AB9.
37. Sauer BG, Gurka MJ, Ellen K, Shami VM, Kahaleh M. Effect of pancreatic duct stent diameter on hospitalization in chronic pancreatitis: does size matter? Pancreas. 2009;38(7):728–31.
38. Morgan DE, Smith JK, Hawkins K, Wilcox CM. Endoscopic stent therapy in advanced chronic pancreatitis: relationships between ductal changes, clinical response, and stent patency. Am J Gastroenterol. 2003;98(4):821–6.
39. Delhaye M, Matos C, Devière J. Endoscopic management of chronic pancreatitis. Gastrointest Endosc Clin N Am. 2003;13(4):717–42.
40. Costamagna G, Bulajic M, Tringali A, Pandolfi M, Gabbrielli A, Spada C, et al. Multiple stenting of refractory pancreatic duct strictures in severe chronic pancreatitis: long-term results. Endoscopy. 2006;38(3):254–9.
41. Park DH, Kim MH, Moon SH, Lee SS, Seo DW, Lee SK. Feasibility and safety of placement of a newly designed, fully covered self-expandable metal stent for refractory benign pancreatic ductal strictures: a pilot study (with video). Gastrointest Endosc. 2008;68(6):1182–9.
42. Sauer B, Talreja J, Ellen K, Ku J, Shami VM, Kahaleh M. Temporary placement of a fully covered self-expandable metal stent in the pancreatic duct for management of symptomatic refractory chronic pancreatitis: preliminary data (with videos). Gastrointest Endosc. 2008;68(6):1173–8.
43. Oh D, Lee JH, Song TJ, Park DH, Lee SK, Kim MH, et al. Long-term outcomes of 6-mm diameter fully covered self-expandable metal stents in benign refractory pancreatic ductal stricture. Dig Endosc. 2018;30:508.
44. Ekkelenkamp VE, de Man RA, Ter Borg F, Borg PC, Bruno MJ, Groenen MJ, et al. Prospective evaluation of ERCP performance: results of a nationwide quality registry. Endoscopy. 2015;47(6):503–7.
45. Williams EJ, Ogollah R, Thomas P, Logan RF, Martin D, Wilkinson ML, et al. What predicts failed cannulation and

therapy at ERCP? Results of a large-scale multicenter analysis. Endoscopy. 2012;44(7):674–83.

46. Itoi T, Kasuya K, Sofuni A, Itokawa F, Kurihara T, Yasuda I, et al. Endoscopic ultrasonography-guided pancreatic duct access: techniques and literature review of pancreatography, transmural drainage and rendezvous techniques. Dig Endosc. 2013;25(3):241–52.
47. Rimbaş M, Larghi A. Endoscopic ultrasonography-guided techniques for accessing and draining the biliary system and the pancreatic duct. Gastrointest Endosc Clin N Am. 2017;27(4):681–705.
48. Tyberg A, Sharaiha RZ, Kedia P, Kumta N, Gaidhane M, Artifon E, et al. EUS-guided pancreatic drainage for pancreatic strictures after failed ERCP: a multicenter international collaborative study. Gastrointest Endosc. 2017;85(1):164–9.
49. Fujii-Lau LL, Levy MJ. Endoscopic ultrasound-guided pancreatic duct drainage. J Hepatobiliary Pancreat Sci. 2015;22(1):51–7.
50. Díte P, Ruzicka M, Zboril V, Novotný I. A prospective, randomized trial comparing endoscopic and surgical therapy for chronic pancreatitis. Endoscopy. 2003;35(7):553–8.
51. Cahen DL, Gouma DJ, Nio Y, Rauws EA, Boermeester MA, Busch OR, et al. Endoscopic versus surgical drainage of the pancreatic duct in chronic pancreatitis. N Engl J Med. 2007;356(7):676–84.
52. Ahmed Ali U, Pahlplatz JM, Nealon WH, van Goor H, Gooszen HG, Boermeester MA. Endoscopic or surgical intervention for painful obstructive chronic pancreatitis. Cochrane Database Syst Rev. 2015;3:CD007884.

Chapter 12 Endoscopic Ampullectomy

Michael B. McCabe and Andrew Y. Wang

Case Presentation

A 65-year-old female with past medical history significant for autoimmune hepatitis treated with azathioprine and unexplained chronic iron deficiency anemia was referred to our center for evaluation of a biopsy-proven ampullary adenoma. She had been followed closely by her local hematologist for iron deficiency anemia, which required prior red blood cell transfusions, with previous endoscopic evaluation including upper endoscopy, colonoscopy, and capsule endoscopy without an identifiable source during the past 3 years. For recurrent symptomatic anemia, she underwent upper endoscopy that found mild nonerosive gastritis and nodular mucosa in the

Electronic Supplementary Material The online version of this chapter (https://doi.org/10.1007/978-3-030-12741-1_12) contains supplementary material, which is available to authorized users.

M. B. McCabe · A. Y. Wang (✉)
Division of Gastroenterology and Hepatology, University of Virginia Health System, Charlottesville, VA, USA
e-mail: ayw7d@virginia.edu

D. K. Mullady (ed.), *Dilemmas in ERCP*,
https://doi.org/10.1007/978-3-030-12741-1_12

second portion of the duodenum, both surrounding and involving the ampulla. This was felt to be morphologically consistent with an ampullary adenoma. Cold forceps biopsies of the lesion were taken, and pathologic assessment revealed tubular adenoma. Her liver function tests were notable for normal AST 38 IU/L, ALT 18 IU/L, and total bilirubin 0.2 mg/dL but with mild elevation in her alkaline phosphatase 155 mg/dL (normal range 39–117 mg/dL). No cross-sectional imaging had been pursued. She was subsequently referred to our institution for consideration of endoscopic ampullectomy.

Ampullary tumors are uncommon lesions with an estimated prevalence of 0.04–0.12% in postmortem studies [1]. Ampullary adenomas are the most common tumor of the ampulla of Vater, arising from either the surface epithelium or the inner lining of the ampulla, with an estimated 3000 cases annually in the United States [2, 3]. These lesions occur sporadically in the general population but are more commonly associated with hereditary syndromes such as familial adenomatous polyposis (FAP) [4]. Historically, these lesions were found in symptomatic patients with resultant underlying malignancy. However, now with more ubiquitous use of endoscopy and cross-sectional imaging, these lesions are being detected incidentally and often times at earlier stages [1]. Furthermore, screening protocols for FAP have also led to increased detection [5].

It is believed that duodenal adenomas follow the adenoma-to-carcinoma sequence, which has been well described in the formation of colonic adenocarcinoma, and as such, resection is recommended [6–9]. The frequency of malignancy is higher for ampullary adenomas when compared to other sporadic non-ampullary duodenal polyps [10]. The incidence of malignancy within ampullary adenomas ranges from 20% to 30% [11–13].

Traditionally surgery, either by transduodenal local resection or pancreatoduodenectomy (Whipple procedure), was the mainstay of treatment of ampullary adenomas [14–16]. However, given advances in therapeutic endoscopy, endoscopic papillectomy has emerged as a minimally invasive, less morbid alternative compared to surgery [11, 16–18]. The endoscopic terms "ampullectomy" and "papillectomy" have been used interchangeably in the literature and in common parlance (as well as in this review). However, papillectomy is the more technically appropriate term for endoscopic resection of an ampullary neoplasm, as complete ampullectomy can only truly be performed by means of surgery [19, 20].

Diagnosis/Assessment

How to Approach an Ampullary Lesion

Although our patient had a biopsy-proven ampullary adenoma, details of the lesion size and morphologic characteristics were not included in the outside gastroenterologist's endoscopy report, possibly owing to the fact that the lesion was assessed by using only a standard forward-viewing gastroscope. While these lesions can be appreciated with the use of a standard forward-viewing endoscope, a side-viewing duodenoscope is optimal and necessary for proper assessment of the ampulla of Vater. Using a duodenoscope, we identified a large, 40-mm sessile, multi-lobulated, laterally spreading polyp in the second portion of the duodenum that involved the ampulla (Fig. 12.1).

Meticulous morphologic assessment of ampullary lesions is important. Even with careful assessment with high-definition white light (HDWL) and narrow-band imaging (NBI), adenomatous changes may be difficult to identify, particularly as NBI for the diagnosis of dysplasia has not been widely validated in the duodenum. Morphologic characteristics including ulceration, excessive friability, and contact bleeding should raise suspicion for malignancy [10]. As such, biopsies of the lesion are recommended and should be obtained prior to attempted resection.

Care should be taken to biopsy away from the ampullary os or pancreatic duct (PD) opening (in the case of separate

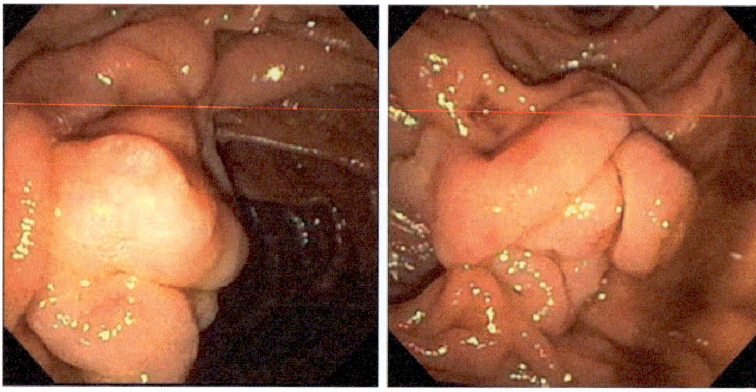

Figure 12.1 Endoscopic appearance of the ampullary adenoma using a side-viewing duodenoscope

biliary and pancreatic ductal orifices) to avoid papillary edema, which may lead to duct obstruction and pancreatitis [21, 22]. While biopsies confirming the diagnosis of an adenoma are helpful, they do not rule out the possibility of a deeper underlying adenocarcinoma [23]. Endoscopic biopsies yielding high-grade dysplasia should raise suspicion for underlying adenocarcinoma [24]. Accuracy of biopsies in diagnosing adenocarcinoma has been reported between 45% and 80%, with false-negative rates of 16–18% [8, 11, 15, 19, 23, 25–29]. This is likely the result of the heterogeneity of malignant tumors and intra-ampullary growth, which may result in sampling error. To obtain deeper biopsies, some have reported increased diagnostic yield with biopsies taken after sphincterotomy is done to expose the deeper ampullary epithelium. While typically done at the time of sphincterotomy, some have advocated obtaining biopsies 48 hours to 1 week after sphincterotomy, as biopsies after a fresh sphincterotomy can be difficult to interpret [30, 31].

The limitations posed by forceps biopsy are overcome by ampullectomy for complete histologic assessment [26]; however, resection of small (<1 cm) asymptomatic papillary lesions, or partial ampullary resection, for the purposes of pathological diagnosis should be avoided. In many instances endoscopists are able to accurately triage patients for endoscopic papillectomy versus surgical management based on the gross endoscopic appearance. Irani et al. [11] demonstrated in a large case series that out of 102 patients believed to have endoscopically resectable adenomas, only 6 patients (5%) who ultimately underwent papillectomy harbored malignancy on final pathology.

Determining Criteria for Endoscopic Papillectomy

Following diagnosis of a biopsy-proven ampullary adenoma, options include endoscopic surveillance versus endoscopic or surgical resection. There are no clinical trials directly comparing these approaches; thus no consensus regarding management exists. Historically local surgical ampullectomy by way of a transduodenal approach was employed; however, high rates of tumor recurrence have given way to pancreaticoduodenectomy as the preferred surgical approach [32, 33]. Pancreaticoduodenectomy offers definitive resection with the lowest recurrence rates but is associated with higher rates of morbidity and mortality [12]. The relatively widespread use of diagnostic upper endoscopy has led to identification of ampullary neoplasms at earlier stages, which has made endoscopic papillectomy an appealing alternative. Relative to surgical options, endoscopic papillectomy has lower morbidity and identical mortality rates. Therefore, endoscopic resection is considered first-line therapy before surgical consideration for benign ampullary lesions in appropriate patients [17].

The criteria of endoscopic papillectomy are not well established, although Binmoeller et al. published an early case series on this topic and recommended endoscopic resection for (1) size <4 cm, (2) no evidence of malignancy on endoscopic inspection (i.e., absence of ulcerations, spontaneous bleeding, and friability), (3) absence of malignancy on biopsy, and (4) lack of intraductal extension as demonstrated on endoscopic retrograde cholangiopancreatography (ERCP)

[34, 35]. These criteria continue to serve as a general guidance when determining a lesion's potential for endoscopic resection, although over time we have witnessed an expansion of criteria in regard to resecting larger lesions that are amenable to wide-field endoscopic mucosal resection techniques [35, 36]. Furthermore, benign adenomas with intraductal extension have been successfully resected, albeit with a lower curative rate relative as compared to lesions without intraductal growth (46% vs 83%) [1]. Controversy exists regarding preferred treatment of pT1 ampullary cancers, as vascular invasion and lymph node metastasis are not seen in lesions confined to the ampulla [8, 37, 38]. There have been reports of successful endoscopic resection of ampullary lesions with in situ carcinoma without recurrence, although this is not universally recommended [39].

Special Population: FAP

Although not applicable to our patient, it is important to consider differences in management of ampullary adenomas in patients with FAP relative to those with sporadic adenomas. It is estimated that 50–90% of FAP patients will develop duodenal adenomas, with the vast majority in the peri-ampullary region [40]. Adenomatous changes of the papilla may not be readily apparent without biopsy [4]. Adenocarcinoma of the peri-ampullary region, arising from duodenal or ampullary adenomas, is the most common site of malignancy and cancer death in FAP patients who have already undergone colectomy [6, 41–45]. The Spigelman staging system was developed to assess degree of duodenal adenomatous polyp burden (size and number), histology, and degree of dysplasia to predict the risk of developing duodenal cancer and to identify high-risk individuals [40].

Management of ampullary adenomas in FAP patients is complicated as the patient's malignancy risk may be affected by the overall degree of polyposis within the duodenum (i.e., the Spigelman score) and not solely their ampullary lesion

[43]. Furthermore, endoscopic resection does not eliminate the risk of recurrence or development of another cancer in the upper gastrointestinal tract. Thus, management of ampullary adenomas in this population is undertaken on a case-by-case basis based on the stage of their disease, with endoscopic treatment being appropriate for selected patients [45].

Burke et al. [44] examined the natural history of untreated duodenal and ampullary adenomas in FAP patients in endoscopic surveillance programs and demonstrated histologic progression in FAP patients is low with only 1 out of 114 patients developing an interval periampullary cancer over 51-month period. Consequently some authors have advocated for surveillance with biopsies in FAP patients with ampullary adenomas without rapid growth or high-grade dysplasia [46], which may be appropriate for small (<1 cm) lesions that are not causing symptoms or evidence of biliary or PD obstruction. Surveillance intervals in this patient population have not been standardized, but frequency should reflect both the Spigelman staging and presence of ampullary involvement [47]. In our institution, our practice is to perform endoscopic surveillance with biopsies every 6–12 months, reserving further interrogation with EUS only if high-risk features (as listed above) are present.

Adjunctive Imaging

Case Presentation (Continued)

Our patient underwent endoscopic ultrasound (EUS) which noted a heterogeneous lobulated mass at the ampulla measuring 25 mm in maximal cross-sectional diameter. The lesion appeared to be confined to the mucosa, without extension into the deeper wall layers, and the muscularis propria was noted to be intact. There was also an intact interface between the mass and the pancreas and bile duct, suggesting lack of invasion (Fig. 12.2).

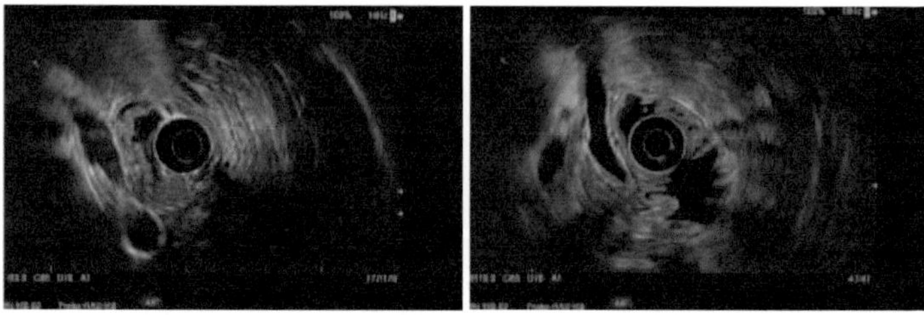

Figure 12.2 EUS assessment of the lesion demonstrated confinement to the mucosa with intact muscularis propria

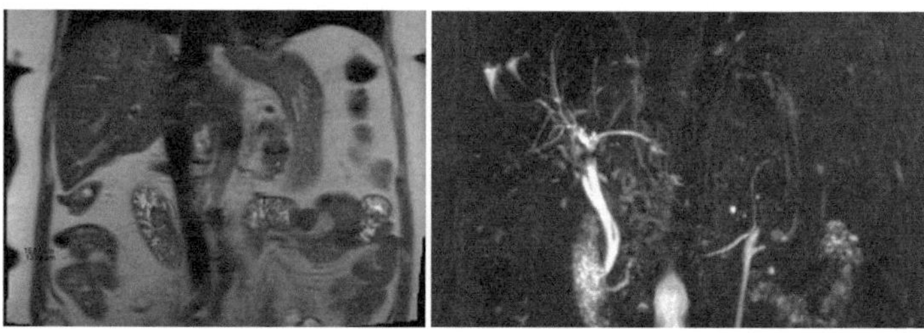

Figure 12.3 MRI/MRCP of lesion arising from the medial wall of the second portion of the duodenum without intraductal involvement

Magnetic resonance imaging (MRI) of the abdomen with and without contrast was obtained and demonstrated a T2-hyperintense lesion measuring 16 mm × 13 mm arising from the medial wall of the second part of the duodenum near the ampulla. There was no evidence of intra- or extrahepatic biliary dilation. The PD was not dilated, and there was no evidence of pancreatic divisum (Fig. 12.3).

Use of adjunctive imaging to aid in accurate tumor staging is critical in guiding therapeutic management regarding ampullary adenomas and neoplasms. Multiple imaging modalities can be employed as adjuncts to aid the endoscopist in staging ampullary tumors. Cross-sectional imaging and EUS can assess for intraductal extension of an ampullary adenoma, and it can also identify invasive cancer as well as potential nodal involvement, which can be critical in choosing between endoscopic papillectomy and surgery [19]. EUS using 7.5–10 MHz was found to be more accurate for T-staging as compared to computed tomography (CT) and MRI, but not for N staging [48–51]. Thus, the use of EUS plus cross-sectional imaging is oftentimes complementary. Although EUS is superior for T-staging, there are some potential caveats. The presence of indwelling stents may compromise accuracy of T-staging by EUS and lead to tumor understaging, although other studies have not found this to be significant [48, 51]. On the contrary, overstaging may occur in the setting of peri-tumoral inflammation and surrounding edema or in fibrosing pancreatitis [52]. Intraductal ultrasound (IDUS) at a frequency of 20–30 MHz offers resolution of 0.07–0.18 mm. IDUS has been reported to be superior to conventional EUS using an dedicated echoendoscope for T-staging, although one prospective study reported a tendency for overstaging [31, 37]. IDUS may serve as a potentially useful adjunct to conventional EUS, although widespread adoption has been limited given the cost and a relatively small number of studies in direct comparison to EUS to date.

There is no consensus regarding whether EUS should be performed routinely for all ampullary adenomas or only in select patients if there is concern for underlying malignancy to include biopsy-proven high-grade dysplasia, features of unresectability (friability, ulceration, fixation), or lesion size >1–2 cm [11, 53]. We believe that EUS has a clear role particularly in patients at risk for malignancy as if evidence of invasive disease or extensive tumor ingrowth (>1.5 cm) is found and then patients can be directed to surgery sparing them the risk of non-curative endoscopic papillectomy [54–56].

ERCP can also be performed prior to endoscopic papillectomy in order to assess for intraductal growth of the adenoma and to delineate ductal anatomy. This is especially important if EUS was not performed prior to attempted papillectomy or if there was ambiguity regarding intraductal involvement on EUS or other adjunctive imaging modalities. Ductal ingrowth (particularly if >1 cm to 1.5 cm) in general should prompt surgical referral, although some groups have reported papillectomy with concomitant successful intraductal ablation of tumor ingrowth [1, 57]. While pancreatography has the added benefit of assessing for pancreas divisum, which would obviate the need for PD stenting following papillectomy of the major papilla, this can be typically determined in a noninvasive fashion via MRCP or EUS at the time of endoscopic staging.

Treatment/Management

Endoscopic Resection

Case Presentation (Continued)

After assessing the lesion with a duodenoscope and having previously employed adjunctive imaging modalities (EUS and MRI) to verify no intraductal involvement or evidence of invasive cancer in this biopsy-proven ampullary adenoma, it was felt the lesion would be amendable to papillectomy and wide-field endoscopic mucosal resection (EMR). We attempted to identify the ampullary orifice, but were not able to clearly see it due to the bulky nature of the adenoma. The area was injected in dynamic fashion with normal saline tinted with methylene blue using a 25-gauge Carr-Locke injection needle (US Endoscopy, Mentor, OH) using the duodenoscope to provide adequate submucosal lifting (Fig. 12.4).

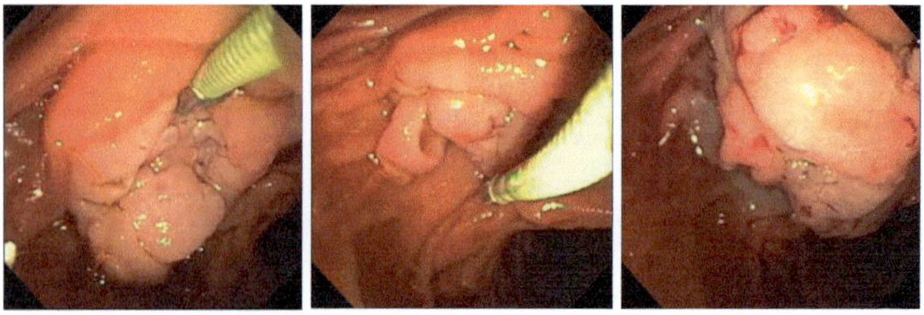

FIGURE 12.4 Submucosal injection

The adenomatous polyp was removed by piecemeal EMR technique by employing a 15-mm Captivator II stiff snare (Boston Scientific, Marlborough, MA) and EndoCut Q (settings, 3–2-1) current, using a VIO 300D generator (ERBE USA, Marietta, GA). The polyp was removed in five pieces (Fig. 12.5). *A small 3-mm focus of tissue remained in the center of the resection base, which was removed using hot biopsy avulsion using EndoCut Q (settings, 3–1-2) with a Radial Jaw 4 hot biopsy forceps (Boston Scientific)* (Fig. 12.6). *Careful inspection of the resection site revealed confirmed complete macroscopic resection. The resected pieces were collected using a retrieval net and sent for histopathological evaluation* (Video 12.1).

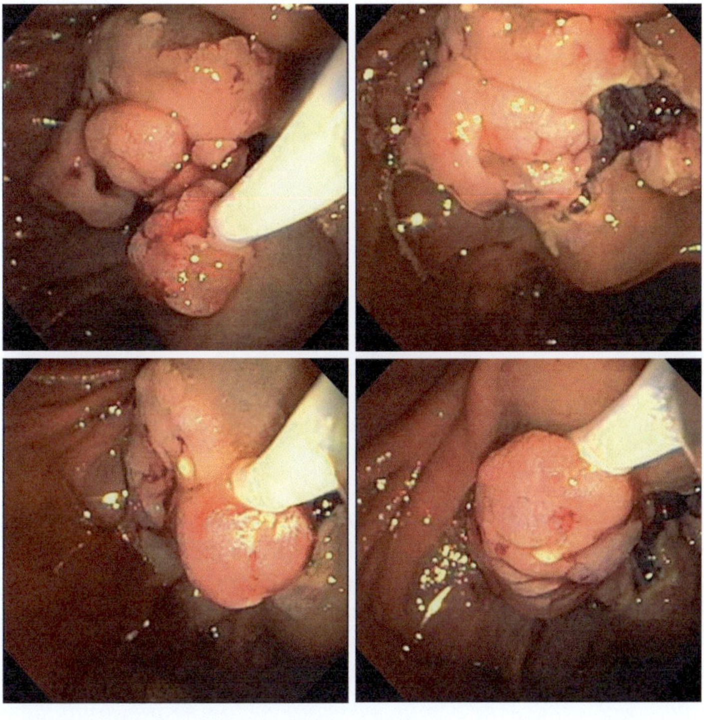

FIGURE 12.5 Piecemeal resection

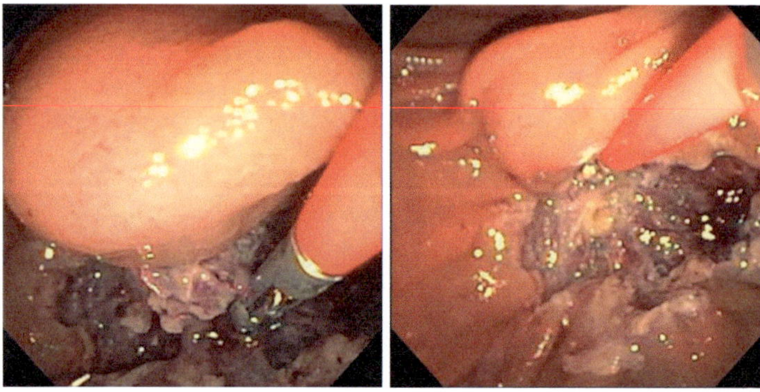

FIGURE 12.6 Hot biopsy avulsion (left panel) of remaining suspected adenomatous tissue foci with resultant complete resection of all macroscopic tissue (right panel)

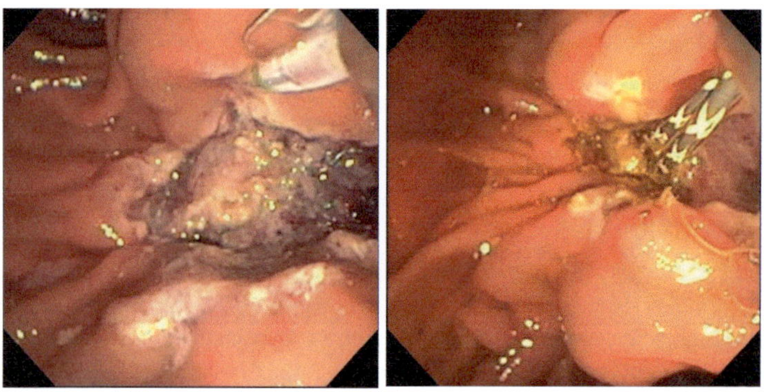

FIGURE 12.7 Accessing the biliary and pancreatic ducts post-resection

Attention was then turned to accessing the biliary and pancreatic ducts (Fig. 12.7). *The ventral PD was accessed using a 0.025 inch × 450 cm VisiGlide wire (Olympus America, Center Valley, PA) passed* via *a tapered-tip sphincterotome (Olympus America). Limited contrast was injected to ascertain absence of intraductal involvement of the PD. The PD in the head and genu was dilated to 5 mm, possibly owing to the ampullary adenoma. A limited ventral pancreatic sphincterotomy was*

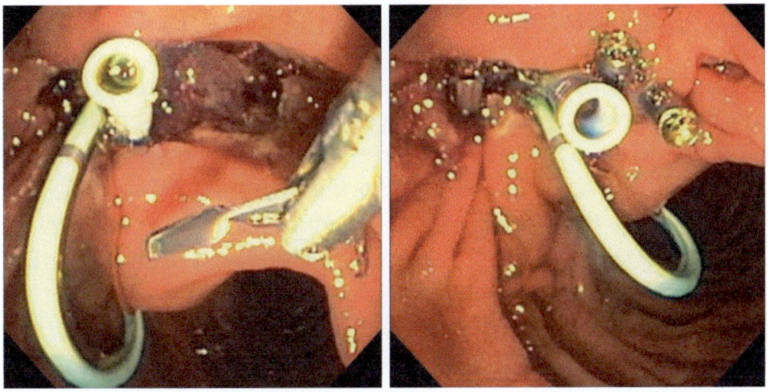

FIGURE 12.8 Biliary and pancreatic duct stents placed followed by mucosal defect closure with endoscopic clips

performed, and the wire in the ventral pancreatic duct was left in place. The bile duct was accessed with a second guide wire loaded into the sphincterotome. Once the bile duct was accessed, a cholangiogram was performed that showed no intraductal tumor ingrowth and a biliary sphincterotomy was performed to reduce the risk of delayed papillary stenosis and possibly cholangitis. A 10 Fr × 7 cm plastic biliary stent was placed into the bile duct to ensure drainage and further decrease the risk of cholangitis. Lastly a 5 Fr × 4 cm plastic stent with an external pigtail was placed into the PD to help mitigate the risk of post-ERCP pancreatitis. Furthermore, indomethacin 100 mg was administered per rectum to further decrease the risk of post-ERCP pancreatitis. The mucosal defect was subsequently closed with five 16-mm-long Duraclips (Conmed Corporation, Utica, NY) to decrease the risk of delayed bleeding (Fig. 12.8).

Technical Aspects of Ampullary Resection

The principles and techniques of endoscopic papillectomy originated from and continue to mirror that of EMR for colon polyps. There are a number of techniques described in the literature with no standardized approach, likely owing the paucity of studies directly comparing different techniques.

Submucosal Injection

There is no consensus regarding whether a submucosal lift is required prior to attempted papillectomy. It has been reported that the absence of an adequate lift may portend underlying malignancy, with one study demonstrating its prognostic significance as the strongest predictor of malignancy followed by EUS T-staging [58, 59]. However, one must remember that the ampulla contains fixed muscular sphincters and ducts that will not lift. The potential space created by the lift can decrease the risk of injury, both mechanical and thermal, to the underlying muscularis propria [60]. Lastly, submucosal injections, especially using an injectate of diluted epinephrine (1:100,000 to 1:200,000), may decrease bleeding risk during papillectomy, particularly if wide-field duodenal EMR is also required [59, 61].

There are drawbacks to submucosal lifting. Submucosal injection can distort the ampullary adenoma secondary to the "anchoring effect" created by the bile duct and PD that course through the lesion, which in turn can create a central depression at the ampullary opening making resection difficult [43]. Others have noted that en bloc resection might be difficult after submucosal lifting as the injectate will increase the volume of the ampullary and peri-ampullary tissue. Lastly, excessive submucosal injection might promote a more superficial resection that can leave the deeper sphincteric musculature intact, and it can also make subsequent PD identification and cannulation more difficult [62].

Snare Resection

Papillectomy is performed with a side-viewing duodenoscope to provide a direct view of the papilla, which with use of the elevator can allow for better access to the lesion with a snare and other endoscopic devices. When possible, en bloc excision of the entire lesion should be pursued. There is no standardization for snare selection, and the size of a snare chosen is often dependent on the size of the lesion. Standard or braided snares are most often used [35, 43, 63, 64]. Fine-wire, flexible snares designed for papillectomy have also been described [60]. Standard snares offer greater flexibility and are easier to maneuver over the elevator. Sniffer snares may allow for easier positioning parallel to the plane of resection [46]. After resection, retrieval of the specimen is critical for histologic assessment. This can be retrieved with the use of the snare or a retrieval net. Antiperistaltic agents, such as glucagon, may be helpful in preventing downstream specimen migration.

There is also no consensus regarding electrosurgical current settings, and so the optimal electrocautery mode is based on expert opinion. Latest-generation adaptive electrosurgical generators, that monitor tissue resistance and only provide the required amount of energy, should be used [19, 64, 65].

If en bloc resection is not feasible, typically because the lesion size is >2 cm (which is around the limit of safe en bloc resection), then piecemeal resection is required. Piecemeal resection is prone to leaving behind mucosal islands that are difficult to remove using a snare. As such, avulsion or adjunctive ablative therapies can be used to ensure removal or destruction of remnant adenomatous tissue. Some authors have even used ablative technology as primary therapy for ampullary and non-ampullary adenomas [66, 67]. Using ablative therapy as the primary therapy has several disadvantages, with the primary shortcoming being lack of histologic examination, which is especially important given risk of occult malignancy in ampullary adenomas. Furthermore, eradication oftentimes requires multiple treatments [67]. As such, we do not recommend primary ablative therapy in most instances for ampullary adenomas, but ablation can play an important adjunctive role in fulgurating small non-ampullary adenomas, particularly in patients with FAP and innumerable small duodenal lesions.

Ablative therapies include argon plasma coagulation (APC) and monopolar or bipolar electrocoagulation. APC is the most commonly used modality owing to its superficial tissue destruction and ubiquity in GI endoscopy suites [34, 35, 64, 68, 69].

Endobiliary radiofrequency ablation (RFA) may play a role in treating limited tumor ingrowth of the bile duct. PD stents are often placed before employing tissue ablative strategies around the PD orifice.

Pancreatic and Biliary Sphincterotomy

Ductal interrogation should be performed to assess for intraductal involvement of the tumor. Cholangiogram and pancreatogram can be performed pre- and/or post-resection [19]. Ductal interrogation prior to resection can aid in post-resection access by creating a road map of ductal anatomy, which anecdotally may allow for easier ductal access after resection. However, some experts believe that post-resection access is often easier after the ampullary mound has been resected and the ductal orifices or deeper muscle complexes are exposed. Post-resection opacification of the ducts is important in order to ensure absence of bile leak or PD leak, as a result of papillary resection. Intraductal involvement (typically >1 cm) previously was a criterion for referral for surgery, although it has been argued that endoscopic papillectomy can still be considered if the intraductal adenomatous tissue is accessible after sphincterotomy [1, 64]. In practice, adenomatous ingrowth of >1.5 cm probably should still prompt operative resection. In the case of pancreas divisum, accessing and studying the ventral PD of Wirsung is not required and may contribute to unnecessary risk.

There is no consensus regarding whether biliary and pancreatic sphincterotomy should be performed routinely and at what stage in the resection process, either pre- or post-papillectomy [1, 53, 58, 59, 63]. The rationale for performing dual sphincterotomies is to ensure drainage given coagulative effect and anatomic distortion following papillectomy, thereby mitigating the risk of post-procedural cholangitis and pancreatitis. Desilets et al. [69] advocated for dual sphincterotomies as well as PD stent placement performed prior to resection to mitigate post-resection complications. Furthermore, PD stenting was felt to protect the PD orifice from thermal injury during electrosurgical resection as well as from adjuvant thermal ablation (if required), thus lessening the risk of pancreatitis and stricturing. As such, some clinicians attempt snare resection of the papilla over a PD stent. However, performing sphincterotomies or placing a PD stent prior to resection may limit the ability to perform an en bloc resection [46, 69].

Other authors have advocated for post-papillectomy sphincterotomy and PD stent placement to allow for en bloc resection [43]. En bloc resection allows for more accurate pathologic examination for the completeness of resection and shortened procedure time [43]. Difficulty identifying the pancreatic orifice after papillectomy can be ameliorated by spraying the presumed area of the PD with methylene blue followed by the use of intravenous secretin [70]. By using this method, the pancreas is stimulated to release pancreatic juice, which makes the area of the orifice appear less blue or even become grossly visible. Alternatively, pancreatogram with injection of methylene blue diluted in contrast (1:2 dilution or even more dilute) prior to papillectomy may aid post-papillectomy access for PD stent placement [70].

Biliary and Pancreatic Stenting

Pancreatitis is a known and dreaded complication of endoscopic papillectomy, and as such prophylactic PD stenting after papillectomy is recommended to reduce the risk of pancreatitis in patients that do not have pancreas divisum anatomy [19]. The benefits of prophylactic PD stenting to prevent post-ERCP pancreatitis are well established [71–73]. Harewood et al. [62] published the first prospective, randomized controlled study that demonstrated that PD stent placement (with 5 Fr × 3 to 5 cm, single flanged stents) reduced post-papillectomy pancreatitis. Some have argued for the need of a larger trial, as this was a small trial with a total of 19 patients enrolled. This study was stopped early given safety concerns after interim analysis demonstrated pancreatitis occurring in 33% of the group without PD stents relative to 0% in the stented group [74]. Others have argued routine prophylactic PD stent placement may not be necessary in all patients and that more studies to clearly ascertain the subgroup that might benefit are needed [75]. Rectal indomethacin is also typically administered given extrapolation from data demonstrating its reduction in risk and severity of post-ERCP pancreatitis in high-risk populations, although no study has looked specifically at risk reduction regarding post-papillectomy pancreatitis [76].

Biliary stenting at the time of papillectomy is often performed. Biliary stenting is particularly indicated if there is concern for poor drainage, as this could predispose the patient to developing cholangitis and biliary sepsis [34, 43, 69].

Adverse Events

Endoscopic papillectomy is one of the highest risk procedures that an advanced endoscopist can perform. Early complications include pancreatitis, bleeding, perforation, cholangitis, and risk of sedation/anesthesia, with late complications including biliary and pancreatic duct stenosis [19, 64]. In a systematic review, Han et al. [77] reported morbidity rates of 23% (range, 10–58%), with the most common complications being bleeding and post-papillectomy pancreatitis.

Given the robust vascular supply of the duodenum, there is an increased risk for both early and delayed bleeding. Bleeding rates have been reported as ranging from 0% to 25%. The vast majority of bleeding can be controlled with endoscopic hemostatic techniques. Post-papillectomy pancreatitis has been reported also ranging from 0% to 25% [77]. In most cases, post-papillectomy pancreatitis was mild to moderate in severity [11]. Again, prophylactic PD stenting has been shown to mitigate the risk of post-papillectomy pancreatitis [62]. Lastly, perforation has a reported frequency of 0–8% [77].

In the event of a complication, early recognition is of paramount importance. As such, the resection site should be carefully inspected to assess for areas of deeper muscle injury or frank perforation. However, endoscopic diagnosis of deeper injury is less reliable relative to other areas of the gastrointestinal tract [63]. Risk of perforation may be higher in cases with extensive lateral extension of the lesion or in invasive cancer [11]. Perforation is typically retroperitoneal, and so the absence of free air in the peritoneum or subdiaphragmatic space on a plain film may provide false reassurance, and cross-sectional imaging is required when the clinical suspicion for a retroperitoneal perforation is high. Thankfully, most retroperitoneal perforations in this setting can be managed conservatively with antibiotics and observation and without the need for surgical repair [35, 60, 77].

Papillary stenosis is a late complication and can occur 7 days to 24 months, or even years later, following endoscopic papillectomy [60, 66, 77]. PD stenosis was less common in those who received a PD stent at the time of resection (15.4% vs. 1.1%) [64, 77]. Routine biliary and pancreatic sphincterotomy and stenting may mitigate the risk of the late complication of papillary stenosis. Mortality from endoscopic papillectomy has been reported as averaging 0.4% (range, 0–7%) [77].

Outcomes

Clinical Presentation (Continued)

The patient was asymptomatic following her ERCP, papillectomy, and wide-field EMR but was admitted to our inpatient service following the procedure for observation, given her comorbidities, and as she did not live close to our medical center. She had no evidence of bleeding or pancreatitis and was subsequently discharged 48 hours later. Final pathology from the resected specimens showed tubular adenoma. There was no evidence of invasive carcinoma. Given this result, we recommend a follow-up ERCP in 3 months for stent removal and ampullary surveillance.

The ultimate goal of endoscopic papillectomy is to achieve curative resection, which can be loosely defined by lack of residual or recurrent dysplastic tissue at subsequent endoscopic follow-up, preferably confirmed by histopathological sampling with cold biopsies. Han et al. [77] performed a systematic review that evaluated the success rates for endoscopic papillectomy, which ranged from 46% to 92%, and recurrence rates which ranged from 0% to 33%. The data regarding overall success rates and recurrence rates were based on multiple small- to medium-sized retrospective case series, but this study was limited due to significant heterogeneity. Catalano et al. [64] found the following factors were significantly associated with success: lesion size <3 cm, older age (defined as >54 years), adjunctive use of thermal ablation, and sporadic adenomas. Irani et al. [11] demonstrated through multivariate analysis that lesion size <2 cm and absence of dilated ducts were the most important factors favoring success.

Surveillance

Case Presentation (Continued)

Despite waiting 3 months, there were mucosal changes that were likely inflammatory and related to the healing process; however, we could not definitively exclude residual adenoma based solely on the endoscopic appearance (Fig. 12.9). *Therefore, extensive biopsies at the time of follow-up ERCP were obtained that showed granulation tissue without evidence of any residual or recurrent adenoma.*

Recurrence rates have been reported between 0% and 33%, and thus endoscopic surveillance is recommended following endoscopic removal of an ampullary adenoma [77]. Surveillance with a duodenoscope is required. Biopsies should be obtained from the resection site even in the absence of morphologic characteristics consistent with residual or recur-

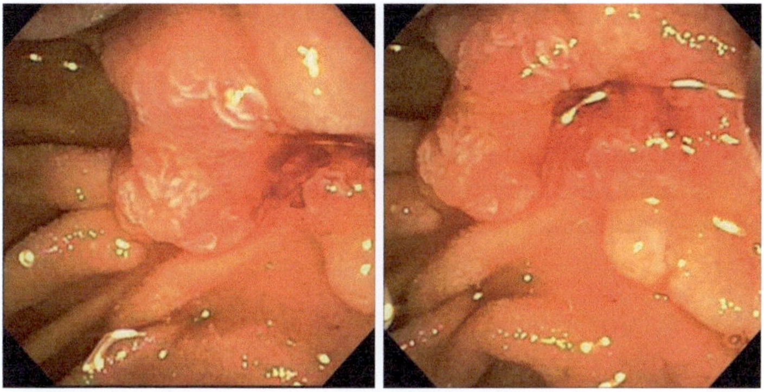

FIGURE 12.9 Endoscopic surveillance was performed 3-month post-resection. While it was difficult to distinguish areas of adenomatous recurrence from inflammatory/granulation tissue, extensive biopsies did not show any residual or recurrent adenoma

rent adenoma. Although there is consensus that a post-papillectomy surveillance strategy should be employed to assess for recurrent or residual adenomatous tissue, consensus regarding posttreatment surveillance intervals is lacking [19].

Many endoscopists follow the surveillance guidelines laid out by Catalano et al. [64] which call for endoscopic surveillance every 2–3 months until complete resection is confirmed with negative biopsies, followed by surveillance every 6–12 months for the next 2 years. After 2 years without recurrence, patients with sporadic adenomas should have repeat endoscopy only if clinical symptoms dictate, whereas patients with FAP should continue surveillance every 2–3 years or as further dictated by their polyp burden in the duodenum (i.e., Spigelman score). Some authors have recommended annual surveillance for 5 years after papillectomy [35]. Factors such as intraductal involvement at the time of resection, piecemeal resection, and histological assessment of degree of dysplasia should be considered when determining case-specific surveillance intervals as well as surveillance duration. Not surprisingly, patients with high-grade dysplasia are at increased risk for recurrence [13].

The need and frequency of follow-up cross-sectional imaging to evaluate for subsequent lymph node metastasis or invasive pancreatic cancer has not been well-defined. In patients who remain free of dysplasia on endoscopic surveillance, it is our practice to obtain follow-up MRI every 1–2 years for up to 5 years to evaluate for the development of regional recurrence or distant metastasis.

Conclusion

Endoscopic management of ampullary adenomas has emerged as the preferred treatment modality, having supplanted surgical resection in many patients. While advancement in endoscopic technologies and refinement of endoscopic techniques continue to push the boundary with respect to what constitutes an endoscopically resectable lesion, enthusiasm should be tempered by the inherent risk and potential adverse outcomes of this procedure. As such, this procedure is best undertaken by experienced pancreaticobiliary endoscopists at large-volume referral centers with sufficient radiological and surgical backup.

Pearls and Pitfalls

- Endoscopic papillectomy requires careful patient selection and appropriate multi-modality staging, especially for larger lesions.
- Biopsies should be pursued prior to attempted resection, as endoscopic morphologic assessment alone is less reliable in predicting deeper invasion relative to other areas in the GI tract. Conversely, one must understand the limitations of superficial biopsies in histologic assessment.
- En bloc resection should be a resection goal whenever possible, as this technique allows for more complete histologic assessment and lower rates of recurrence.

- Ampullary resection techniques merge those of luminal EMR and advanced ERCP. There are a myriad of endoscopic techniques that can be used with no standardized approach.
- Pancreatic duct stenting should be performed post-papillectomy to mitigate the risk of post-procedure pancreatitis. Identifying pancreas divisum can obviate the need for attempted pancreatic duct stenting.
- Numerous techniques have been described to aid in pancreatic duct orifice identification/cannulation and stenting following papillectomy. These include pre-papillectomy pancreatogram to obtain a road map of ductal anatomy, obtaining a pancreatogram with contrast tinted with diluted methylene blue for easier endoscopic identification after tissue resection, or spraying the presumed area of the pancreatic duct orifice with methylene blue post-resection and then administering intravenous secretin to look for clearance of the blue dye.
- Given the high-risk nature of this procedure, the endoscopy team should monitor vigilantly for both early and delayed complications.

Disclosures Dr. Wang has received research support from Cook Medical on the topic of covered metal biliary stents. Dr. McCabe has nothing to disclose.

References

1. Bohnacker S, Seitz U, Nguyen D, Thonke F, Seewald S, deWeerth A, et al. Endoscopic resection of benign tumors of the duodenal papilla without and with intraductal growth. Gastrointest Endosc. 2005;62(4):551–60.
2. Patel R, Varadarajulu S, Wilcox CM. Endoscopic ampullectomy: techniques and outcomes. J Clin Gastroenterol. 2012;46(1):8–15.

3. Posner S, Colletti L, Knol J, Mulholland M, Eckhauser F. Safety and long-term efficacy of transduodenal excision for tumors of the ampulla of Vater. Surgery. 2000;128(4):694–701.
4. Offerhaus GJ, Giardiello FM, Krush AJ, Booker SV, Tersmette AC, Kelley NC, et al. The risk of upper gastrointestinal cancer in familial adenomatous polyposis. Gastroenterology. 1992;102(6):1980–2.
5. Lindor NM, Greene MH. The concise handbook of family cancer syndromes. Mayo Familial Cancer Program. J Natl Cancer Inst. 1998;90(14):1039–71.
6. Spigelman AD, Talbot IC, Penna C, Nugent KP, Phillips RK, Costello C, et al. Evidence for adenoma-carcinoma sequence in the duodenum of patients with familial adenomatous polyposis. The Leeds Castle Polyposis Group (Upper Gastrointestinal Committee). J Clin Pathol. 1994;47(8):709–10.
7. Baczako K, Buchler M, Beger HG, Kirkpatrick CJ, Haferkamp O. Morphogenesis and possible precursor lesions of invasive carcinoma of the papilla of Vater: epithelial dysplasia and adenoma. Hum Pathol. 1985;16(3):305–10.
8. Yamaguchi K, Enjoji M. Carcinoma of the ampulla of vater. A clinicopathologic study and pathologic staging of 109 cases of carcinoma and 5 cases of adenoma. Cancer. 1987;59(3):506–15.
9. Takashima M, Ueki T, Nagai E, Yao T, Yamaguchi K, Tanaka M, et al. Carcinoma of the ampulla of Vater associated with or without adenoma: a clinicopathologic analysis of 198 cases with reference to p53 and Ki-67 immunohistochemical expressions. Mod Pathol. 2000;13(12):1300–7.
10. Culver EL, McIntyre AS. Sporadic duodenal polyps: classification, investigation, and management. Endoscopy. 2011;43(2):144–55.
11. Irani S, Arai A, Ayub K, Biehl T, Brandabur JJ, Dorer R, et al. Papillectomy for ampullary neoplasm: results of a single referral center over a 10-year period. Gastrointest Endosc. 2009;70(5):923–32.
12. Cahen DL, Fockens P, de Wit LT, Offerhaus GJ, Obertop H, Gouma DJ. Local resection or pancreaticoduodenectomy for villous adenoma of the ampulla of Vater diagnosed before operation. Br J Surg. 1997;84(7):948–51.
13. Heidecke CD, Rosenberg R, Bauer M, Werner M, Weigert N, Ulm K, et al. Impact of grade of dysplasia in villous adenomas of Vater's papilla. World J Surg. 2002;26(6):709–14.

14. Farnell MB, Sakorafas GH, Sarr MG, Rowland CM, Tsiotos GG, Farley DR, et al. Villous tumors of the duodenum: reappraisal of local vs. extended resection. J Gastrointest Surg. 2000;4(1):13–21.. discussion 2-3.
15. Clary BM, Tyler DS, Dematos P, Gottfried M, Pappas TN. Local ampullary resection with careful intraoperative frozen section evaluation for presumed benign ampullary neoplasms. Surgery. 2000;127(6):628–33.
16. Onkendi EO, Naik ND, Rosedahl JK, Harmsen SW, Gostout CJ, Baron TH Sr, et al. Adenomas of the ampulla of Vater: a comparison of outcomes of operative and endoscopic resections. J Gastrointest Surg. 2014;18(9):1588–96.
17. Ceppa EP, Burbridge RA, Rialon KL, Omotosho PA, Emick D, Jowell PS, et al. Endoscopic versus surgical ampullectomy: an algorithm to treat disease of the ampulla of Vater. Ann Surg. 2013;257(2):315–22.
18. De Palma GD. Endoscopic papillectomy: indications, techniques, and results. World J Gastroenterol. 2014;20(6):1537–43.
19. Chathadi KV, Khashab MA, Acosta RD, Chandrasekhara V, Eloubeidi MA, Faulx AL, et al. The role of endoscopy in ampullary and duodenal adenomas. Gastrointest Endosc. 2015;82(5):773–81.
20. Beger HG, Staib L, Schoenberg MH. Ampullectomy for adenoma of the papilla and ampulla of Vater. Langenbeck's Arch Surg. 1998;383(2):190–3.
21. Morales TG, Hixson LJ. Acute pancreatitis following endoscopic biopsy of the ampulla in a patient with Gardner's syndrome. Gastrointest Endosc. 1994;40(3):367–9.
22. Gincul R, Ciocirlan M, Dumortier J, Guerrier B, Comte JM, Faure A, et al. Severe acute pancreatitis following endoscopic biopsy of the minor duodenal papilla. Endoscopy. 2009;41(Suppl 2):E195–6.
23. Yamaguchi K, Enjoji M, Kitamura K. Endoscopic biopsy has limited accuracy in diagnosis of ampullary tumors. Gastrointest Endosc. 1990;36(6):588–92.
24. Meneghetti AT, Safadi B, Stewart L, Way LW. Local resection of ampullary tumors. J Gastrointest Surg. 2005;9(9):1300–6.
25. Schwarz M, Pauls S, Sokiranski R, Brambs HJ, Glasbrenner B, Adler G, et al. Is a preoperative multidiagnostic approach to predict surgical resectability of periampullary tumors still effective? Am J Surg. 2001;182(3):243–9.

26. Elek G, Gyori S, Toth B, Pap A. Histological evaluation of preoperative biopsies from ampulla vateri. Pathol Oncol Res. 2003;9(1):32–41.
27. Yamaguchi K, Enjoji M. Adenoma of the ampulla of Vater: putative precancerous lesion. Gut. 1991;32(12):1558–61.
28. Ryan DP, Schapiro RH, Warshaw AL. Villous tumors of the duodenum. Ann Surg. 1986;203(3):301–6.
29. Martin JA, Haber GB. Ampullary adenoma: clinical manifestations, diagnosis, and treatment. Gastrointest Endosc Clin N Am. 2003;13(4):649–69.
30. Bourgeois N, Dunham F, Verhest A, Cremer M. Endoscopic biopsies of the papilla of Vater at the time of endoscopic sphincterotomy: difficulties in interpretation. Gastrointest Endosc. 1984;30(3):163–6.
31. Menzel J, Hoepffner N, Sulkowski U, Reimer P, Heinecke A, Poremba C, et al. Polypoid tumors of the major duodenal papilla: preoperative staging with intraductal US, EUS, and CT--a prospective, histopathologically controlled study. Gastrointest Endosc. 1999;49(3 Pt 1):349–57.
32. Bohra AK, McKie L, Diamond T. Transduodenal excision of ampullary tumours. Ulster Med J. 2002;71(2):121–7.
33. Di Giorgio A, Alfieri S, Rotondi F, Prete F, Di Miceli D, Ridolfini MP, et al. Pancreatoduodenectomy for tumors of Vater's ampulla: report on 94 consecutive patients. World J Surg. 2005;29(4):513–8.
34. Binmoeller KF, Boaventura S, Ramsperger K, Soehendra N. Endoscopic snare excision of benign adenomas of the papilla of Vater. Gastrointest Endosc. 1993;39(2):127–31.
35. Cheng CL, Sherman S, Fogel EL, McHenry L, Watkins JL, Fukushima T, et al. Endoscopic snare papillectomy for tumors of the duodenal papillae. Gastrointest Endosc. 2004;60(5):757–64.
36. Zadorova Z, Dvofak M, Hajer J. Endoscopic therapy of benign tumors of the papilla of Vater. Endoscopy. 2001;33(4):345–7.
37. Ito K, Fujita N, Noda Y, Kobayashi G, Horaguchi J, Takasawa O, et al. Preoperative evaluation of ampullary neoplasm with EUS and transpapillary intraductal US: a prospective and histopathologically controlled study. Gastrointest Endosc. 2007;66(4):740–7.
38. Yamashita Y, Ito K, Fujita N, Noda Y, Kobayashi G, Obana T, et al. A case of early carcinoma of the papilla of Vater confined to the mucosa and continuative epithelium of glands in Oddi's

sphincter (m-God) treated by endoscopic papillectomy. Intern Med. 2010;49(22):2447–50.
39. Ponchon T, Berger F, Chavaillon A, Bory R, Lambert R. Contribution of endoscopy to diagnosis and treatment of tumors of the ampulla of Vater. Cancer. 1989;64(1):161–7.
40. Spigelman AD, Williams CB, Talbot IC, Domizio P, Phillips RK. Upper gastrointestinal cancer in patients with familial adenomatous polyposis. Lancet. 1989;2(8666):783–5.
41. Sato T, Konishi K, Kimura H, Maeda K, Yabushita K, Tsuji M, et al. Adenoma and tiny carcinoma in adenoma of the papilla of Vater--p53 and PCNA. Hepato-Gastroenterology. 1999;46(27):1959–62.
42. Griffioen G, Bus PJ, Vasen HF, Verspaget HW, Lamers CB. Extracolonic manifestations of familial adenomatous polyposis: desmoid tumours, and upper gastrointestinal adenomas and carcinomas. Scand J Gastroenterol Suppl. 1998;225:85–91.
43. Chini P, Draganov PV. Diagnosis and management of ampullary adenoma: the expanding role of endoscopy. World J Gastrointest Endosc. 2011;3(12):241–7.
44. Burke CA, Beck GJ, Church JM, van Stolk RU. The natural history of untreated duodenal and ampullary adenomas in patients with familial adenomatous polyposis followed in an endoscopic surveillance program. Gastrointest Endosc. 1999;49(3 Pt 1):358–64.
45. Hirota WK, Zuckerman MJ, Adler DG, Davila RE, Egan J, Leighton JA, et al. ASGE guideline: the role of endoscopy in the surveillance of premalignant conditions of the upper GI tract. Gastrointest Endosc. 2006;63(4):570–80.
46. Baron TH, Kozarek RA, Carr-Locke DL. ERCP. Philadelphia, PA: Elsevier; 2019.
47. Latchford AR, Neale KF, Spigelman AD, Phillips RK, Clark SK. Features of duodenal cancer in patients with familial adenomatous polyposis. Clin Gastroenterol Hepatol. 2009;7(6):659–63.
48. Chen CH, Yang CC, Yeh YH, Chou DA, Nien CK. Reappraisal of endosonography of ampullary tumors: correlation with transabdominal sonography, CT, and MRI. J Clin Ultrasound. 2009;37(1):18–25.
49. Chen CH, Tseng LJ, Yang CC, Yeh YH. Preoperative evaluation of periampullary tumors by endoscopic sonography, transabdominal sonography, and computed tomography. J Clin Ultrasound. 2001;29(6):313–21.
50. Rivadeneira DE, Pochapin M, Grobmyer SR, Lieberman MD, Christos PJ, Jacobson I, et al. Comparison of linear array

endoscopic ultrasound and helical computed tomography for the staging of periampullary malignancies. Ann Surg Oncol. 2003;10(8):890–7.
51. Cannon ME, Carpenter SL, Elta GH, Nostrant TT, Kochman ML, Ginsberg GG, et al. EUS compared with CT, magnetic resonance imaging, and angiography and the influence of biliary stenting on staging accuracy of ampullary neoplasms. Gastrointest Endosc. 1999;50(1):27–33.
52. Maluf-Filho F, Sakai P, Cunha JE, Garrido T, Rocha M, Machado MC, et al. Radial endoscopic ultrasound and spiral computed tomography in the diagnosis and staging of periampullary tumors. Pancreatology. 2004;4(2):122–8.
53. Baillie J. Endoscopic ampullectomy. Am J Gastroenterol. 2005;100(11):2379–81.
54. Ridtitid W, Schmidt SE, Al-Haddad MA, LeBlanc J, DeWitt JM, McHenry L, et al. Performance characteristics of EUS for locoregional evaluation of ampullary lesions. Gastrointest Endosc. 2015;81(2):380–8.
55. Gaspar J, Shami VM. The role of EUS in ampullary lesions: is the answer black and white? Gastrointest Endosc. 2015;81(2):389–90.
56. Gaspar JP, Stelow EB, Wang AY. Approach to the endoscopic resection of duodenal lesions. World J Gastroenterol. 2016;22(2):600–17.
57. Kim JH, Moon JH, Choi HJ, Lee HS, Kim HK, Cheon YK, et al. Endoscopic snare papillectomy by using a balloon catheter for an unexposed ampullary adenoma with intraductal extension (with videos). Gastrointest Endosc. 2009;69(7):1404–6.
58. Kahaleh M, Shami VM, Brock A, Conaway MR, Yoshida C, Moskaluk CA, et al. Factors predictive of malignancy and endoscopic resectability in ampullary neoplasia. Am J Gastroenterol. 2004;99(12):2335–9.
59. Eswaran SL, Sanders M, Bernadino KP, Ansari A, Lawrence C, Stefan A, et al. Success and complications of endoscopic removal of giant duodenal and ampullary polyps: a comparative series. Gastrointest Endosc. 2006;64(6):925–32.
60. Norton ID, Gostout CJ, Baron TH, Geller A, Petersen BT, Wiersema MJ. Safety and outcome of endoscopic snare excision of the major duodenal papilla. Gastrointest Endosc. 2002;56(2):239–43.
61. Pandolfi M, Martino M, Gabbrielli A. Endoscopic treatment of ampullary adenomas. JOP. 2008;9(1):1–8.

62. Harewood GC, Pochron NL, Gostout CJ. Prospective, randomized, controlled trial of prophylactic pancreatic stent placement for endoscopic snare excision of the duodenal ampulla. Gastrointest Endosc. 2005;62(3):367–70.
63. Bassan M, Bourke M. Endoscopic ampullectomy: a practical guide. J Interv Gastroenterol. 2012;2(1):23–30.
64. Catalano MF, Linder JD, Chak A, Sivak MV Jr, Raijman I, Geenen JE, et al. Endoscopic management of adenoma of the major duodenal papilla. Gastrointest Endosc. 2004;59(2):225–32.
65. Norton ID, Geller A, Petersen BT, Sorbi D, Gostout CJ. Endoscopic surveillance and ablative therapy for periampullary adenomas. Am J Gastroenterol. 2001;96(1):101–6.
66. Saurin JC, Chavaillon A, Napoleon B, Descos F, Bory R, Berger F, et al. Long-term follow-up of patients with endoscopic treatment of sporadic adenomas of the papilla of vater. Endoscopy. 2003;35(5):402–6.
67. Lienert A, Bagshaw PF. Treatment of duodenal adenomas with endoscopic argon plasma coagulation. ANZ J Surg. 2007;77(5):371–3.
68. Vogt M, Jakobs R, Benz C, Arnold JC, Adamek HE, Riemann JF. Endoscopic therapy of adenomas of the papilla of Vater. A retrospective analysis with long-term follow-up. Dig Liver Dis. 2000;32(4):339–45.
69. Desilets DJ, Dy RM, Ku PM, Hanson BL, Elton E, Mattia A, et al. Endoscopic management of tumors of the major duodenal papilla: refined techniques to improve outcome and avoid complications. Gastrointest Endosc. 2001;54(2):202–8.
70. Poincloux L, Scanzi J, Goutte M, Pereira B, Devaud H, Joubert J, et al. Pancreatic intubation facilitated by methylene blue injection decreases the risk for postpapillectomy acute pancreatitis. Eur J Gastroenterol Hepatol. 2014;26(9):990–5.
71. Singh P, Das A, Isenberg G, Wong RC, Sivak MV Jr, Agrawal D, et al. Does prophylactic pancreatic stent placement reduce the risk of post-ERCP acute pancreatitis? A meta-analysis of controlled trials. Gastrointest Endosc. 2004;60(4):544–50.
72. Fazel A, Quadri A, Catalano MF, Meyerson SM, Geenen JE. Does a pancreatic duct stent prevent post-ERCP pancreatitis? A prospective randomized study. Gastrointest Endosc. 2003;57(3):291–4.
73. Freeman ML. Role of pancreatic stents in prevention of post-ERCP pancreatitis. JOP. 2004;5(5):322–7.

74. Baillie J. Endoscopic ampullectomy: does pancreatic stent placement make it safer? Gastrointest Endosc. 2005;62(3):371–3.
75. Chang WI, Min YW, Yun HS, Lee KH, Lee JK, Lee KT, et al. Prophylactic pancreatic stent placement for endoscopic duodenal ampullectomy: a single-center retrospective study. Gut Liver. 2014;8(3):306–12.
76. Elmunzer BJ, Scheiman JM, Lehman GA, Chak A, Mosler P, Higgins PD, et al. A randomized trial of rectal indomethacin to prevent post-ERCP pancreatitis. N Engl J Med. 2012;366(15):1414–22.
77. Han J, Kim MH. Endoscopic papillectomy for adenomas of the major duodenal papilla (with video). Gastrointest Endosc. 2006;63(2):292–301.

Chapter 13
Cholangioscopy

Cassandra Fritz and Gabriel D. Lang

Introduction

Cholangioscopy has been increasingly used in evaluation of biliary pathology. It allows for direct visualization and sampling of biliary abnormalities that asre concerning for malignancy, such as dilated and tortuous blood vessels, villous mucosal projections, ulcerated strictures, and intraductal nodules [1]. Cholangioscopy is also instrumental in the management of both large bile duct stones and pancreatic duct stones. Recently, cholangioscopy has also been utilized to access difficult-to-approach targets within the biliary tree and retrieve migrated stents.

Initially, cholangioscopy did not garner widespread use due to the cumbersome two-person operating system, small working

---

Electronic Supplementary Material The online version of this chapter (https://doi.org/10.1007/978-3-030-12741-1_13) contains supplementary material, which is available to authorized users.

C. Fritz
Internal Medicine, Washington University School of Medicine/Barnes Jewish Hospital, Saint Louis, MO, USA

G. D. Lang (✉)
Division of Gastroenterology, Washington University in Saint Louis, Saint Louis, MO, USA
e-mail: gabriellang@wustl.edu

D. K. Mullady (ed.), *Dilemmas in ERCP*,
https://doi.org/10.1007/978-3-030-12741-1_13

channel, and high rates of complications [2]. The initial approach, the mother-daughter cholangioscopy (MDC), provides a high visual sensitivity and accuracy. Unfortunately, the reusable scope is easily damaged and requires two operators, two light sources, and two video monitors [3].

Direct peroral cholangioscopy (DPOC), which is a single-operator system, provides the highest-resolution images, precise tip control, and larger working channel but has been reported to be operationally challenging [3].

Single-operator cholangioscopy (SOC) requires only one endoscopist, allows for visually directed biopsies, and is reported to be easier to use due to its four-way tip deflection of at least 30 degrees in all directions [4] . The single-operator cholangioscope is passed through the working channel (4.2 mm) of a standard therapeutic duodenoscope. The device is approved by the Food and Drug Administration for both biliary and pancreatic indications. The scope uses 10 French access, a 1.2 mm working channel (for passing guidewires, lithotripsy probes, and miniature forceps), and two irrigation channels. Moreover, the scope is disposable, which mitigates concerns about scope damage and scope sterilization. Initially, this modality was noted to have lower resolution due to the fiber-optic probe and limited durability [3], but more recent versions with digital imaging have significantly improved image quality. These innovations have demonstrated an improved detection of malignancy over combination endoscopic retrograde cholangiopancreatography (ERCP) techniques [5, 6].

In this chapter we will focus on the use of cholangioscopy in the evaluation of indeterminate biliary strictures, stone disease, and alternative uses of cholangioscopy including challenging wire placement during ERCP.

Case 1

A 48-year-old male presents with biliary colic for 1 month and was found to have elevated liver function tests, most notably a total bilirubin of 2.3 mg/dL. An ERCP was performed, which revealed a dilated common bile duct and

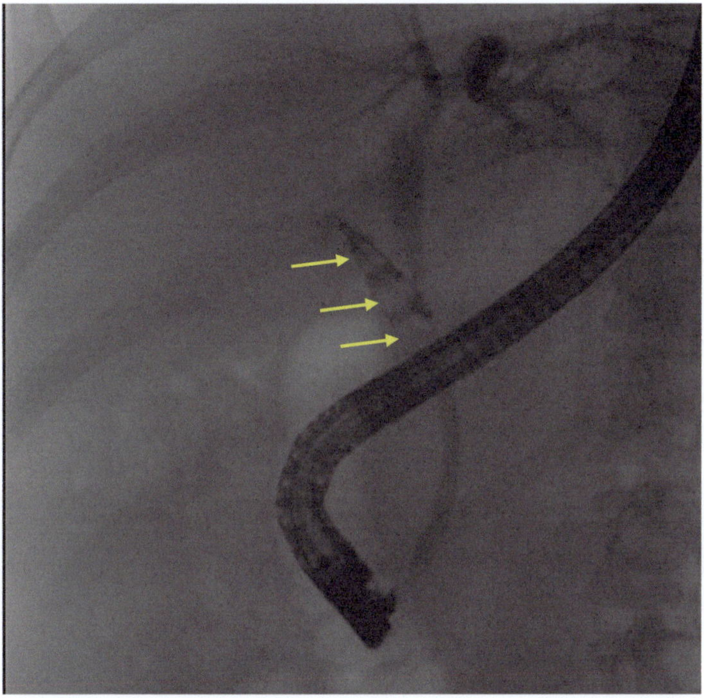

FIGURE 13.1 Cholangiogram revealing extrinsic compression of common hepatic duct by multiple stones in the cystic duct (arrows) consistent with Mirizzi syndrome

numerous cystic duct stones concerning for Mirizzi syndrome (Fig. 13.1). Due to a small distal common bile duct, the stones were unable to be removed, and a plastic biliary stent was placed. Subsequently, the patient was taken for a cholecystectomy. The gallbladder was contracted, necrotic, and highly inflamed. As such, complete dissection of the cystic duct could not be performed, and the patient was referred following cholecystectomy for a second ERCP with stone removal. ERCP was performed with the assistance of SOC and electrohydraulic lithotripsy (EHL). The stones were fragmented and removed (Video 13.1). The patient tolerated the procedure well and was discharged on 5 days of ciprofloxacin.

Diagnosis and Assessment

Patients with large bile duct stones most commonly present with biliary colic and elevated liver function tests. They may also present with cholangitis or acute pancreatitis. MRCP and endoscopic ultrasound (EUS) are more sensitive for the detection of common bile duct stones compared to transabdominal ultrasound or computed tomography (CT) scans. Unfortunately, it is challenging to determine if a stone will be difficult to remove until visualized by ERCP. Factors that may make a bile duct stone difficult to remove include large size, small size of downstream bile duct, stacked stones, impacted stones, those located proximal to a bile duct stricture, and inability to perform a large sphincterotomy. The treatment aim for these patients is to decompress the bile duct in as few procedures as possible. If the patient is hemodynamically unstable or has cholangitis, a stent can be placed to temporize the situation until the patient is stable enough to endure a longer endoscopic procedure.

Treatment and Management

Common bile duct stones have typically been treated with biliary sphincterotomy and extraction of stones with a balloon catheter or basket. Unfortunately, 10–15% of stones are unable to be removed with standard techniques [7]. Although there is no standard defining size for large bile duct stones, stones larger than 15 mm have proven to be difficult to extract [8]. Stone fragmentation improves duct clearance and stone removal, which traditionally has been accomplished with mechanical lithotripsy. Endoscopic papillary large balloon dilation (EPLBD) has also been utilized as an alternative or adjunct to endoscopic sphincterotomy.

In the past, a failed conventional ERCP would have led to a common bile duct exploration. Patients with previous cholecystectomy would have had an additional surgery for a common bile duct exploration and stone removal. Although surgical intervention has historically been required, the use of cholangioscopy has significantly improved the treatment of difficult biliary stones. Peroral cholangioscopy can be combined with laser lithotripsy (LL) or EHL to effectively treat complicated or large bile duct stones [9]. The stone clearance rate with the use of cholangioscopy is cited to be 88% from a pooled analysis [10].

Single-operator cholangioscopy (SOC) with lithotripsy provides direct visualization of stone fragmentation during each procedure and minimizes bile or pancreatic duct injury. EHL uses saline irrigation to complete shock wave energy transmission, while LL uses laser light to induce wave-mediated fragmentation [8]. Either mechanism is enhanced by the direct visualization of SOC as to confirm that shock waves are directed appropriately at the stone and not the bile duct wall. Overall, the adverse event rate is cited to be 7% [8].

In order to perform SOC, copious amounts of water may need to be instilled. Therefore, it is recommended that patients are intubated prior to the procedure. Of note, many practitioners caution against the instillation of a large amount of contrast prior to performing cholangioscopy as this may inhibit full visualization, although these concerns seem to have been diminished with newer iterations of this device. Next, cannulation of the CBD with the cholangioscope can be performed with or without the use of a guidewire. Instillation of 0.9% normal saline helps conduct an electrical impulse necessary for EHL. The cholangioscope is then advanced to the level of the stone via both fluoroscopy and direct visualization. Once the stone is visualized, the EHL probe can be advanced out of the cholangioscope and into direct contact with the stone and then pulled back ever so slightly. The optimal distance between EHL tip and the stone is 2–3 mm. There may be difficulty in advancing the EHL probe out of the cholangioscope. If difficulties are encountered, one can consider unlocking all wheels. Second, the EHL probe can to be advanced out of the cholangioscope while in the duodenum and left at the tip of the cholangioscope prior to entering the bile duct. Simultaneous saline instillation and application of current is then performed. Initial power and frequency are set to the lowest settings and can be increased as needed for effective fragmentation. During the procedure, shocks are created that produce high-amplitude hydraulic pressure waves for stone fragmentation. The generator produces high-voltage electrical impulses at a frequency of 1–20 per second at a power range of 50–100 watts. After the stone is fragmented, the cholangioscope is withdrawn, and fragments are removed via traditional ERCP methods. Due to fragility of the probe, it may take more than one EHL probe to fragment a stone. Once stone debris is removed, the cholangioscope can be reinserted into the duct to confirm stone clearance. If the stones cannot be completely removed, a stent is reinserted until re-treatment. With laser lithotripsy, light of a particular wavelength is focused on the stone to induce a wave-mediated fragmentation. It must be noted that this technique is less efficacious on stones which are mobile within the common bile duct, as a stable position for lithotripsy is difficult to achieve.

Outcomes

A multicenter retrospective analysis compared LL to EHL with regard to procedure time and stone clearance rate. Procedure time was found to be longer in EHL, but stone clearance rate was similar (around 80%) for both groups [11]. Fewer than 5% of patients from either group required additional surgical intervention [11]. Moreover, a randomized study compared conventional therapies (mechanical lithotripsy and endoscopic papillary large balloon dilation) to cholangioscopy-guided LL and found that cholangioscopy-guided LL had longer procedural times, but increased stone clearance rates with similar adverse event rates [11]. Therefore, SOC-guided LL and EHL are thought to be useful for clearance of difficult bile duct stones with similar rates of adverse events.

Interestingly, a meta-regression analysis demonstrated a statistically significant difference between stone clearance rate and type of cholangioscope used; specifically the highest rates of success have been achieved with single-operator cholangioscopy [10]. In this meta-analysis the overall stone clearance for SOC-guided therapy was 88% (95% CI [85%–91%]) [10]. The adverse event rate was 7% with a severe adverse event rate of 1%. A retrospective study evaluating 306 patients with SOC at 22 tertiary care centers found that ducts were completely cleared in 97.3% of patients and 77.4% had duct clearance in a single session. The authors concluded that this procedure was safe in greater than 95% of patients with difficult or large biliary stones [11]. A multicenter experience of 69 patients utilizing LL in patients who had a minimum of one failed ERCP for stone extraction required a mean of 1.2 LL sessions to achieve a 97% clearance rate and a 4% adverse event rate [12].

In a similar manner to SOC with EHL or LL in the bile duct, peroral pancreatoscopy can be performed instead of extracorporeal shock wave lithotripsy (ESWL) as a primary modality in patients with large main pancreatic duct stones. A study involving 39 patients who underwent peroral pancreatoscopy demonstrated complete or partial stone clearance in 91%, with complete clearance in 70%. There was no difference between groups who underwent SOC or endoscope-based pancreatoscopy. The overall clinical success at median follow-up of 15 months was 74% [13]. In addition, a retrospective study at 4 tertiary care centers found 28 patients who underwent peroral pancreatoscopy. Technical success occurred in 22 patients (79%) with complete ductal clearance. Clinical success at a median of 13 months was noted in 25/28 (89%) as judged by an improvement in pain, decreased narcotic use, or reduced hospitalizations [14].

Case 2

A 74-year-old female with no significant past medical history presents with painless jaundice (total bilirubin of 13.6 mg/dL). An ERCP was performed at an outside hospital, which

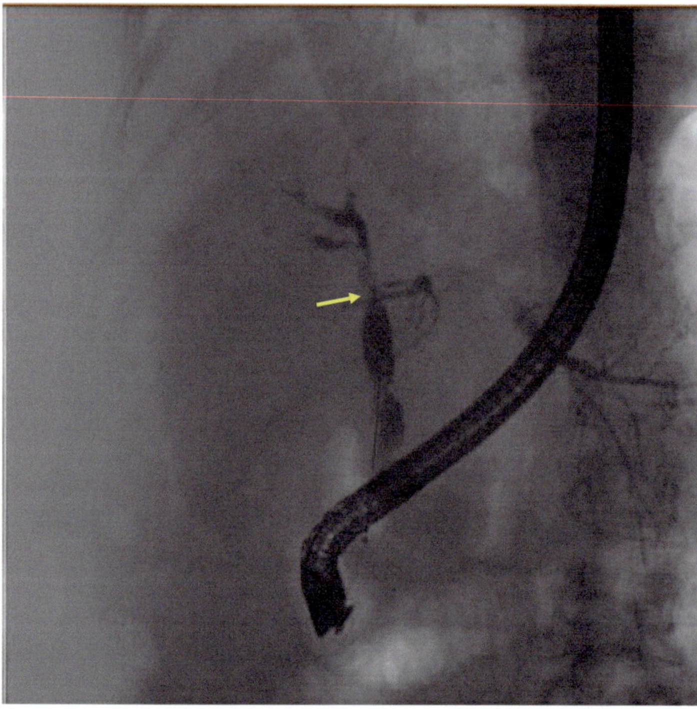

FIGURE 13.2 Malignant-appearing hilar stricture (arrow)

revealed a hilar stricture. Brushings of the stricture were performed which revealed atypical cells. Bilateral plastic stents were placed. She was referred to our center for ERCP, which re-demonstrated the stricture (Fig. 13.2). Brushings for cytology and FISH were obtained from the stricture. SOC showed dilated and tortuous blood vessels as well as areas of ulceration (Fig. 13.3). Brushings again returned negative, but SOC-assisted biopsies demonstrated adenocarcinoma (Video 13.2).

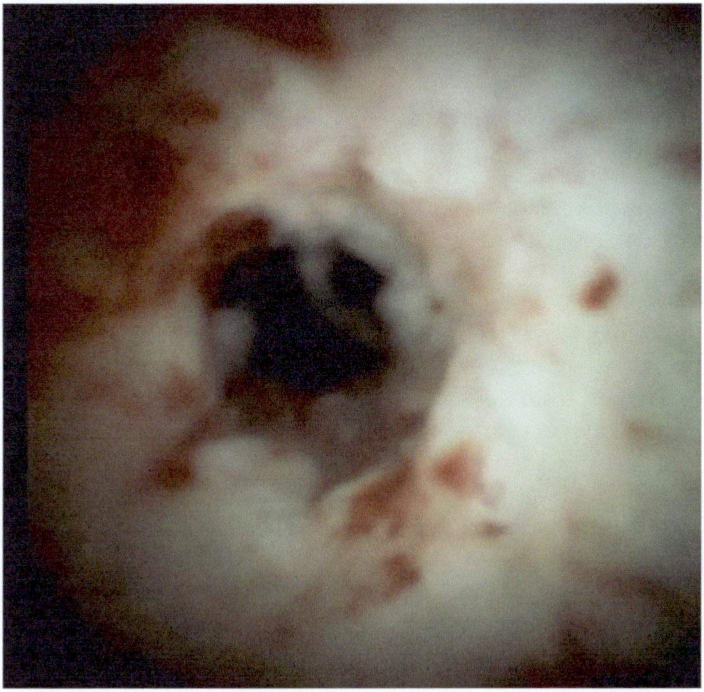

FIGURE 13.3 Cholangioscopic appearance of stricture with friable, ulcerated tissue and tortuous blood vessels, all consistent with malignancy

Diagnosis/Assessment

Biliary strictures are considered indeterminate after basic laboratory work-up, cross-sectional imaging, and ERCP with biliary sampling are all nondiagnostic. Unfortunately, there are no perfect clinical or radiologic features to distinguish benign from malignant strictures. A cholestatic pattern of liver chemistries, especially those with very abnormal liver chemistries, has a higher likelihood of malignancy. Serum CA 19-9 and CEA levels have been used in clinical practice to help identify those with hepatobiliary malignancies. Yet CA

19-9 levels can be elevated in patients with any cause of biliary obstruction, as well as cirrhosis and gastric cancer.

Furthermore, many of the benign etiologies, including primary sclerosing cholangitis and IgG4-related sclerosing cholangitis, place patients at increased risk for developing malignancy, which only complicates the diagnostic process [15]. Cholangiocarcinoma and pancreatic adenocarcinoma are the most common causes of biliary strictures [15]. Yet previous studies have demonstrated that 5% to 15% of patients who undergo surgical resection prove to have benign pathology [16, 17]. Unfortunately, there is a lack of consensus on pre-surgical resection features to confirm benign etiology [18]. Therefore, determining benign from malignant etiologies is of the utmost importance given the morbidity and mortality associated with surgery, chemotherapy, and radiation.

Historically, ERCP has been the primary pre-surgical technique to determine biliary pathology. Tissue sampling with ERCP is safe and inexpensive and therefore can be widely used. Yet obtaining adequate specimen cellularity with ERCP tissue sampling has proved difficult in a number of situations including severely narrowed strictures, proximal lesions, tumors associated with ulceration or fibrosis, lesions with submucosal spread, and extrinsic mass lesions [4].

ERCP with intraductal brush cytology is still the first-line approach for specimen sampling. While this approach is the most convenient for tissue sampling and has a high specificity at 99%, its sensitivity has been cited to be as low as 36% to 45% [5, 19].

Although a number of factors including the experience of the pathologist can affect sensitivity [20], cancer detection rates using brush cytology can vary drastically depending on the type of cancer. Cancer detection rates with brush cytology are reportedly the highest for cholangiocarcinoma at 63% while cited to be only 37% for pancreatic cancer detection from a pooled analysis [19]. Other technical modifications have been attempted to increase sensitivity. For example, repeat brushing has been shown to increase diagnostic yield by about 9% [4]. Overall, ERCP with brush cytology is safe and provides excellent specificity but lacks adequate sensitivity.

Sampling using intraductal biopsy forceps is a more challenging and time-consuming procedure and therefore is used less frequently. This procedure generally requires a sphincterotomy to allow passage of the forceps through the papilla. Fluoroscopy is used to advance the forceps to the distal area of the stricture where blind specimen collection can be obtained. There is consensus that at least three specimens should be obtained during this procedure to increase sensitivity [21]. Similar to ERCP with brush cytology, specificity is high at 99% [5]. Yet even with a deeper tissue sample, ERCP fluoroscopic-guided forceps biopsy continues to be limited by low sensitivity at 48% [5]. ERCP with forceps biopsy is a relatively safe procedure, and adverse events are rarely reported in the literature. Of the few adverse reports, bleeding and perforation have been documented [22, 23]. Although sampling with ERCP biopsy allows for increased tissue sampling, this procedure is still limited by sensitivity and technical difficulty and appears to have more adverse events than ERCP with brush cytology.

When ERCP with brush cytology and forceps biopsy are combined, sensitivity improves to 70% [23]. Combination sampling has also been shown to have a higher cancer detection rate than either single modality.

FISH is a cytogenetic technique that requires fewer cells than cytology and capitalizes on the increased aneuploidy of cancer cells. When FISH is used as a single modality, sensitivity is only 52%; but when used in concert with brush cytology, sensitivity increases to 89% [24].

Although ERCP and MRCP are the primary methods for determining biliary strictures, it is important to mention EUS as an important modality when the work-up for a biliary stricture is nondiagnostic. A study in 2014 directly compared EUS-FNA and ERCP tissue sampling in a prospective, single-blind study [25]. This study demonstrated that sensitivity of EUS-FNA was 80% for biliary strictures, which was greater than the sensitivity reported from ERCP with cytology and forceps at 67%. Of note, EUS is more likely to detect a distal than proximal cholangiocarcinoma [26]. EUS has a sensitivity of 53% when utilized to determine unresectability for preoperative planning. Although EUS-FNA can provide increased sensitivity and is becoming more widespread in use, it is important to remember that EUS-FNA is less sensitive for proximal bile duct lesions and sampling should not be obtained in all cases, as it can preclude patients from future transplantation [27].

Treatment/Management

Improvements in cholangioscopy technology are increasingly important for indeterminate biliary strictures, especially when the clinical suspicion for malignancy is high. When reviewing all biliary strictures evaluated by cholangioscopy prior to the newest generation of SOC in 2015, a pooled analysis found cholangioscopy-guided biopsies had a sensitivity of 60% and specificity of 98%, which is a significant improvement when compared to conventional ERCP techniques [5].

The newest generation SOC has the ability to diagnosis biliary disease through visual impression (VI) and miniature forceps biopsies (MFB) with further improved sensitivity. In a meta-analysis including older and newer generation SOC, VI and MFB demonstrated high combined sensitivity at 90% with a slight reduction in specificity at 87% [28]. Utilizing a combined approach is best for diagnosing malignancy. By using VI to potentially detect malignancy and MFB to help confirm malignancy [28], it is important to note that even with combining modalities, clinical suspicion for malignancy should remain high.

SOC has a 1.2 mm accessory channel that permits passage of miniature forceps (width of 4.1 mm) as well as a 6000-pixel optical probe providing a 70-degree field of view, as well as a high definition resolution for optimum visualization.

Maneuvering the SOC for the evaluation of indeterminate strictures is similar to the technique used for large bile duct stones. The SOC system is advanced into the bile duct over a guidewire or in a freehand fashion. The probe is then advanced under direct and fluoroscopic visualization to the level of the stricture. Locking the dials of the cholangioscope can help stabilize the position. Irrigating the bile duct with water helps with visualization. Once in position, biopsies of the affected mucosa can be obtained. It is helpful to deflect the probe tip to try and sample the stricture or abnormal mucosa in four quadrants. Prior studies have found that exophytic lesions, papillary mucosal projections, ulceration, and dilated tortuous vessels are suggestive of malignancy [29]. Some centers have direct on-site pathology available for immediate evaluation of biopsies. This is usually achieved by smearing a sample between two slides ("smash protocol") followed by staining similar to immediate cytologic evaluation. This may improve the diagnostic yield of sampling.

Outcomes

When only assessing studies utilizing newer generation SOC, sensitivity was improved to 95.5% while maintaining specificity at 94.5% [9]. The improvements in sensitivity are attributed to the improvements in visualization with the newer scopes. Meaning, newer SOC has the highest rates of sensitivity and specificity for diagnosis of malignancy to date.

Although VI demonstrates high sensitivity, currently there is no standard classification system for malignancy utilizing visual impression as a stand-alone technique. Sampling indeterminate biliary strictures with SOC has its challenges and limitations, but acquiring multiple biopsies appears to improve rates of sensitivity. A recent study suggests at least five biopsies for each lesion should be obtained to improve histologically diagnosis [9].

As far as safety, SOC provides more detailed information about indeterminate biliary strictures without significant increased procedural risk when compared to ERCP [30]. The adverse event rate has been cited to be between 7% and 13%, including pancreatitis, cholangitis, and perforation [9, 30]. The severe adverse event rate is cited to be only 1%, which included perforation [10]. A recent multicenter analysis found mortality after SOC to be 0% [9]. This study also reiterated the use of single-shot peri-interventional antibiotic as a best practice. When comparing patients who received antibiotics to those who did not, rates of cholangitis increased from 1% to 12.8% [9].

Pooled studies have shown that the sensitivity of cholangioscopy with intraductal biopsy has a sensitivity of 92%, specificity of 93%, and diagnostic accuracy of 93% compared to 66%, 51%, and 55%, respectively, with standard ERCP brush cytology. MFB associated with SOC allows for adequate histologic specimens in >95% of cases. Navaneethan et al. prospectively studied 36 patients with indeterminate strictures who underwent SOC and MFB [5]. Four biopsy specimens were obtained in 33 cases. Twenty-two patients were diagnosed with malignancy, and SOC biopsies yielded diagnoses in 18 of those 22 patients. In this study, the overall sensitivity and specificity for visual impression were 95% and 79%, while SOC biopsies had a sensitivity of 82% [5].

The first US multicenter study using the new SOC included 85 patients for stricture or ductal evaluation. Eight of these patients underwent cholangioscopy to assess the extent of tumor, while the remaining 77 has indeterminate strictures. Forty percent of these patients had neoplasia of which 81% were confirmed with SOC biopsies. In this study, the sensitivity, specificity, positive predictive value, and negative predictive value of SOC biopsies were 97%, 96%, 94%, and 98% [31].

In a systematic review involving 10 studies and 456 patients, the pooled sensitivity and specificity of cholangioscopy-assisted biopsies were 60.1% and 98%, respectively. Among studies in which patients had nondiagnostic work-up including imaging, brushing, or biopsies, the pooled sensitivity and specificity were 74.7% and 93.3%. The pooled sensitivity and specificity to detect CCA were 66.2% and 97% [32].

Case 3

A 67-year-old female with metastatic breast cancer presented with jaundice secondary to biliary obstruction. The patient had a metallic biliary stent and enteral stent placed 5 months ago for malignant biliary obstruction and gastric outlet obstruction. After cannulating the biliary stent through the interstices of the enteral stent, contrast was injected, and a completely obstructed bile duct was encountered (Fig. 13.4). Despite pressure injection and the use of multiple slim and angled wires, the obstruction could not be traversed.

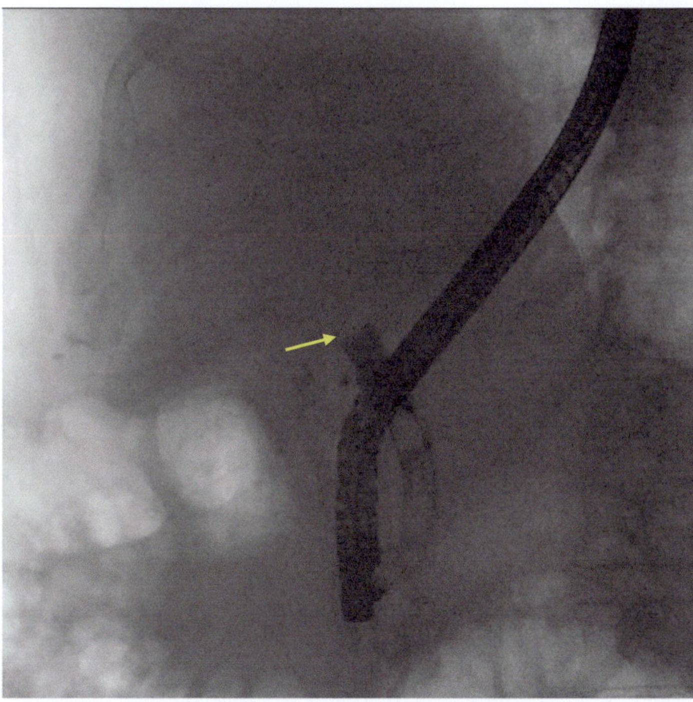

FIGURE 13.4 Completely obstructed bile duct (arrow) at proximal aspect of previously placed metallic biliary stent

Ultimately, DPOC was utilized. The upper endoscope was advanced to the level of the stricture. At this level, there was dense tissue ingrowth, and the bile duct appeared completely obstructed. Again, multiple unsuccessful attempts were made to probe the stricture with the guidewire under direct endoscopic visualization with the choledochoscope. The mucosa in this area was edematous from previous attempts at guidewire passage as well as a submucosal injection. Then, a punctate area of bile staining was noted (Fig. 13.5). Once the bile stain was probed with the guidewire, there was no resistance in

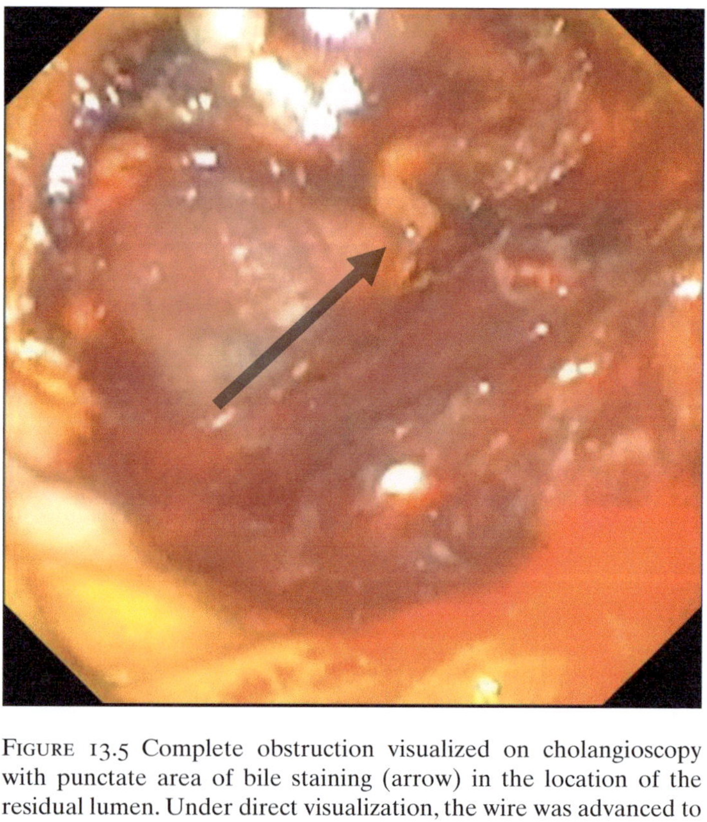

Figure 13.5 Complete obstruction visualized on cholangioscopy with punctate area of bile staining (arrow) in the location of the residual lumen. Under direct visualization, the wire was advanced to this area and into the intrahepatic ducts

guidewire passage up the biliary tree. The choledocoscope was then removed and the wire left in place. The bile duct was then cannulated with a balloon over a wire, and a cholangiogram was obtained, which demonstrated a single severe stenosis in the upper third of the bile duct. Then, a 10 mm × 8 cm uncovered metal stent was placed (Video 13.3). Ultimately, the jaundice resolved.

Diagnosis/Assessment

Manipulating a guidewire to reach difficult to access targets can be one of the most technically challenging aspects of ERCP. Generally, when ERCP is unsuccessful, it's because the guidewire is unable to cross an obstructed or difficult to opacify bile duct, especially in cases of hilar cholangiocarcinoma or transpapillary cystic duct stents. When an obstructed bile duct is encountered, diagnostic maneuvers are limited to blind passaging of the guidewire and performing an occlusion cholangiogram to look for a trickle of contrast in order to mark the area of interest. If these maneuvers fail, EUS-guided access or percutaneous transhepatic cholangiography in interventional radiology can be attempted.

Proximally migrated biliary and pancreatic duct stents can be an immediate problem of stent mal-deployment during ERCP or occur as a late complication. It is important to remove migrated stents as the stent itself, or the buildup that occurs around these stents, can lead to pancreatitis or jaundice.

Treatment/Management

Cholangioscopy can be used to help gain access to difficult biliary targets. The cholangioscope is maneuvered within the bile duct, and the specific target is directly visualized. The duct itself or bile staining can be used to probe with a guidewire under both direct endoscopic and fluoroscopic guidance. Once the wire is in position, the cholangioscope can be removed, and the remainder of the ERCP can be performed in a traditional fashion.

Migrated stents are typically removed via balloon sweeps or with the aid of a basket. If this approach fails, biopsy forceps can be utilized under fluoroscopic visualization to grasp and remove the stent. Oftentimes, the migrated stents can move proximally as further attempts are made to retrieve them. Care should be taken to avoid causing a bile/pancreatic duct leak in the process of stent removal. If other measures fail, a cholangioscope can be inserted and the miniature forceps can be utilized to grasp the stent under direct visualization. In the near future, a small basket will be available to use with the single-operator cholangioscope.

Outcomes

Published literature is sparse in this area, but the authors' experience with the use of cholangioscopy for accessing difficult targets and removing migrated stents has been encouraging.

Pearls and Pitfalls

- Given the water insufflation that is needed to achieve good visualization with SOC, we recommend elective intubation of patients undergoing this procedure.
- Due to the risk of cholangitis with cholangioscopy, we recommend intraprocedure antibiotic administration as well as post-procedure antibiotics.
- Cholangioscopy with EHL/LL is a very effective treatment for difficult biliary stones. This technique may take numerous sessions to achieve ductal clearance. Placing the lithotripter catheter within 2–3 mm of the stone optimizes stone destruction.
- Cholangioscopy-assisted treatment of difficult bile duct stones works best for stones which are not mobile within the common bile duct. Mobile stones will cause the practitioner to "chase" the stone up the bile duct.

- Use lithotripsy to help fragment the stone, and then use balloons and baskets to clear the duct. Once the duct appears clear, reinsert the cholangioscope to ensure ductal clearance.
- Cholangioscopy should be a part of the algorithm in the work-up of indeterminate strictures. The use of cholangioscopy can occur either concomitantly with cytology and intraductal biopsies or at the second ERCP after traditional sampling techniques have failed to yield a diagnosis.
- Taking many four quadrant biopsies helps in obtaining a diagnosis. While studies suggest greater than four passes, it has been the authors' experience that eight or more biopsies are often needed.
- Avoid using water insufflation when taking biopsies as the water will knock the specimen off the forceps.
- Using cholangioscopy for reaching difficult to access targets is easy and clinically useful. Searching for minute areas of bile staining can be helpful. Cases in which this may be of use are hilar strictures, completely obstructed bile ducts, and finding the cystic duct when placing transpapillary gallbladder stents.

References

1. Anderson MA, et al. The role of endoscopy in the evaluation and treatment of patients with biliary neoplasia. Gastrointest Endosc. 2013;77(2):167–74.
2. Laleman W, Verraes K, Steenbergen W, et al. Usefulness of the single-operator cholangioscopy system SpyGlass in biliary disease: a single-center prospective cohort study and aggregated review. Surg Endosc. 2017;31:2223–32.
3. Thaker A, Muthusamy VR. The role and utility of cholangioscopy for diagnosing indeterminate biliary strictures. Gastrointest Interv. 2017;6(1):2–8.

4. Korc P, Sherman S. ERCP tissue sampling. Gastrointest Endosc. 2016;84(4):557–71.
5. Navaneethan U, Njei B, Lourdusamy V, et al. Comparative effectiveness of biliary cytology and intraductal biopsy for detection of malignant biliary strictures: a systematic review and meta-analysis. Gastrointest Endosc. 2015;81:168–76.
6. Draganov PV, Chauhan S, Wagh MS. Diagnostic accuracy of conventional and cholangioscopy-guided sampling of indeterminate biliary lesions at the time of ERCP: a prospective, long-term follow-up study. Gastrointest Endosc. 2012;75(2):347–53.
7. McHenry L, Lehman G. Difficult bile duct stones. Curr Treat Options Gastroenterol. 2006;9:123–32.
8. Doshi B, Yasuda I, Ryozawa S, et al. Current endoscopic strategies for managing large bile duct stones. Dig Endosc. 2018;30(Suppl. 1):59–66.
9. Turowski F, Hügle U, Dormann A, et al. Diagnostic and therapeutic single-operator cholangiopancreatoscopy with SpyGlassDS: results of a multicenter retrospective cohort study. Surg Endosc. 2018;32(9):3981–8.
10. Korrapati P, Ciolino J, Wani S, et al. The efficacy of peroral cholangioscopy for difficult bile duct stones and indeterminate strictures: a systematic review and meta-analysis. Endosc Int Open. 2016;4:E263–75.
11. Brewer G, Bekkali NLH, Raijman I, et al. Efficacy and safety of digital single-operator cholangioscopy for difficult biliary stones. Clinc Gastroenterol Hepatol. 2017;16(6):918–26.
12. Patel SN, Rosenkranz L, Hooks B, et al. Holmium-yttrium aluminum garnet laser lithotripsy in the treatment of biliary calculi using single-operator cholangioscopy: a multicenter experience (with video). Gastrointest Endosc. 2014;79(2):344–8.
13. Attwell AR, Brauer BC, Chen YK, et al. Endoscopic retrograde cholangiopancreatography with per oral pancreatoscopy for calcific chronic pancreatitis using endoscope and catheter-based pancreatoscopes: a 10-year single-center experience. Pancreas. 2014;43(2):268–74.
14. Attwell AR, Patel S, Kahaleh M, et al. ERCP with per-oral pancreatoscopy–guided laser lithotripsy for calcific chronic pancreatitis: a multicenter US experience. Gastrointest Endosc. 2015;82(2):311–8.
15. Bowlus CL, Olson KA, Gershwin ME. Evaluation of indeterminate biliary strictures. Nat Rev Gastroenterol Hepatol. 2016;13(1):28–37.

16. Wakai T, Shirai Y, Sakata J, et al. Clinicopathological features of benign biliary strictures masquerading as biliary malignancy. Am Surg. 2012;78(12):1388–91.
17. Gerhards M, Vos P, van Gulik TM, et al. Incidence of benign lesions in patients resected for suspicious hilar obstruction. Br J Surg. 2002;88(1):48–51.
18. Corvera C, Blumgart LH, Darvishian F, et al. Clinical and pathologic features of proximal biliary Stricuters masquerading as hilar cholangiocarcinoma. J Am Coll Surg. 2005;201(6):862–9.
19. Fukuda Y, Tsuyuguchi T, Sakai Y, et al. Diagnostic utility of peroral cholangioscopy for various bile-duct lesions. Gastrointest Endosc. 2005;62(3):374 to 382.
20. Stewart CJR, Mills PR, Garter R. Brush cytology in the assessment of pancreatico-biliary strictures: a review of 406 cases. J Clin Pathol. 2001;54(6):449–55.
21. Kimura H, Matsubayashi H, Saski K, et al. Factors affecting the yield of endoscopic transpapillary bile duct biopsy for the diagnosis of pancreatic head cancer. Pancreatology. 2013;13(5):524–9.
22. Pugliese V, Conio M, Nicolo G. Endoscopic retrograde forceps biopsy and brush cytology of biliary strictures: a prospective study. Gastrointest Endosc. 1995;42(6):520–6.
23. Schoefl R, Haefner M, Wrba F. Forceps biopsy and brush cytology during endoscopic retrograde cholangiopancreatography for the diagnosis of biliary stenosis. Scand J Gastroenterol. 1997;32(4):363–8.
24. Smoczynski M, Jablonska A, Matyskiel A. Routine brush cytology and fluorescence in situ hybridization for assessment of pancreatobiliary strictures. Gastrointest Endosc. 2012;75(1):65–73.
25. Weilert F, Bhat YM, Binmoeller KF. EUS-FNA is superior to ERCP-based tissue sampling in suspected malignant biliary obstruction: results of a prospective, single-blind, comparative study. Gastrointest Endosc. 2014;80(1):97–104.
26. Mohamadnejad M, JM DW, Sherman S, et al. Role of EUS for preoperative evaluation of cholangiocarcinoma: a large single-center experience. Gastrointest Endosc. 2011;73(1):71–8.
27. Heimbach JK, Sanchez W, Rosen CB. Trans-peritoneal fine needle aspiration biopsy of hilar cholangiocarcinoma is associated with disease dissemination. HPB. 2011;12(5):356–60.
28. Sun X, Zhou Z, Tian J, et al. Is single-operator peroral cholangioscopy a useful tool for the diagnosis of indeterminate biliary lesion? A systematic review and meta-analysis. Gastrointest Endosc. 2015;82:79–87.

29. Shah RJ, Langer DA, Antillon MR. Cholangioscopy and cholangioscopic forceps biopsy in patients with indeterminate pancreaticobiliary pathology. Clin Gastroenterol Hepatol. 2006;4(2):219–25.
30. Hammerle CW, Haider S, Chung M, et al. Endoscopic retrograde cholangiopancreatography complications in the era of cholangioscopy: is there an increased risk? Dig Liver Dis. 2012;44(9):754–8.
31. Shah R, Robert H, Brauer BC, et al. 346 a US multi-center first human use experience using the fully disposable, digital single-operator cholangiopancreatoscope (DSOCP). Gastrointest Endosc. 2016;83(5):AB141.
32. Navaneethan U, Hasan MK, Lourdusamy V, et al. Single-operator cholangioscopy and targeted biopsies in the diagnosis of indeterminate biliary strictures: a systematic review. Gastrointest Endosc. 2015;82(4):608–14.

Chapter 14
Post-ERCP Pancreatitis

Ernesto M. Llano and Christopher G. Chapman

Case Presentation

A 36-year-old woman presents with a history of recurrent acute pancreatitis. She has had three episodes of documented acute pancreatitis confirmed by the revised Atlanta classification. She does not drink alcohol or smoke cigarettes and has normal serum triglyceride levels and liver enzymes. She has a history of obesity, hypertension, and gastroesophageal reflux disease – treated with amlodipine and pantoprazole, respectively. She has no family history of pancreatitis.

During her prior admissions, the episodes of pancreatitis were uncomplicated and resolved with supportive care. CT examinations demonstrated peripancreatic fat stranding without biliary dilation or pancreatic fluid collections. MRCP demonstrated no anatomic ductal variants.

Electronic Supplementary Material The online version of this chapter (https://doi.org/10.1007/978-3-030-12741-1_14) contains supplementary material, which is available to authorized users.

E. M. Llano · C. G. Chapman (✉)
University of Chicago Medicine, Center for Endoscopic Research and Therapeutics (CERT), Chicago, IL, USA
e-mail: christopher.chapman@uchospitals.edu

D. K. Mullady (ed.), *Dilemmas in ERCP*,
https://doi.org/10.1007/978-3-030-12741-1_14

She undergoes an endoscopic ultrasound (EUS) at an outside hospital facility, which identifies a small, 2 mm stone that is seen in a 4 mm main pancreatic duct. Thought to be contributing to her symptoms, she undergoes ERCP for removal of this stone. Rectal indomethacin is administered for pharmacoprophylaxis of post-ERCP pancreatitis. During the ERCP, the ventral pancreatic duct is deeply cannulated, contrast is injected, and a single stone is seen. A ventral pancreatic sphincterotomy is made using electrocautery. The ventral pancreatic duct is swept with an 8.5 mm balloon, and a 5 Fr by 5 cm plastic pancreatic stent is placed into the ventral pancreatic duct. After the procedure, the patient has significant epigastric pain with an elevated serum lipase and is admitted for post-ERCP pancreatitis. She is managed with aggressive intravenous hydration, nutritional support, and pain control and is discharged home after 3 days.

She transfers care to our institution for further assessment and management of her recurrent acute pancreatitis. Abdominal X-ray confirms retained pancreatic duct stent, and she undergoes endoscopy for pancreatic duct stent removal. During the endoscopy, her stent is removed, and she is noted to have a mildly prominent ampulla. Biopsies are performed and are consistent with a villous adenoma.

The ampullary adenoma is determined to be the likely cause of her recurrent acute pancreatitis, and the patient returns for ERCP and endoscopic ampullectomy (Video 14.1). Upon initial inspection, a 12 mm villous mass is seen at the major papilla. A 0.025 inch guidewire is passed into the biliary tree, and a sphincterotome is passed over the guidewire to deeply cannulate the bile duct, contrast is injected, and a sphincterotomy is made with electrocautery. Next, the 0.025 guidewire is passed into the ventral pancreatic duct. This is also deeply cannulated with the sphincterotome, and contrast is injected. Using a 15 mm snare, the major papilla is grasped and then resected using electrocautery. A small villous area is noted at the pancreatic duct orifice and is biopsied. After resection, a guidewire is again passed into the ventral pancreatic duct, and a 5 Fr by 3 cm plastic pancreatic stent with a full external pigtail and a single internal flap is placed. Similarly, a guidewire is passed into the bile duct, and a 7 Fr by 7 cm plastic biliary stent with a single external flap and a single internal flap is placed with fluid flowing through both stents. Pathologic analysis confirms a diagnosis of ampullary adenoma but unfortunately with residual adenoma at the pancreatic duct orifice. The patient is initially discharged home after 24-hour observation but admitted 2 days later for another episode of post-ERCP pancreatitis. Abdominal radiograph confirms premature pancreatic duct stent migration. She receives supportive care and is discharged home 2 days later.

Introduction

Endoscopic retrograde cholangiopancreatography (ERCP) provides the ability to detect, classify, and provide therapy for diseases involving the pancreaticobiliary system. Despite being introduced in the late 1960s, it remains one of the most technically challenging and high-risk endoscopic procedures performed. Complications arising from ERCP can include post-ERCP pancreatitis (PEP), bleeding, perforation, cholecystitis, and cholangitis. Of these complications, PEP is the most frequent and can lead to significant morbidity and occasionally mortality.

Due in part to the risk of complications and the advancements in EUS and cross-sectional radiologic imaging techniques, namely, magnetic resonance cholangiopancreatography (MRCP), ERCP has transitioned primarily to pancreatobiliary therapeutics. However, advances in technology built on the scaffold of ERCP, including intraductal ultrasound, direct cholangioscopy, and pancreatoscopy, have secured ERCP as an obligate endoscopic procedure for clinical problems involving the pancreatic duct and hepatobiliary system. Therefore, understanding the definition, patient and procedural risk factors, and preventative management strategies for PEP are critical for any therapeutic endoscopist practicing ERCP.

Diagnosis/Assessment

Incidence and Definition

Post-ERCP pancreatitis (PEP) is the most common complication of ERCP (Table 14.1). Prospective, multicenter studies have examined the frequency of PEP and found incidence rates ranging from 3% to 15% for the average-risk population with approximately 5% of patients developing a severe course [1–9]. In high-risk stratified cohorts, the risk of PEP has been reported to range from 15% to 25%.

Two recent large cohort studies evaluate the incidence of PEP in which the reported incidence rate of PEP has been estimated to be 3.5% and 9.7%. Andriulli et al. [10] conducted a systematic review of 21 prospective studies, including 16,855 ERCPs for PEP incidence, and found that post-procedural pancreatitis occurred in 3.5% of all patients undergoing ERCP with approximately 90% being mild or moderate in severity (Table 14.1). This was followed in 2015 by Kochal et al. who conducted a systematic review of the control groups (placebo or no-stent arms) of 108 randomized, controlled trials (RCTs) to determine the incidence, severity, and mortality of PEP [11]. Evaluating 13,296 control patients that underwent ERCP for both diagnostic and therapeutic purpose, the overall rate of PEP was 9.7%, with a mortality rate of 0.7% and incidence of severe PEP of 0.5%.

The definition of PEP includes the consensus PEP-specific diagnostic and grading severity criteria, proposed by Cotton et al. in 1991 [12], and the revised 2012 Atlanta international classification [13]. The proposed consensus PEP-specific diagnostic criteria includes new or increased abdominal pain

Table 14.1 Incidence and mortality of ERCP complications

Complication	Pancreatitis	Bleeding	Perforation	Infection
Incidence (%)	3.47	1.34	0.60	1.43
Mortality (%)	0.11	0.05	0.06	0.11

Adapted from Andriulli et al. [10]

characteristic of pancreatitis, serum amylase ≥3 times the upper limit of normal at ≥24 hours after ERCP, and requirement of hospital admission or a prolongation of planned admission of at least two nights. Cotton et al. [12] also propose a PEP severity grading system to differentiate between mild, moderate, and severe PEP (Table 14.2). While providing a standardized reporting method of PEP, this criterion is limited by the decreased use of serum amylase and subjective nature of defining post-procedure pain and requirement for hospitalization. To address these limitations, Freeman et al. have proposed modifying the criteria to include serum lipase and defining clinical pancreatitis as "new or worsened abdominal pain."

Although not designed specifically for PEP, the revised Atlanta classification provides a clear classification for acute pancreatitis that can be extrapolated for use in diagnosing PEP. According to the revised Atlanta classification, acute pancreatitis can be diagnosed if two of the following three criteria are present: (1) abdominal pain consistent with acute pancreatitis (epigastric, radiating to the back), (2) serum amylase and/or lipase ≥3 times the upper limit of normal, and (3) CT or MRI findings characteristic of acute pancreatitis [11]. The revised Atlanta classification system is limited for PEP evaluation in that the utility of contrast-enhanced cross-section imaging in the PEP setting has not been extensively studied.

Table 14.2 Grading system for severity of post-ERCP pancreatitis

Criteria	**Mild**	**Moderate**	**Severe**
Length of hospitalization (days)	2–3	4–10	>10
Other complications	None	None	Hemorrhagic pancreatitis Phlegmon Pseudocyst Percutaneous drainage Surgery

Adapted from Cotton et al. [12]

Case Discussion

In the case presented above, the patient met criteria for acute pancreatitis as she had characteristic abdominal pain and lipase ≥3 times the upper limit of normal. Demonstrating the limitations of the consensus criteria for PEP, she cannot be evaluated by the criteria proposed by Cotton et al. [12] as our institution does not routinely test serum amylase to diagnose acute pancreatitis. The recommendation by multiple societies [14–18] to preferentially use serum lipase over serum amylase in the diagnosis of acute pancreatitis may be a barrier to widespread use of the Cotton et al. [12] criteria, as it was in our case. By the Cotton et al. [12] grading system, our patient met criteria for mild PEP given that she was hospitalized for 3 days and had no other complications.

Risk Factors for Post-ERCP Pancreatitis

The mechanism through which ERCP causes pancreatitis is multifactorial. Most evidence points to increased hydrostatic pressure and mechanical obstruction due to post-procedural papillary edema as the primary mechanisms. However, the risk for PEP can be influenced by multiple patient, procedural, and operator characteristics, and the key factor to preventing PEP is pre-procedural careful selection of patients and identification of high-risk patients. Identification of these factors is necessary for risk-stratification, informed consent, and implementation of preventative measure to reduce the incidence and severity of PEP.

Patient-Related Risk Factors

Patient characteristics associated with an increased risk of PEP include sphincter of Oddi dysfunction, female gender, younger age, history of recurrent pancreatitis, prior history of PEP, normal serum bilirubin, non-dilated bile ducts, and absence of common bile duct stones.

Patients with sphincter of Oddi dysfunction are unequivocally at higher risk for PEP, though the mechanism is unknown. Prospective, multicenter studies have found odds ratio (OR) for PEP of 5.0 [2] and 2.6 [1]. A meta-analysis of 15 prospective studies found an OR of 4.1 [19]. These patients also tend to have more severe PEP [2]. Female sex, for unknown reasons, is an independent risk factor for PEP (OR 2.5) [2]. Younger age is a PEP risk factor. One prospective, multicenter study found that a 30-year-old has an OR of 2.1 of PEP compared to a 70-year-old [3]. Another prospective, multicenter study found that patients age <60 have an OR of 2.1 compared to patients age >0 [20]. Patients with a history of recurrent pancreatitis had PEP at a rate of 16% versus 6% for those without it [21]. Another study found an OR of 2.5 [19]. Prior history of PEP strongly predicts future risk of PEP (OR 5.3) [2]. Normal serum bilirubin doubles the risk of PEP [2]. Absence of common bile duct stones is also a risk factor [22].

Procedural-Related Risk Factors

The methods utilized in attempting selective cannulation can have a significant impact on the risk of developing PEP. Cannulation techniques (guidewire assisted vs. contrast assisted), pancreatic duct contrast injection (OR 1.4–2.7), difficult cannulation (OR 2.4–14.9), pancreatic sphincterotomy (OR 1.7–3.1), minor papillotomy (Video 14.2), failed pancreatic stenting, balloon dilation of an intact sphincter, advanced cannulation techniques, and self-expanding metal biliary stent placement (Fig. 14.1) have all been associated with increased risk of PEP [23, 24].

Difficult cannulation, frequently referred to as the failure to obtain selective deep access of the duct of interest using standard cannulation techniques, has been demonstrated to be one of the strongest independent risk factors for PEP (OR 2.4–14.9) [23]. Repeated (>5) attempts at cannulation carry a 11.9% risk of PEP as opposed to a 0.6% risk with a single cannulation attempt [23]. Therefore in the case of difficult cannulation, typically defined as >5 attempts or >10 minutes of

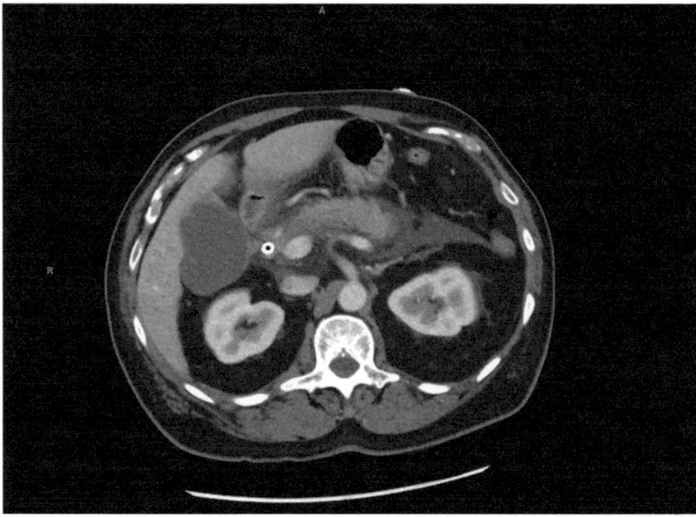

FIGURE 14.1 CT scan showing changes of post-ERCP pancreatitis (PEP) after self-expandable metal stent placement. After placement of an 8 mm × 8 cm uncovered metal biliary stent for the treatment of cholangiocarcinoma, the patient developed acute interstitial pancreatitis. CT examination revealed new marked peripancreatic stranding and fluid. Extending in the mesenteric root and bilateral anterior pararenal space. Rectal indomethacin and aggressive fluid hydration were administered during ERCP as part of routine practice. The pancreatic duct was neither cannulated nor injected during the ERCP

attempting to cannulate (OR 1.76) [8] a native papilla, some experts advocate early utilization (after 2–3 attempts) of advanced access techniques, consideration for repeat attempt in 24–48 hours, or referral to another endoscopist [25]. The advanced techniques commonly include the double-wire technique (Fig. 14.2), biliary cannulation adjacent to a pancreatic duct stent, needle-knife precut sphincterotomy (+/− over a pancreatic duct stent) (Video 14.3), transpancreatic septotomy, and biliary fistulotomy. While these advanced techniques may increase the likelihood of achieving biliary access, they can also increase the risk of PEP. Precut sphincterotomy has been associated with a higher risk of pancreatitis (OR 3.6) [3], though this risk can be mitigated with pancreatic duct stenting

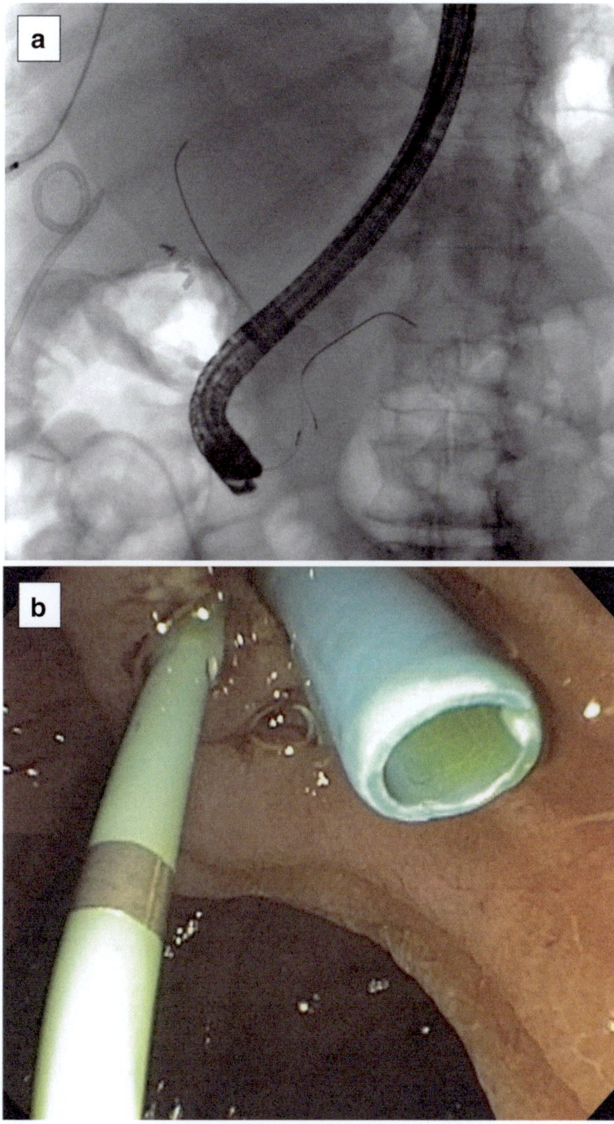

FIGURE 14.2 Double-wire technique to aid biliary cannulation. (**a**) Guidewire placement in the PD can help aid in subsequent cannulation of the common bile duct (CBD) and (**b**) can then be used for PD stent placement to prevent PEP

[26], and it is possible that some of the risk attributed to precut sphincterotomy is confounded by the PEP risk of difficult cannulation. Precut sphincterotomy is usually used after failed cannulation, at which point the papilla may have been sufficiently traumatized to cause PEP.

Operator-Related Risk Factors

Some evidence points to experience, as determined by case volume, to influence PEP risk [3]. Loperfido et al. [5] found that centers performing <200 ERCPs per year had increased rates of PEP. However, other studies have not found a significant difference [2, 27]. It is likely that endoscopists with lower case volumes choose to perform fewer risky cases than high-volume endoscopists, confounding complication rates for each group [27]. There is mixed evidence on effect of trainee involvement on PEP risk. Cheng et al. found increased risk when trainees participated in the case (OR 1.5) [1]. However, Schulman et al. showed that PEP risk does not vary throughout the year at academic institutions, suggesting that trainee experience, at least, does not influence risk [28] and Freeman et al. [3] did not find increased risk with trainee involvement.

One important finding regarding PEP risk factors is that the risk is not simply additive but rather synergistic. For example, Freeman et al. [2] found that a woman with normal serum bilirubin, suspected sphincter of Oddi dysfunction, and a difficult cannulation would have a PEP risk greater than 40%.

Diagnostic Evaluation: Clinical Assessment

Although patients are most frequently identified as having clinical findings suspicious for PEP in the post-procedure recovery unit, the diagnostic consideration and evaluation for PEP should begin prior to the procedure, be maintained throughout the duration of the procedure, and continued until discharged. Even before the procedure is initiated, the indication for the procedure, determination of independent patient and procedure-related risk factors for PEP, and consideration for procedural techniques and pharmacologic intervention should be assessed.

Early recognition of possible PEP is important to initiate the appropriate medical management. Throughout the duration of the ERCP, patient vital signs should be continuously monitored for acute changes. New-onset tachycardia intraoperatively, while under anesthesia, should raise concern for possible impending or developing complication including PEP. In our practice, if these changes are identified in the setting of difficult biliary cannulation, inadvertent pancreatic duct cannulation, and/or contrast injection, we initiate therapeutic maneuvers including intensifying IV hydration with Lactated Ringer's solution, ensuring placement of prophylactic pancreatic stents and delivering rectal NSAIDs (if not already given).

Given the diagnosis of acute pancreatitis can be confounded with benign etiologies of abdominal discomfort such as insufflation-related discomfort and there is significant morbidity for delay in initiation of therapy, the treatment team should have a very low threshold for considering PEP. In our clinical practice, when patients have post-ERCP abdominal pain, we routinely look for objective signs to supplement subjective reports of abdominal pain including changes in vital signs and laboratory testing. Use of radiologic imaging, including plain films or cross-sectional imaging, is not routinely performed in the immediate (2–4 hour post-procedure) period for assessment of PEP and, however, should be considered in cases of suspected perforation.

Similar to the intraoperative assessment, post-procedure vital signs changes including tachycardia in the setting of new or worsening abdominal pain increase our suspicion for PEP. However, while assessing the vital signs, it is important to review the medical record for use of any heart rate controlling agents such as beta-blockers or calcium channel blockers which may provide a false-negative assessment for possible inflammatory conditions such as PEP.

In addition to observing vital signs, it is our practice to obtain a serum amylase and lipase level 2–4 hours post-procedure on patients with post-ERCP abdominal pain. Although studies have primarily evaluated the predictive value of amylase for PEP, including a recent study from Brazil that identified negative predictive value of 94% with an amylase level <1.5 times the ULN at 4 hours [29], a single study evaluating lipase identified a level of <4 times the ULN was associated with a negative predictive value for PEP of 99% [30]. As recommended by the European Society for Gastrointestinal Endoscopy (ESGE), if a serum amylase level is less than 1.5 times the ULN or serum lipase level is less than 4 times the ULN obtained 2–4 hours, the PEP risk is sufficiently low to safely discharge the patient without risk for PEP [31].

Case Discussion

The patient in this case was at very high risk for post-ERCP pancreatitis with multiple patient and procedural risk factors that likely acted in a synergistic manner. Regarding patient risk factors, our patient (1) was a woman (2) of young age (3) with a history of recurrent pancreatitis and (4) a history of prior PEP and (5) normal liver function tests and non-dilated bile ducts. There were also procedural technical factors that contributed to an increased risk of PEP including pancreatic duct contrast injection. Further the procedure itself, an ampullectomy, is associated with an increased risk of PEP (~15%) [26].

Treatment/Management

The management of PEP is not different than that of acute pancreatitis from other causes and consists of early, aggressive intravenous fluid resuscitation, pain control, early implementation of enteral nutrition, and monitoring for severe complications such as necrosis or cholangitis [3, 16, 32].

Prevention Strategies

There is strong interest in developing preventive measures for PEP, and these can be divided into procedural interventions and chemopreventive interventions.

Procedural Prevention Strategies

Guidewire-Assisted Cannulation

Conventional contrast-assisted bile duct cannulation consists of inserting a cannula or papillotome into the papilla and advanced into the bile duct using contrast injection for confirmation. Guidewire cannulation is thought to potentially prevent PEP by decreasing papillary trauma and contrast injections into the pancreatic duct in comparison to conventional cannulation (Fig. 14.3). In this technique, the tip of a dual-lumen catheter is inserted 2–3 mm into the ampulla, and a guidewire, usually 0.035 or 0.025 inches in diameter, is advanced under fluoroscopy into the bile duct and the catheter then advanced over the guidewire with contrast injection used for confirmation [33]. If the guidewire is inadvertently inserted into the pancreatic duct, it can be withdrawn and redirected – though repeated guidewire insertion into the pancreatic duct is associated with increased of PEP (OR 2.25) [34].

In cases of difficult bile duct cannulation, a guidewire can also be inserted into the pancreatic duct first; this alters the anatomy in a way that facilitates insertion of a second guidewire into the bile duct. In one study, this technique led to successful selective cannulation of the bile duct in 73% of patients in which a 15-minute attempt at conventional cannulation had been unsuccessful [35]. A meta-analysis of 12 RCTs found that guidewire cannulation of the bile duct decreased incidence of PEP by 49% (NNT = 31) and improved cannulation success (84% vs. 77%) without increased complications when compared to conventional cannulation [36]. Based on this data, guidewire cannulation is considered standard of care for PEP prevention and recommended by both the ASGE and ESGE [31, 37].

Prophylactic Pancreatic Duct Stent Placement

Placement of prophylactic pancreatic stents is another technique that has been successful in preventing PEP. As discussed earlier in this chapter, mechanical outflow obstruction of pancreatic secretions due to papillary edema and injury due

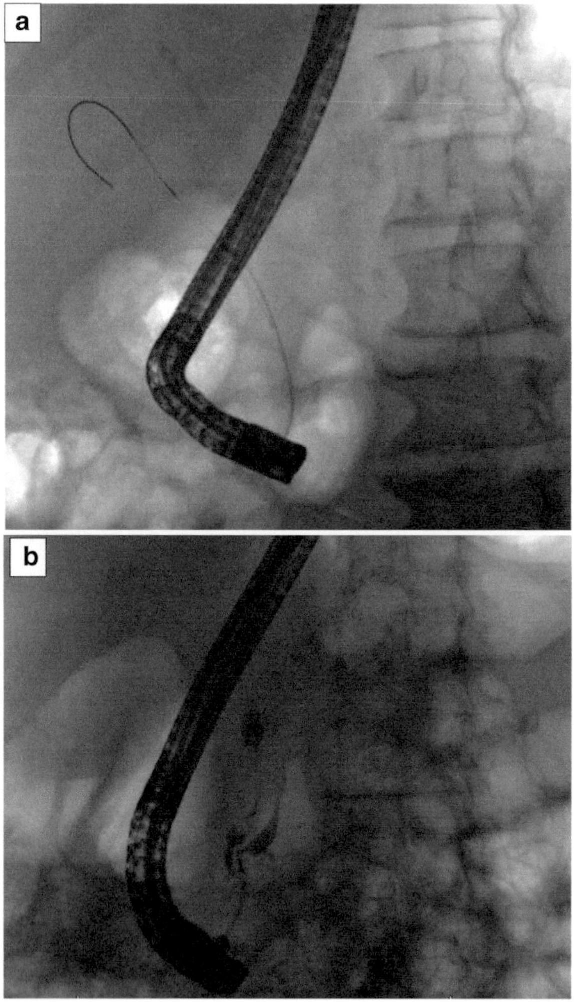

FIGURE 14.3 Guidewire-assisted cannulation vs. contrast-assisted cannulation. (**a**) Guidewire cannulation is thought to potentially prevent PEP by decreasing papillary trauma and contrast injections into the pancreatic duct and is considered standard of care for PEP prevention. (**b**) Contrast-assisted cannulation may be beneficial in cases of difficult cannulation; however repeated injection of the pancreatic duct can increase the risk of PEP

to increased hydrostatic pressure are thought to be the most important mechanisms in the pathogenesis of PEP. Placement of pancreatic duct stents in theory should lead to appropriate drainage and decompression of the duct even in the setting of papillary edema. A recent meta-analysis of 14 RCTs pooling 1541 patients found that prophylactic pancreatic stent placement after ERCP decreased the risk of pancreatitis by 61% (NNT = 8) [38]. The benefit was seen in both mild to moderate PEP and severe PEP (55% and 74% relative risk reduction, respectively). Given the strong benefit seen in these trials, prophylactic pancreatic stent placement after ERCP for PEP prevention is recommended by the ASGE and ESGE [42, 43]. There is little evidence regarding optimal stent choice. Chahal et al. showed no difference in PEP or stent dislodgement between long 3 Fr and short 5 Fr stents in an RCT [39]. One expert reports using 4-Fr, 11-cm, soft, unflanged, single-pigtail stent in cases when the guidewire can easily be passed to the pancreatic tail and a 5-Fr, double-inner and double-outer flanged, ultrasoft stent if the wire does not pass beyond the genu [40]. Spontaneous stent passage can be assessed with an abdominal radiograph 2–3 weeks post-procedure; if a stent does not pass spontaneously, it should be endoscopically removed. There is some evidence that if a patient who underwent prophylactic pancreatic duct stent placement develops severe PEP, it may be due to premature stent migration, and outcomes may improve with prompt replacement of the stent. Similarly, if a patient did not have a prophylactic pancreatic stent placed and subsequently develops severe PEP, prompt placement of a stent may improve outcomes [41].

Pharmacologic Prevention Strategies

Rectal Nonsteroidal Anti-Inflammatory Drugs

Nonsteroidal anti-inflammatory drugs (NSAIDs) are the most effective PEP chemopreventive agents to date. Elmunzer et al. [42] demonstrated, in a meta-analysis pooling 912 patients from four RCTs, that prophylactic administration of rectal NSAIDs decreased the incidence of PEP by

64% and of moderate or severe PEP by 90%. This study was followed by a multicenter, double-blind RCT [43] that tested rectal indomethacin versus placebo in 602 patients, showing that patients who received indomethacin were 46% less likely to develop pancreatitis (NNT = 13) and 50% less likely to develop moderate or severe pancreatitis (NNT = 23). Despite these strongly positive results, there is conflicting evidence. Levenick et al. [44] conducted a single-center RCT also administering 100 mg of rectal indomethacin or a placebo suppository and found no difference between the two groups in the incidence or severity of PEP. Of note, this trial contained more patients of average-risk, as opposed to high-risk patients than prior RCTs. This suggested that perhaps NSAID chemoprevention was only effective in high-risk patient populations. However, a subgroup meta-analysis pooling 2450 average-risk patients from five RCTs (including the Levenick et al. [44] study) still found a relative PEP risk reduction of 28% [45]. As of the time of this writing, both the American Society for Gastrointestinal Endoscopy (ASGE) and the European Society of Gastrointestinal Endoscopy (ESGE) recommend rectal NSAID administration (100 mg of indomethacin or diclofenac) for PEP prophylaxis [31, 37].

In regard to the timing of the delivery of rectal NSAIDs, Yu et al. performed a meta-analysis which showed effectiveness prior to ERCP as well as after ERCP [46]. Additional experts have supported delivering the rectal NSAIDs prior to the procedure, as the initiation of the inflammatory cascade of pancreatitis may be early in the procedure [23, 47]. In our practice, we deliver rectal NSAIDs to all of our patients prior to the beginning of the ERCP unless there is a documented allergy.

Protease Inhibitors

Protease inhibitors are another class of drugs that may have a role in PEP chemoprevention. Like NSAIDs, protease inhibitors attempt to interrupt the inflammatory reaction that leads to PEP but in this case through inhibition of trypsin activation as opposed to inhibition of prostaglandin and phospholipase A-2 signaling. Nafamostat mesylate has been the most promising protease inhibitor thus far. In a meta-analysis, pooling 2956 patients from 7 RCTs showed a 53% decrease in PEP incidence compared to controls [48], though it is likely more helpful for low-risk rather than high-risk patients [49]. Despite this significant chemopreventive effect, nafamostat mesylate is not widely used due to high costs and the logistical inconvenience of needing to administer a lengthy intravenous infusion, sometimes lasting up to 24 hours, and is not recommended in the ASGE or ESGE guidelines [31, 37]. Two other protease inhibitors have been thoroughly studied, gabexate and ulinastatin, but have overall been less effective and more cumbersome than nafamostat mesylate [50–52]. Other drug classes are also being investigated with mixed results to date, as shown on Table 14.3.

Table 14.3 Classes of chemopreventive agents under investigation and recommendation status in society guidelines [31, 37]

PEP chemopreventive agents under investigation		
Drug class	**Mechanism**	**ASGE or ESGE recommendation**
Rectal NSAIDs [42–45]	Anti-inflammatory effect through prostaglandin and phospholipase A-2 inhibition	Yes
Protease inhibitors [48, 49]	Trypsin activation inhibition	No
Sublingual nitroglycerin [62]	Sphincter of Oddi relaxation	No
Topical epinephrine [63–65]	Papillary edema reduction through vasoconstriction	No
Somatostatin and analogues [66]	Inhibition of pancreatic exocrine secretion	No

Somatostatin and Nitroglycerin

Somatostatin and nitroglycerin have been investigated as potential pharmacological interventions to prevent PEP. Somatostatin, a suppressor of pancreatic exocrine function, has been studied for PEP prevention in at least 15 RCTs. A meta-analysis of these trials found that somatostatin significantly decreased the incidence of PEP in high-risk patients when administered as a long-term infusion (0.25 mg/h intravenously for >10 hours) initiated 0–60 minutes prior to ERCP; unfortunately no preventive effect was seen with less burdensome delivery regimens or in patients who were not at high risk [53]. However, this long-term delivery is not practical for outpatient ERCP procedures. Another meta-analysis found the evidence for somatostatin to be inconclusive [54].

Nitroglycerin may prevent PEP by promoting relaxation of the sphincter of Oddi and outflow of pancreatic secretions; however the published data to date has been conflicting. Four RCTs – two using transdermal nitroglycerin, one intravenous, and one sublingual – were examined in a meta-analysis; this study suggested some reduction in PEP but did not achieve statistical significance [55]. However, three additional placebo-controlled RCTs have demonstrated a significant reduction in PEP [56–58]. Further, a double-blind RCT combination study by Sotoudehmanesh et al. [59] reported that the rates of PEP were significantly decreased in patients who received combination indomethacin-nitroglycerin therapy compared with the indomethacin-placebo cohort (6.7% vs. 15.3%).

Therefore, while somatostatin and nitroglycerin both show some promise as agents for pharmacological prevention of PEP and can be considered in certain cases, current data remains inconclusive, and larger trials are necessary before widespread clinical adoption.

Aggressive Periprocedural Lactated Ringer's Solution

Early aggressive intravenous hydration provides support to the microcirculation of the pancreas, reducing tissue ischemia, and thereby aids in the prevention of severe pancreatitis.

Lactated Ringer's (LR) solution is currently the favored crystalloid solution for fluid resuscitation as it reduced the likelihood for metabolic acidosis and has been found to decrease systemic inflammation and serum C-reactive protein levels in patients with acute pancreatitis more effectively than normal saline (NS). In addition to the treatment of acute pancreatitis, LR can also be used as a preventive measure against PEP. Two RCTs demonstrated that aggressive LR administration resulted in lower incidence of PEP when compared to standard LR administration (defined as 1.5 ml/kg/hr. during and 8 hours post-ERCP) [60, 61]. The optimal LR administration strategy for PEP prevention is unknown; both a regimen of 10 ml/kg bolus pre-ERCP, 3 ml/kg/hr. during, and 8 hours post-ERCP and a regimen of 3 ml/kg/hr. during, 20 ml/kg bolus post-ERCP, and 3 ml/kg/hr. for 8 hours post-ERCP were found to significantly decrease rates of PEP compared to the standard regimen without causing volume overload.

Case Discussion

Despite identifying the patient in this case to be high risk for PEP and undertaking maneuvers to reduce the likelihood of PEP, the patient still developed PEP on two different occasions. In the two instances that this patient developed PEP, she received standard of care PEP prevention measures discussed above, including administration of rectal indomethacin, guidewire cannulation, and prophylactic pancreatic stent placement.

Although these cases are challenging, acknowledgment of the patient's risk factors allows for a thorough, pre-procedure informed consent process prior to completing the ampullectomy. It also raises the question whether or not combination therapy to target different components of the pancreatitis inflammatory cascade should be considered. In addition to the aforementioned RCT demonstrating superior PEP prevention in patients receiving rectal indomethacin and sublingual nitroglycerine, a recently published RCT compared combination therapies of different IV crystalloid fluids and rectal indomethacin. In this study, Mok et al. [67] reported that the combination of LR and rectal indomethacin was associated with a lower rate of PEP than NS and placebo (6% vs. 21%). However, there was no statistical difference between LR alone and LR with rectal indomethacin. Some experts have questioned whether rectal indomethacin can decrease the need for pancreatic duct stenting, as one post hoc analysis demonstrated that after adjusting for risk using two different logistic regression models, rectal indomethacin alone appeared to be more cost-effective and possibly more clinically effective for preventing PEP than a pancreatic duct stent alone and the combination of indomethacin and a pancreatic duct stent [68]. A comparative effectiveness, multicenter, randomized, double-blind, non-inferiority study of rectal indomethacin alone versus the combination of rectal indomethacin and pancreatic stenting for preventing PEP in high-risk cases is ongoing [69].

Her recurrent episode of PEP after the ampullectomy and noted premature/early passage (48 hours) of the short 5 Fr × 3 cm pancreatic duct stent also warrants discussion. There is limited data on (1) the optimal stent size and length for prophylactic pancreatic duct stenting or (2) the optimal duration required for effective prophylaxis.

Of the available data published on pancreatic duct stents, larger stents (5 Fr stents) have been demonstrated to have higher rate of successful placement and in theory may better facilitate pancreatic pressure reduction, but also a higher rate of pancreatic duct injury when compared to smaller stents (3 or 4 Fr stents) [39, 70]. There is limited data available on optimal stent length. Chahal et al. reported no particular advantage of long (>8 cm) 3 Fr stents over short (3 cm) 5 Fr stents, including no difference in PEP incidence, increased rate of spontaneous dislodgement with short 5 Fr stents, and increased rate of stent placement failure in the long, 3 Fr cohort [39]. This suggests that the added manipulation required for deep guidewire cannulation into the pancreatic tail is not necessarily warranted to place a long stent. In our practice, we favor placing short, 3 cm stents (occasionally with the inner flange removed) to facilitate this passage and decrease the need for repeat endoscopy for removal.

Although most stents pass spontaneously on their own within a few weeks of placement, there remains minimal data regarding optimal duration of pancreatic duct stenting for prophylaxis. Some experts have hypothesized that early salvage ERCP to replace prematurely migrated pancreatic stents might reduce the severity of PEP. In a study of 3216 ERCPs, Kerdsirichairat et al. [41] performed urgent salvage ERCP to place or replace a pancreatic stent in 14/57 patients with PEP, including 7 with premature pancreatic duct stent migration. In this small cohort, very early outward stent migration was temporally associated with moderately delayed onset PEP, and stent reinsertion improved the severity of pancreatitis. Further investigation is required before recommending salvage ERCP for stent replacement in cases of early migration and delayed onset PEP.

In our patient, given (1) the nature of increased thermal injury to the pancreatic sphincter from the ampullectomy and (2) the synergistic high-risk patient risk factors for PEP, a more prolonged duration of prophylactic stenting with a longer, more stable stent may have been a better choice to ensure complete pancreatic duct decompression until the trauma and edema of the ampullectomy had resolved.

Outcomes

Despite PEP being the most frequent complication of ERCP, the majority of patients will have a mild to moderate course with approximately 5% of patients developing a severe course requiring prolonged hospitalization or additional interventions [11]. Early identification and management with aggressive intravenous fluid resuscitation, pain control, early implementation of enteral nutrition, and monitoring for severe complications are required to limit the severity of PEP.

Case Discussion

Six weeks after her ampullectomy, the patient presented for an EGD for biliary stent removal. A small pancreatic orifice lesion is again seen, concerning for recurrent adenoma; this is confirmed through pathologic analysis. The patient is further evaluated with an EUS, which demonstrated a 4 mm frond-like projection into the main pancreatic duct suspicious for tissue in-growth from external papillary adenoma. Given her young age, intraductal extension of her adenoma, and recurrent pancreatitis history, she is referred to a pancreatic surgeon who recommended elective pancreaticoduodenectomy (Whipple) procedure to prevent further episodes of pancreatitis or malignant transformation of adenoma. The patient underwent the Whipple procedure and has not had any further episodes of acute pancreatitis.

Pearls and Pitfalls

- Pancreatitis is the most common complication of ERCP (3–15% of patients) and results in significant cost, morbidity, and occasionally mortality.
- Post-ERCP pancreatitis occurs as an inflammatory reaction and is activated by increased hydrostatic pressure in the pancreatic duct and/or outflow obstruction of pancreatic juices due to post-procedural papillary edema.
- A complete understanding of patient- and procedural-related risk factors for PEP informs pre-, mid-, and post-procedural management strategies, including informed consent and use of procedural and pharmacotherapy prevention strategies.
- The patient- and procedural-related risk factors for PEP may have a synergistic effect.
- The most important factor in preventing post-ERCP pancreatitis is careful and appropriate selection of patients with adherence to the evidence-based indications for ERCP.

- In addition to new-onset abdominal pain, new-onset vital sign changes, particularly intra-procedure or post-procedure tachycardia, should raise suspicion of possible PEP. Watch for false negatives in patients on beta-blockers.
- After >10 minutes or >3 attempts, if standard cannulation techniques remain unsuccessful at selective biliary cannulation, consider alternative more advanced cannulation techniques.
- Guidewire cannulation, rectal NSAID administration, and prophylactic pancreatic duct stent placement are all standard of care measures to prevent PEP in high-risk cases and should be considered in average-risk patients.
- In our practice, unless a documented allergy, we give rectal NSAIDs to all patients undergoing ERCP.
- Aggressive, liberal delivery of intravenous hydration with lactated Ringer's solution (1 liter in pre-op, 150 mL/hour after) should be considered for patients undergoing ERCP.
- Pancreatic duct stents (typically short, 5 Fr soft stents) placed for PEP prevention must be documented to spontaneously have passed (abdominal X-ray) or be removed endoscopically.

References

1. Cheng CL, Sherman S, Watkins JL, et al. Risk factors for post-ERCP pancreatitis: a prospective multicenter study. Am J Gastroenterol. 2006;101:139–47.
2. Freeman ML, DiSario JA, Nelson DB, et al. Risk factors for post-ERCP pancreatitis: a prospective, multicenter study. Gastrointest Endosc. 2001;54:425–34.
3. Freeman ML, Nelson DB, Sherman S, et al. Complications of endoscopic biliary sphincterotomy. N Engl J Med. 1996;335:909–18.

4. Glomsaker T, Hoff G, Kvaloy JT, et al. Patterns and predictive factors of complications after endoscopic retrograde cholangiopancreatography. Br J Surg. 2013;100:373–80.
5. Loperfido S, Angelini G, Benedetti G, et al. Major early complications from diagnostic and therapeutic ERCP: a prospective multicenter study. Gastrointest Endosc. 1998;48:1–10.
6. Masci E, Toti G, Mariani A, et al. Complications of diagnostic and therapeutic ERCP: a prospective multicenter study. Am J Gastroenterol. 2001;96:417–23.
7. Rabenstein T, Schneider HT, Bulling D, et al. Analysis of the risk factors associated with endoscopic sphincterotomy techniques: preliminary results of a prospective study, with emphasis on the reduced risk of acute pancreatitis with low-dose anticoagulation treatment. Endoscopy. 2000;32:10–9.
8. Wang P, Li ZS, Liu F, et al. Risk factors for ERCP-related complications: a prospective multicenter study. Am J Gastroenterol. 2009;104:31–40.
9. Williams EJ, Taylor S, Fairclough P, et al. Risk factors for complication following ERCP; results of a large-scale, prospective multicenter study. Endoscopy. 2007;39:793–801.
10. Andriulli A, Loperfido S, Napolitano G, et al. Incidence rates of post-ERCP complications: a systematic survey of prospective studies. Am J Gastroenterol. 2007;102:1781–8.
11. Kochar B, Akshintala VS, Afghani E, et al. Incidence, severity, and mortality of post-ERCP pancreatitis: a systematic review by using randomized, controlled trials. Gastrointest Endosc. 2015;81:143–9.. e9
12. Cotton PB, Lehman G, Vennes J, et al. Endoscopic sphincterotomy complications and their management: an attempt at consensus. Gastrointest Endosc. 1991;37:383–93.
13. Banks PA, Bollen TL, Dervenis C, et al. Classification of acute pancreatitis--2012: revision of the Atlanta classification and definitions by international consensus. Gut. 2013;62:102–11.
14. Pezzilli R, Zerbi A, Di Carlo V, et al. Practical guidelines for acute pancreatitis. Pancreatology. 2010;10:523–35.
15. Tenner S, Baillie J, DeWitt J, et al. American College of Gastroenterology guideline: management of acute pancreatitis. Am J Gastroenterol. 2013;108:1400–15, 1416
16. Working Group IAPAPAAPG. IAP/APA evidence-based guidelines for the management of acute pancreatitis. Pancreatology. 2013;13:e1–15.

17. Working Party of the British Society of Gastroenterology, Association of Surgeons of Great Britain and Ireland, et al. UK guidelines for the management of acute pancreatitis. Gut. 2005;54 Suppl 3:iii1–9.
18. Yokoe M, Takada T, Mayumi T, et al. Japanese guidelines for the management of acute pancreatitis: Japanese Guidelines 2015. J Hepatobiliary Pancreat Sci. 2015;22:405–32.
19. Masci E, Mariani A, Curioni S, et al. Risk factors for pancreatitis following endoscopic retrograde cholangiopancreatography: a meta-analysis. Endoscopy. 2003;35:830–4.
20. Sherman SLG, Earle D, et al. Risk factors for post-ERCP pancreatitis: a prospective multicenter study. Gastrointest Endosc. 1997;45:AB165.
21. Vandervoort J, Soetikno RM, Tham TC, et al. Risk factors for complications after performance of ERCP. Gastrointest Endosc. 2002;56:652–6.
22. Mehta SN, Pavone E, Barkun JS, et al. Predictors of post-ERCP complications in patients with suspected choledocholithiasis. Endoscopy. 1998;30:457–63.
23. Zhang H, Cho J, Buxbaum J. Update on the prevention of post-ERCP pancreatitis. Curr Treat Options Gastroenterol. 2018;16(4):428–40.
24. Kawakubo K, Isayama H, Nakai Y, et al. Risk factors for pancreatitis following transpapillary self-expandable metal stent placement. Surg Endosc. 2012;26:771–6.
25. Morales SJ, Sampath K, Gardner TB. A review of prevention of post-ERCP pancreatitis. Gastroenterol Hepatol (NY). 2018;14:286–92.
26. Cha SW, Leung WD, Lehman GA, et al. Does leaving a main pancreatic duct stent in place reduce the incidence of precut biliary sphincterotomy-associated pancreatitis? A randomized, prospective study. Gastrointest Endosc. 2013;77:209–16.
27. Testoni PA, Mariani A, Giussani A, et al. Risk factors for post-ERCP pancreatitis in high- and low-volume centers and among expert and non-expert operators: a prospective multicenter study. Am J Gastroenterol. 2010;105:1753–61.
28. Schulman AR, Abougergi MS, Thompson CC. Assessment of the July effect in post-endoscopic retrograde cholangiopancreatography pancreatitis: Nationwide Inpatient Sample. World J Gastrointest Endosc. 2017;9:296–303.

29. Artifon EL, Chu A, Freeman M, et al. A comparison of the consensus and clinical definitions of pancreatitis with a proposal to redefine post-endoscopic retrograde cholangiopancreatography pancreatitis. Pancreas. 2010;39:530–5.
30. Gottlieb K, Sherman S, Pezzi J, et al. Early recognition of post-ERCP pancreatitis by clinical assessment and serum pancreatic enzymes. Am J Gastroenterol. 1996;91:1553–7.
31. Dumonceau JM, Andriulli A, Elmunzer BJ, et al. Prophylaxis of post-ERCP pancreatitis: European Society of Gastrointestinal Endoscopy (ESGE) Guideline - updated June 2014. Endoscopy. 2014;46:799–815.
32. Banks PA, Freeman ML, Practice Parameters Committee of the American College of Gastroenterology. Practice guidelines in acute pancreatitis. Am J Gastroenterol. 2006;101:2379–400.
33. Tarnasky PR. ERCP cannulation may come down to the wire. Am J Gastroenterol. 2007;102:2154–6.
34. Nakai Y, Isayama H, Sasahira N, et al. Risk factors for post-ERCP pancreatitis in wire-guided cannulation for therapeutic biliary ERCP. Gastrointest Endosc. 2015;81:119–26.
35. Ito K, Fujita N, Noda Y, et al. Pancreatic guidewire placement for achieving selective biliary cannulation during endoscopic retrograde cholangio-pancreatography. World J Gastroenterol. 2008;14:5595–600; discussion 5599
36. Tse F, Yuan Y, Moayyedi P, et al. Guide wire-assisted cannulation for the prevention of post-ERCP pancreatitis: a systematic review and meta-analysis. Endoscopy. 2013;45:605–18.
37. ASGE Standards of Practice Committee, Chandrasekhara V, Khashab MA, et al. Adverse events associated with ERCP. Gastrointest Endosc. 2017;85:32–47.
38. Mazaki T, Mado K, Masuda H, et al. Prophylactic pancreatic stent placement and post-ERCP pancreatitis: an updated meta-analysis. J Gastroenterol. 2014;49:343–55.
39. Chahal P, Tarnasky PR, Petersen BT, et al. Short 5Fr vs long 3Fr pancreatic stents in patients at risk for post-endoscopic retrograde cholangiopancreatography pancreatitis. Clin Gastroenterol Hepatol. 2009;7:834–9.
40. Freeman ML. Use of prophylactic pancreatic stents for the prevention of post-ERCP pancreatitis. Gastroenterol Hepatol (NY). 2015;11:420–2.
41. Kerdsirichairat T, Attam R, Arain M, et al. Urgent ERCP with pancreatic stent placement or replacement for salvage of post-ERCP pancreatitis. Endoscopy. 2014;46:1085–94.

42. Elmunzer BJ, Waljee AK, Elta GH, et al. A meta-analysis of rectal NSAIDs in the prevention of post-ERCP pancreatitis. Gut. 2008;57:1262–7.
43. Elmunzer BJ, Scheiman JM, Lehman GA, et al. A randomized trial of rectal indomethacin to prevent post-ERCP pancreatitis. N Engl J Med. 2012;366:1414–22.
44. Levenick JM, Gordon SR, Fadden LL, et al. Rectal indomethacin does not prevent post-ERCP pancreatitis in consecutive patients. Gastroenterology. 2016;150:911–7; quiz e19
45. Elmunzer BJ, Foster LD, Durkalski V. Should we still administer prophylactic rectal NSAIDs to average-risk patients undergoing ERCP? Gastroenterology. 2016;151:566–7.
46. Yu LM, Zhao KJ, Lu B. Use of NSAIDs via the rectal route for the prevention of pancreatitis after ERCP in all-risk patients: an updated meta-analysis. Gastroenterol Res Pract. 2018;2018:1027530.
47. Katsinelos P, Fasoulas K, Paroutoglou G, et al. Combination of diclofenac plus somatostatin in the prevention of post-ERCP pancreatitis: a randomized, double-blind, placebo-controlled trial. Endoscopy. 2012;44:53–9.
48. Yu G, Li S, Wan R, et al. Nafamostat mesilate for prevention of post-ERCP pancreatitis: a meta-analysis of prospective, randomized, controlled trials. Pancreas. 2015;44:561–9.
49. Park KT, Kang DH, Choi CW, et al. Is high-dose nafamostat mesilate effective for the prevention of post-ERCP pancreatitis, especially in high-risk patients? Pancreas. 2011;40:1215–9.
50. Andriulli A, Leandro G, Federici T, et al. Prophylactic administration of somatostatin or gabexate does not prevent pancreatitis after ERCP: an updated meta-analysis. Gastrointest Endosc. 2007;65:624–32.
51. Taenaka N, Shimada Y, Hirata T, et al. New approach to regional anticoagulation in hemodialysis using gabexate mesilate (FOY). Crit Care Med. 1982;10:773–5.
52. Yoo JW, Ryu JK, Lee SH, et al. Preventive effects of ulinastatin on post-endoscopic retrograde cholangiopancreatography pancreatitis in high-risk patients: a prospective, randomized, placebo-controlled trial. Pancreas. 2008;37:366–70.
53. Wang G, Xiao G, Xu L, et al. Effect of somatostatin on prevention of post-endoscopic retrograde cholangiopancreatography pancreatitis and hyperamylasemia: a systematic review and meta-analysis. Pancreatology. 2018;18:370–8.
54. Kubiliun NM, Adams MA, Akshintala VS, et al. Evaluation of pharmacologic prevention of pancreatitis after endoscopic

retrograde cholangiopancreatography: a systematic review. Clin Gastroenterol Hepatol. 2015;13:1231–9; quiz e70–1
55. Shao LM, Chen QY, Chen MY, et al. Nitroglycerin in the prevention of post-ERCP pancreatitis: a meta-analysis. Dig Dis Sci. 2010;55:1–7.
56. Hao JY, Wu DF, Wang YZ, et al. Prophylactic effect of glyceryl trinitrate on post-endoscopic retrograde cholangiopancreatography pancreatitis: a randomized placebo-controlled trial. World J Gastroenterol. 2009;15:366–8.
57. Moreto M, Zaballa M. Prospective randomized double-blind placebo-controlled trial of glyceryl trinitrate in endoscopic retrograde cholangiopancreatography-induced pancreatitis. Br J Surg. 2002;89:628; author reply 629
58. Moreto M, Zaballa M, Casado I, et al. Transdermal glyceryl trinitrate for prevention of post-ERCP pancreatitis: a randomized double-blind trial. Gastrointest Endosc. 2003;57:1–7.
59. Sotoudehmanesh R, Eloubeidi MA, Asgari AA, et al. A randomized trial of rectal indomethacin and sublingual nitrates to prevent post-ERCP pancreatitis. Am J Gastroenterol. 2014;109:903–9.
60. Buxbaum J, Yan A, Yeh K, et al. Aggressive hydration with lactated Ringer's solution reduces pancreatitis after endoscopic retrograde cholangiopancreatography. Clin Gastroenterol Hepatol. 2014;12:303–7.. e1
61. Choi JH, Kim HJ, Lee BU, et al. Vigorous periprocedural hydration with lactated ringer's solution reduces the risk of pancreatitis after retrograde cholangiopancreatography in hospitalized patients. Clin Gastroenterol Hepatol. 2017;15:86–92.. e1
62. Ding J, Jin X, Pan Y, et al. Glyceryl trinitrate for prevention of post-ERCP pancreatitis and improve the rate of cannulation: a meta-analysis of prospective, randomized, controlled trials. PLoS One. 2013;8:e75645.
63. Akshintala VS, Hutfless SM, Colantuoni E, et al. Systematic review with network meta-analysis: pharmacological prophylaxis against post-ERCP pancreatitis. Aliment Pharmacol Ther. 2013;38:1325–37.
64. Matsushita M, Takakuwa H, Shimeno N, et al. Epinephrine sprayed on the papilla for prevention of post-ERCP pancreatitis. J Gastroenterol. 2009;44:71–5.

65. Xu LH, Qian JB, Gu LG, et al. Prevention of post-endoscopic retrograde cholangiopancreatography pancreatitis by epinephrine sprayed on the papilla. J Gastroenterol Hepatol. 2011;26:1139–44.
66. Omata F, Deshpande G, Tokuda Y, et al. Meta-analysis: somatostatin or its long-acting analogue, octreotide, for prophylaxis against post-ERCP pancreatitis. J Gastroenterol. 2010;45:885–95.
67. Mok SRS, Ho HC, Shah P, et al. Lactated Ringer's solution in combination with rectal indomethacin for prevention of post-ERCP pancreatitis and readmission: a prospective randomized, double-blinded, placebo-controlled trial. Gastrointest Endosc. 2017;85:1005–13.
68. Elmunzer BJ, Higgins PD, Saini SD, et al. Does rectal indomethacin eliminate the need for prophylactic pancreatic stent placement in patients undergoing high-risk ERCP? Post hoc efficacy and cost-benefit analyses using prospective clinical trial data. Am J Gastroenterol. 2013;108:410–5.
69. Elmunzer BJ, Serrano J, Chak A, et al. Rectal indomethacin alone versus indomethacin and prophylactic pancreatic stent placement for preventing pancreatitis after ERCP: study protocol for a randomized controlled trial. Trials. 2016;17:120.
70. Rashdan A, Fogel EL, McHenry L Jr, et al. Improved stent characteristics for prophylaxis of post-ERCP pancreatitis. Clin Gastroenterol Hepatol. 2004;2:322–9.

Chapter 15
ERCP-Related Perforations

Jason G. Bill and Vladimir M. Kushnir

Case 1

An 84-year-old female with history of peptic ulcer disease s/p Billroth II gastrectomy presents with right upper quadrant pain. Laboratory evaluation demonstrated a white blood cell count of 15.3, total bilirubin of 2.5, alkaline phosphatase of 221, aspartate transaminase (AST) of 857, and alanine transaminase (ALT) of 386. CT scan of the abdomen and pelvis revealed multiple common bile duct stones associated with intrahepatic and extrahepatic ductal dilatation. ERCP was performed. The scope was advanced through the gastroenterostomy several centimeters to the opening of the afferent limb. Upon withdrawing the endoscope slightly, a 2 cm tear was noted in the proximal afferent limb (Fig. 15.1a, b). Free air was seen under the diaphragm on fluoroscopy, and abdominal decompression was performed (Fig. 15.1c). Endoscopic closure with hemoclips was performed. Nasogastric tube was placed, and IV antibiotics were given, and surgical consultation was obtained.

J. G. Bill
Division of Gastroenterology, Washington University School of Medicine in St. Louis, St. Louis, MO, USA

V. M. Kushnir (✉)
Division of Gastroenterology, Washington University School of Medicine in St. Louis, St. Louis, MO, USA
e-mail: vkushnir@wustl.edu

D. K. Mullady (ed.), *Dilemmas in ERCP*,
https://doi.org/10.1007/978-3-030-12741-1_15

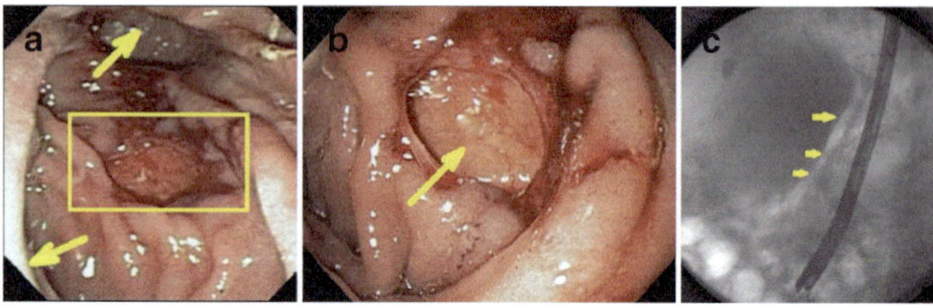

Figure 15.1 Afferent loop of the jejunum: perforation (box), diverticulum (top arrow), afferent limb (bottom arrow) (**a**). Afferent loop of the jejunum perforation (**b**), fluoroscopy revealing free air under the liver margin (**c**)

Case 2

A 78-year-old female with chronic right upper quadrant pain was referred to our institution for ERCP for possible biliary obstruction and sphincter of Oddi dysfunction after magnetic resonance cholangiopancreatography (MRCP) revealed biliary dilatation without evidence of stones or sludge. ERCP revealed a large periampullary diverticulum (Fig. 15.2a, b), diffuse dilation of the common bile duct, and biliary papillary stenosis. The patient was treated with biliary sphincterotomy and placement of a biliary stent. The sphincterotomy site was inspected and suspicious for duodenal perforation (Fig. 15.2c). This was treated with placement of two biliary stents and three hemoclips placed at the apex of the biliary sphincterotomy (Fig. 15.2d). Subsequently a CT scan of the abdomen and pelvis revealed retroperitoneal free fluid adjacent to the duodenum which tracked into the perirenal fat. A nasogastric (NG) tube was placed and intravenous (IV) antibiotics were started.

Diagnosis and Assessment

While ERCP-related perforation is a dreaded complication for any endoscopist, having the knowledge and confidence that allows quick recognition and appropriate management decisions will ensure the best possible outcome. The endosco-

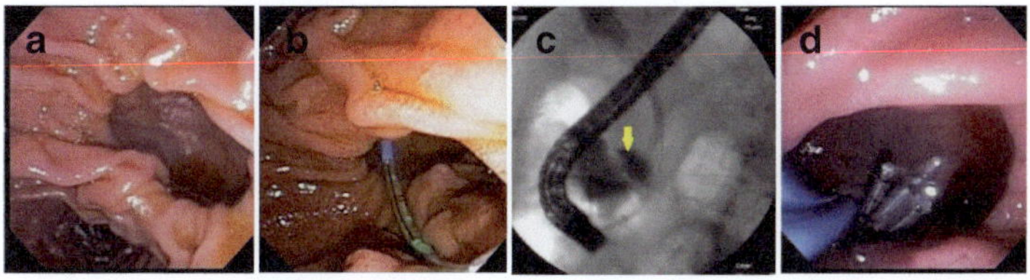

FIGURE 15.2 Presence of a large periampullary diverticulum as seen in (**a**) with attempted cannulation (**b**). Following sphincterotomy, contrast-injected images obtained were concerning for perforation (**c**). Repair was performed with multiple through the scope clips (**d**)

pist must have an extremely high index of suspicion in order to recognize, attempt repair, and obtain appropriate surgical consultation when needed. Multiple risk factors have been reported in the literature, and a thorough pre-procedural evaluation identifying these factors may allow the endoscopist to better prepare for or prevent potential adverse events. Risk factors that have been reported include postsurgical anatomy (Billroth II gastrectomy, Roux-en-Y gastric bypass, and Whipple procedure), presence of a periampullary diverticulum (PAD), and the use of pre-cut sphincterotomy techniques. In the analysis of over 11,497 procedures over a 12-year period, 16 were identified to have perforations related to ERCP. Virtually all of the patients with duodenal perforation were found in those with foregut surgery [1]. Therefore, prior to performing ERCP on patients with difficult anatomy, extreme care must be taken with advancement of the endoscope with most endoscopists favoring use of a forward viewing gastroscope prior to attempting passage of the duodenoscope.

While postsurgical anatomy seems to be risk factor for ERCP-related perforation, the presence of a PAD (Fig. 15.3a, b) as a risk factor is less clear [2–4]. Multiple prospective studies have demonstrated that ERCP is effective and safe; however, a more recent study noted higher rates of bleeding, infection, and pancreatitis when a PAD is present [5]. Given the rarity of ERCP-related perforations, it is difficult to definitively establish PAD as a risk factor.

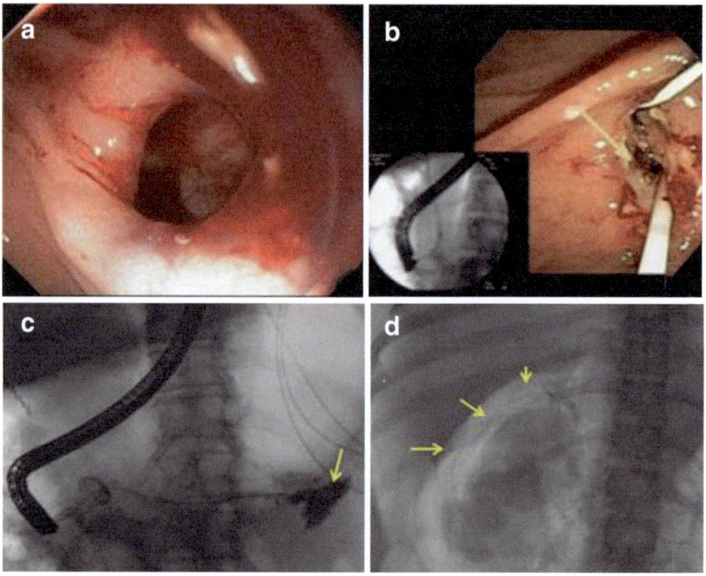

FIGURE 15.3 Definitions with endoscopic and fluoroscopic examples of ERCP-related perforations: (**a**) Type I – Defect seen in lateral/medial duodenal wall secondary to endoscope trauma. (**b**) Type II – Sphincterotomy-related perforation (arrow) with presence of pancreatic duct stent. (**c**) Type III – Ductal or duodenal perforations secondary to instruments (i.e., guidewires, baskets, stents). Pancreatic duct leak seen on pancreatogram (arrow). (**d**) Type IV – presence of retroperitoneal air seen on fluoroscopy (arrows)

Often, the papilla remains accessible on the side wall of the diverticulum, but difficulty can arise when the papilla lies deep within a diverticulum or if the orientation is unfavorable. Performance of a safe sphincterotomy can be difficult due to the inability to visualize the proper axis to guide the sphincterotome. In this setting placement of a protective pancreatic duct stent followed by pre-cut technique or balloon sphincteroplasty should be considered [6]. There are no specific comparative data favoring sphincterotomy versus endoscopic papillary balloon dilation in this setting. Perforation may also occur due to the tip of the duodenoscope negotiating the inside of the diverticulum when cannulation is attempted.

Due to a higher risk of bleeding and perforation, needle-knife sphincterotomy should be performed only by experienced endoscopists. This was emphasized in a review which compared those who performed more than one sphincterotomy per week versus those who performed fewer. Success rate using pre-cut technique was 90% for higher-volume providers and 52% for low-volume providers. Therefore, given the higher risk of perforation and lower success rate, referral to higher-volume centers should be considered [7]. As mentioned performance of a pre-cut technique in the setting of a periampullary diverticulum is possible in experienced hands but should be performed following placement of a protective pancreatic duct stent when possible [8]. Further procedural-related risk factors include common bile duct dilatation, sphincter of Oddi dysfunction, longer duration of procedure, biliary stricture dilatation, and performance of sphincterotomy (Table 15.1) [9].

The diagnosis of ERCP-related perforations can be classified based on location and timing of recognition (early vs late). The most widely used system was developed by Stapfer et al., characterizing perforations based on mechanism and location [10]. Type I perforations are due to endoscope trauma of the lateral duodenal wall, type II are related to sphincterotomy, type III are due to perforation of the bile duct with endoscopic tools, and type IV are usually minuscule

Table 15.1 Adapted from Enns et al. Procedural factors related to increase risk for ERCP-related perforations

Factors	OR (95% CI)
Dilated CBD	2.32 (1.02–5.03)
Sphincter of Oddi dysfunction	3.20 (1.64–8.94)
Longer duration of procedure	1.02 (1.0–1.04)
Biliary stricture dilation	7.29 (1.84–28.11)
Performance of sphincterotomy	6.94 (2.43–19.77)

and only identified by free air on fluoroscopic imaging (Fig. 15.3). Early recognition often requires a high index of suspicion with the ability to recognize the complication visually or through the use of fluoroscopy. The authors recommend defining early recognition as "during endoscopy," as this definition has the most clinical relevance, allowing the endoscopist to attempt repair when appropriate.

Most type I perforations can be definitively visualized during endoscopy, whereas type II, III, and IV perforations may be more difficult, demonstrating only retroperitoneal fat or mucosal bleeding on endoscopic inspection. In the latter cases, fluoroscopy can be very helpful to identify free intraperitoneal air or leakage of contrast (Fig. 15.3c, d). Additionally, the use of a "safety injection" (injection of contrast while withdrawing a cannula through the sphincterotomy incision over a guidewire) can aid the recognition of occult type II perforations [11] (Fig. 15.2c). Early recognition is of utmost importance as studies have demonstrated that this may lead to improved outcomes (less systemic inflammatory response syndrome (SIRS), shorter hospital stay, shorter number of ICU days) and allow the endoscopist an attempt at endoscopic repair when deemed appropriate [12].

The prognosis is generally worse for any gastrointestinal perforation with a delay in diagnosis [12–14]. Presenting signs or symptoms can be non-specific and may be mistaken for other complications including post-ERCP-related pancreatitis [11]. It is important to consider the retroperitoneal location of the duodenum which may mask immediate peritoneal signs and symptoms leading to an even greater delay in diagnosis. Therefore, endoscopists should have a low threshold to perform cross-sectional imaging in post-ERCP patients, especially those with associated risk factors.

Physical exam is generally non-specific with fevers, tachycardia, hypotension, and diffuse abdominal tenderness. The presence of SIRS and presence of peritoneal signs are generally poor prognostic indicators and have been predictive of requiring operative repair [13]. Laboratory evaluation may reveal a leukocytosis, anion gap metabolic acidosis with an elevated lactic acid. Given the retroperitoneal location of the duodenum, free air may not be visualized with plain abdominal radiography, and therefore, cross-sectional imaging is the gold standard in making the diagnosis (Fig. 15.4) demonstrating free air within the peritoneum or retroperitoneum. Importantly, the amount of air does not necessarily correlate with the severity of the complication as 29% of asymptomatic patients can have retroperitoneal air revealed on CT scan performed 24 hours post-ERCP. This suggests that air in the absence of symptoms does not indicate perforation [15].

Treatment and Management

Principles regarding management of luminal perforations throughout the gastrointestinal tract apply to perforations related to ERCP. The use of carbon dioxide rather than air is

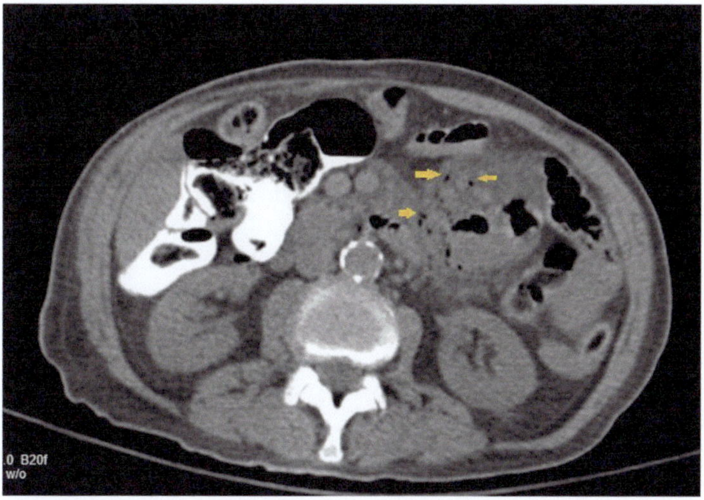

FIGURE 15.4 CT imaging of endoscopic-related perforation evidenced by free air (arrows)

important and should be standard. It remains true that abdominal air under pressure is an emergency and therefore palpation of the abdomen should be performed with abdominal decompression when appropriate [16].

Historically, management of ERCP-related perforations tends to depend on institutional preference and endoscopist experience rather than on evidence-based approach. Experts have based the decision to pursue surgical repair on a patient's dynamic markers including radiographic findings or vital signs. More recently, however, an algorithmic approach based on the classification system proposed by Stapfer et al. has gained relevance (Table 15.2) [11]. General principles include the following:

1. Type I perforations: Immediate attempt at endoscopic repair if recognized during ERCP, surgical consultation, and urgent repair if endoscopic repair failed or if patient's clinical status (SIRS, peritoneal signs) warrants.
2. Type II perforations: When recognized immediately, biliary diversion (stenting) and repair of the defect should be

Table 15.2 Classification of ERCP-related perforations and initial management

Type I	Lateral duodenal wall perforation secondary to endoscope trauma	Attempt at endoscopic repair only if recognized immediately. Immediate surgical consultation as the majority of cases will require operative repair
Type II	Sphincterotomy-related perforation	Performance of biliary diversion therapy or local repair with hemoclips
Type III	Perforation of the bile duct with endoscopic tools (guidewires, stents, baskets)	Biliary or pancreatic diversion therapy is favored over conservative treatment alone
Type IV	Usually minuscule and identified with free air on fluoroscopic imaging	Conservative management

attempted. When delayed the decision to pursue surgery should be based on the presence of SIRS or peritoneal signs.
3. Type III: Generally do not require surgical repair. We would advocate biliary diversion therapy (FCSEMS or plastic biliary stent) vs conservative therapy.
4. Type IV: Generally require no endoscopic or surgical intervention.

It is our practice that all patients with type I and II perforations receive IV antibiotics, bowel rest, and NG tube placement. The decision to pursue endoscopic management vs surgical management is based on timing and location of the perforation along with the patient's clinical status. Khumbari et al. were able to retrospectively validate an algorithmic approach, noting that type I perforations were better managed surgically and type II perforations managed medically unless they were deemed to clinically worsen.

In our experience, if the perforation is recognized immediately and the endoscopist is experienced, an attempt at repair with the use of through the scope clips, endoscopic suturing, or over the scope clips (OTSC) should be performed [17]. The decision to select which repair method is beyond the scope of this chapter, but repair methods are chosen based on experience, location of perforation, and size of perforation [16, 18]. The most commonly used methods are through the scope clips or OTSC. Deployment of the OTSC in the duodenum can be extremely challenging due to the size of the outer diameter of the clip and sharp angulation in the duodenal sweep. Even if endoscopic repair is attempted, a multidisciplinary approach in conjunction with hepatobiliary surgery remains extremely important in type I perforations. The patient must be continually monitored for signs of clinical deterioration. Predictors of needing operative repair include (1) late identification of perforation, (2) location of perforation, and (3) the presence of SIRS or peritoneal signs [13].

Type II perforations are most commonly encountered in clinical practice. Older studies describe high failure rates of conservative management in this patient population, with up to 30% of patients requiring operative intervention [19].

However, recent studies have demonstrated that the overwhelming majority of patients with type II perforations can be successfully managed with biliary diversion (nasobiliary drain, plastic or covered metal stent) and antibiotics, particularly if the perforation is recognized during ERCP [11, 12, 20]. To date, the superiority of plastic vs FCSEMS remains to be determined. Furthermore, if a large periampullary defect is seen, the use of hemoclips can also be helpful [21]. If clip placement is necessary, placement of protective stents into the bile duct and pancreatic duct may be necessary in order to minimize the risk of duct obstruction.

Type III perforations generally have a good prognosis. Recent literature demonstrates success rates (defined by avoidance of surgery) nearing 100% with biliary diversion therapy alone [12, 20]. Type IV perforations tend to do well with biliary diversion therapy or conservative management [11, 12].

Outcomes

Overall mortality as a result of ERCP-related perforations is reported up to 8%. This varies significantly depending on timing of recognition and location of perforation [22]. A recent study demonstrated that immediate recognition (during endoscopy) led to more favorable patient-related outcomes, with a lower incidence of SIRS, less need for ICU care, and an overall shorter hospital stay [12]. Additionally, immediate recognition of Stapfer type I and II perforations was associated with a decreased perforation-associated mortality. Thus emphasizing the importance of training endoscopists in the recognition and therapy of ERCP related perforations.

In regard to location, Stapfer type I perforations are the most serious and are associated highest rate of operative repair, morbidity, and mortality [9–13]. While endoscopic repair methods have shown to be efficacious in the setting of colon or rectal perforations related to endoscopic mucosal resection, there are limited data given the rarity of duodenal perforations that endoscopist can use to guide in decision-making. As experience with novel endoscopic repair methods increases, endoscopists may have the potential to repair a significant portion of duodenal perforations related to ERCP and therefore prevent surgical intervention and a significant portion of patient-related morbidity.

Outcomes of type II perforations vary greatly in the literature. A recently published meta-analysis demonstrated a failure rate of non-operative management nearing 30% with conservative management alone [19]. This differs from other recent data demonstrating 100% success, defined by avoidance of surgery, with biliary diversion therapy (FCSEMS or plastic stents) [12, 20]. Given this favorable data, we favor biliary diversion therapy for all immediately recognized sphincterotomy-related perforations. Furthermore, literature recently has demonstrated excellent outcomes in type III perforations with biliary diversion therapy [12, 20]. Type IV perforations generally have a good prognosis with conservative management.

Case Follow-Up

Case 1

The first case highlights a patient with a history of Billroth II gastrectomy with a technically difficult to access afferent limb with significant looping noted prior to recognition of the perforation. The patient was admitted with hepatobiliary surgery following in consultation. She was made NPO, given IV antibiotics, and did well with conservative management. Forty-eight hours post-procedure, the patient underwent an upper GI series with water-soluble contrast demonstrating no intestinal leak. Her diet was advanced, and she was eventually discharged home. Interventional radiology was contacted to assist in management of her choledocholithiasis and performed a percutaneous transhepatic cholangiogram with internal/external biliary drainage and subsequent stone extraction.

Case 2

The second case highlights a patient with a large periampullary diverticulum with resultant sphincterotomy-related perforation. Following endoscopy the patient was admitted to the hepatobiliary surgical service. She continued to have intermittent abdominal pain, and therefore repeat CT scans continued to show stable and eventually improving size of her retroperitoneal fluid collections. After a few days, she was tolerating PO intake and eventually was discharged home without further intervention.

Pearls and Pitfalls

- Extreme care should be taken when performing ERCP in patients with surgically altered anatomy, those with a large periampullary diverticulum, and when pre-cut access is needed.
- Diagnosis of ERCP-related perforation requires a high index of suspicion, and early detection is key in achieving favorable outcome.
- Endoscopic repair with hemoclips or OTSC should be strongly considered when perforation is detected early.
- All patients with type I and II perforations require close observation and surgical consultation.
- We would recommend biliary diversion therapy in all patients with type II and type III perforations.
- A multidisciplinary approach in close coordination with hepatobiliary surgery is a key to a successful outcome.
- Know when to refer complex cases to expert/high-volume centers, either prior to performing ERCP or after a perforation has occurred.

References

1. Cotton PB, et al. Risk factors for complications after ERCP: a multivariate analysis of 11,497 procedures over 12 years. Gastrointest Endosc. 2009;70(1):80–8.

2. Katsinelos P, et al. Impact of periampullary diverticula on the outcome and fluoroscopy time in endoscopic retrograde cholangiopancreatography. Hepatobiliary Pancreat Dis Int. 2013;12(4):408–14.
3. Panteris V, et al. Influence of juxtapapillary diverticula on the success or difficulty of cannulation and complication rate. Gastrointest Endosc. 2008;68(5):903–10.
4. Tyagi P, et al. Periampullary diverticula and technical success of endoscopic retrograde cholangiopancreatography. Surg Endosc. 2009;23(6):1342–5.
5. Karaahmet F, Kekilli M. The presence of periampullary diverticulum increased the complications of endoscopic retrograde cholangiopancreatography. Eur J Gastroenterol Hepatol. 2018;30:1009.
6. Baillie J. Difficult biliary access for ERCP. Curr Gastroenterol Rep. 2012;14(6):542–7.
7. Freeman ML, et al. Complications of endoscopic biliary sphincterotomy. N Engl J Med. 1996;335(13):909–18.
8. Testoni PA, et al. Papillary cannulation and sphincterotomy techniques at ERCP: European Society of Gastrointestinal Endoscopy (ESGE) clinical guideline. Endoscopy. 2016;48(7):657–83.
9. Enns R, et al. ERCP-related perforations: risk factors and management. Endoscopy. 2002;34(4):293–8.
10. Stapfer M, et al. Management of duodenal perforation after endoscopic retrograde cholangiopancreatography and sphincterotomy. Ann Surg. 2000;232(2):191–8.
11. Kumbhari V, et al. Algorithm for the management of ERCP-related perforations. Gastrointest Endosc. 2016;83(5):934–43.
12. Bill JG, et al. The importance of early recognition in management of ERCP-related perforations. Surg Endosc. 2018;32:4841.
13. Jin YJ, et al. Clinical course and proposed treatment strategy for ERCP-related duodenal perforation: a multicenter analysis. Endoscopy. 2013;45(10):806–12.
14. La Torre M, et al. Promptness of diagnosis is the main prognostic factor after colonoscopic perforation. Color Dis. 2012;14(1):e23–6.
15. Ruiz-Tovar J, et al. Case series: pneumoretroperitoneum secondary to duodenal perforation after endoscopic retrograde cholangiopancreatography. Can J Surg. 2009;52(1):68–9.
16. Baron TH, et al. A comprehensive approach to the management of acute endoscopic perforations (with videos). Gastrointest Endosc. 2012;76(4):838–59.

17. Hyun JJ. Endoscopic Suturing of a large type I duodenal perforation. VideoGIE. 2018;17;4(2):78–80.
18. Baron TH, et al. Use of an over-the-scope clipping device: multicenter retrospective results of the first U.S. experience (with videos). Gastrointest Endosc. 2012;76(1):202–8.
19. Cirocchi R, et al. A systematic review of the management and outcome of ERCP related duodenal perforations using a standardized classification system. Surgeon. 2017;15(6):379–87.
20. Tringali A, et al. Type II-III ERCP-related perforations treated with temporary fully covered self-expandable stents. Dig Liver Dis. 2017;49(10):1169–70.
21. Howard TJ, et al. Classification and management of perforations complicating endoscopic sphincterotomy. Surgery. 1999;126(4):658–63; discussion 664-5.
22. Machado NO. Management of duodenal perforation post-endoscopic retrograde cholangiopancreatography. When and whom to operate and what factors determine the outcome? A review article. JOP. 2012;13(1):18–25.

Chapter 16
ERCP-Related Bleeding Adverse Events

Jennifer M. Kolb and Sachin Wani

Introduction

Since the first bile duct cannulation in 1968, the technical approach and practice of endoscopic retrograde cholangiopancreatography (ERCP) have rapidly flourished alongside technological advancements. ERCP has evolved from a diagnostic tool to a primary therapy in the endoscopic management of pancreaticobiliary disorders. As our techniques and technology improve, so too does the complexity of the cases and subsequently adverse events. ERCP-related adverse events occur in about 5–10% of cases. The most common events are post-ERCP pancreatitis (5–10%), cholangitis/cholecystitis (1–2%), hemorrhage (0.1–2.0%), perforation (0.3–0.6%), and sedation-related cardiopulmonary events (0.9–1.33%) [1, 2]. Less frequently encountered adverse events include impaction of a stone retrieval basket, systemic air and bile embolism, reaction to contrast, cannulation/opacification of the portal vein or hepatic artery, gallstone ileus, and pneumothorax or pneumoperitoneum [3]. It is critical for the endoscopist to understand how to avoid and treat adverse events. This chapter will focus on bleeding-related

J. M. Kolb · S. Wani (✉)
Division of Gastroenterology and Hepatology, University of Colorado Anschutz Medical Center, Aurora, CO, USA

D. K. Mullady (ed.), *Dilemmas in ERCP*,
https://doi.org/10.1007/978-3-030-12741-1_16

adverse events, including risk factors, prevention, and management.

The most common cause of ERCP-related bleeding is endoscopic biliary and/or pancreatic sphincterotomy, which has been reported in as few as 0.1 but up to 2% of cases [4]. The true incidence is unknown, and variable rates are described due to retrospective study design, lack of standardized definitions, and insufficient data on relevant patient and physician factors. Immediate oozing after sphincterotomy that resolves is not considered an adverse event. Less common etiologies of ERCP-related bleeding include splenic injury, hepatic injury, pseudoaneurysm, and vascular injury. The bleeding can be immediate (intraprocedure or immediately after) or delayed (hours to weeks post procedure with late being any time after 14 days) and can range in severity from minor to clinically significant.

The initial grading system proposed by Cotton et al. defined the severity of ERCP-related adverse events according to the intervention required [5]. For example, bleeding was defined as mild if only blood transfusion was provided, moderate if angiographic intervention needed, and severe if necessitating surgery. A more recent statement by the American Society for Gastrointestinal Endoscopy (ASGE) defines bleeding as hematemesis and/or melena or a hemoglobin drop >2 g following a procedure (Table 16.1) [6]. Hospital admission and level of acuity are also critical descriptors. An adverse event that requires an unplanned hospital admission or prolongation of hospital stay for <3 nights is graded mild in severity compared to severe if requiring >10 nights or >1 night in ICU. Bleeding that requires transfusion or a repeat endoscopy is graded as moderate severity.

Bleeding in the post-ERCP patient requires attention to patient and procedure-related factors, a thoughtful approach to diagnosis, consideration for multiple endoscopic treatment modalities, and access to radiographic or surgical salvage therapies.

Table 16.1 Common adverse events and consensus definitions

Category Adverse event	**Definition**
Bleeding	Hematemesis and/or melena or hemoglobin drop >2 g
Pancreatitis	Typical pain with amylase/lipase >3 times upper limit of normal
Cardiovascular	
Hypotension	<90/50 or 20% decrease
Hypertension	>190/130 or 20% increase
Dysrhythmia, cardiac arrest, myocardial infarction, cerebrovascular event	
Pulmonary	
Hypoxia	$O_2 < 85\%$
Hypopnea, laryngospasm, Bronchospasm, pneumonia	
Thromboembolic	
Deep venous thrombosis, pulmonary embolus	
Instrumental	
Perforation	Evidence of air or luminal contents outside the GI tract
Penetration	Visual or radiographic evidence of unintended penetration beyond the mucosa or duct, without perforation
Impaction	Unable to remove instrument or device
Infection	
Cholangitis	Temperature >38C >24 h with cholestasis
Pancreatic infection	Temperature >38C >24 h with collection
Pain	Not caused by pancreatitis or perforation
Integument	Damage to skin, eyes, bones, muscles

Adapted from Cotton et al. [6]

Case Presentations

Case 1

A 37-year-old female with a history of a deep venous thrombosis on anticoagulation with warfarin is evaluated in the clinic for abnormal liver function tests, typical biliary pain, and mild dilation of biliary ducts suspicious for papillary stenosis. She is bridged with low molecular weight heparin and undergoes ERCP. A 5 mm precut biliary sphincterotomy was performed with a needle knife followed by extension using a freehand technique with electrocautery. The pancreatic duct followed by the common bile duct was cannulated, and injection of contrast showed a diffusely dilated common bile duct up to 8 mm diameter. The biliary sphincterotomy was extended to 10 mm with a traction (standard) sphincterotome using electrocautery. There was no bleeding at the end of the procedure. This was an elective ambulatory case, and the patient was discharged in stable condition.

The next day she returned with abdominal pain and a lipase of 1262 U/L consistent with post-ERCP pancreatitis requiring admission for pain control. Her labs also showed AST 300 U/L, ALT 673 U/L, alkaline phosphatase 129 U/L, and total bilirubin 1.4 mg/dL. She had a leukocytosis of 10,600 10^9/L. She resumed anticoagulation with low molecular weight heparin as a bridge to warfarin. On hospital day 3 (post-procedure day 4), she had an acute drop in her hemoglobin from 11.5 to 7.9 g/dL. A computed tomography angiography (CTA) was performed which revealed slightly high attenuation content surrounding the loop of the pancreatic stent terminating in the duodenal second portion and in the proximal jejunum possibly representing hematoma or blood clot; however, there was no evidence of active extravasation (Fig. 16.1). She subsequently had melena so her anticoagulation was held. The following day, ERCP was performed to investigate the source of bleeding. The major papilla appeared ulcerated (Fig. 16.2a, b). Oozing from a visible vessel was seen inferior to the pancreatic orifice. Previous biliary and pancreatic sphincterotomy

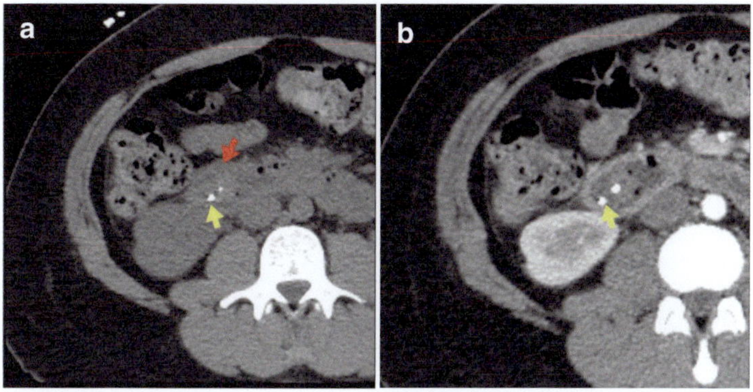

Figure 16.1 Computed tomography angiography (CTA). (**a**) Non-contrast image demonstrates slight hyperattenuation around the pancreatic stent terminating in the second portion of the duodenum, suspicious for blood clot. (**b**) Arterial contrast phase image demonstrates no change in attenuation, suggesting no active extravasation. Red arrow – region of hyperattenuation. Yellow arrow – pancreatic duct plastic stent

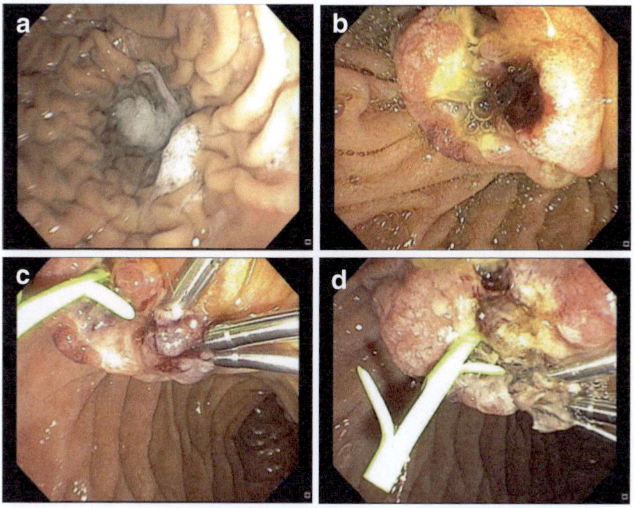

Figure 16.2 Case 1. (**a**) Stomach without blood. (**b**) Ampulla – area of oozing. (**c**) Pancreatic duct stent and three hemostatic clips in place. (**d**) After application of bipolar therapy

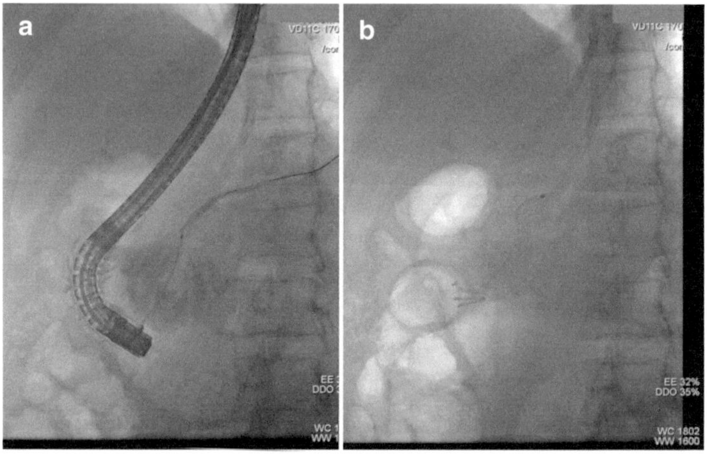

FIGURE 16.3 Case 1. (**a**) Pancreatogram. (**b**) Final film after placement of pancreatic stent

sites appeared open. Blood was coming from adjacent to the major papilla. The ventral pancreatic duct was cannulated and pancreatogram was normal. For pancreatitis prophylaxis, a single 7 Fr by 9 cm pancreatic stent with two external flaps and a single internal flap was placed 9 cm into the ventral pancreatic duct with return of clear fluid (Fig. 16.3). Three hemostatic clips were successfully placed adjacent to the ampulla at the oozing vessel (Fig. 16.2c, d). Bipolar coagulation was applied to additional areas adjacent to the ampulla for hemostasis. The patient had no further episodes of bleeding, and the pancreatic duct stent was removed a few weeks later.

Case 2

An 80-year-old male with a history of diabetes mellitus, hypertension, and hyperlipidemia presented with 2 days of non-radiating epigastric pain. He was afebrile, was hemodynamically stable, and had laboratory studies and imaging findings suggestive of biliary pancreatitis. He was not taking any aspirin or anticoagulants at the time.

The patient underwent ERCP notable for a dilated common bile duct of 8 mm with a 3 mm stone in the distal duct and normal intrahepatic biliary ducts. A 8 mm short-nosed monofilament traction biliary sphincterotomy using electrocautery was performed. The biliary tree was swept with a 12 mm balloon, and three small stone fragments and sludge were found. There was no bleeding at the end of the procedure.

The next day, the patient developed hypoxemic respiratory failure, and electrocardiogram showed a non-ST-elevation myocardial infarction (NSTEMI) with corresponding positive troponin value and echocardiogram showing ejection fraction of 12%. He was given aspirin 325 mg, started on a heparin drip, and underwent cardiac catheterization that showed severe three-vessel coronary artery disease. No coronary stents were placed, and he was discharged to a nursing home on aspirin 81 mg daily and clopidogrel 75 mg daily.

Two days later (post-ERCP day 11), he presented to the hospital with three episodes of dark tarry stools and hemoglobin drop from 10.1 to 6.9 g/dL. An urgent ERCP was performed (Fig. 16.4). Dark-colored and fresh blood was

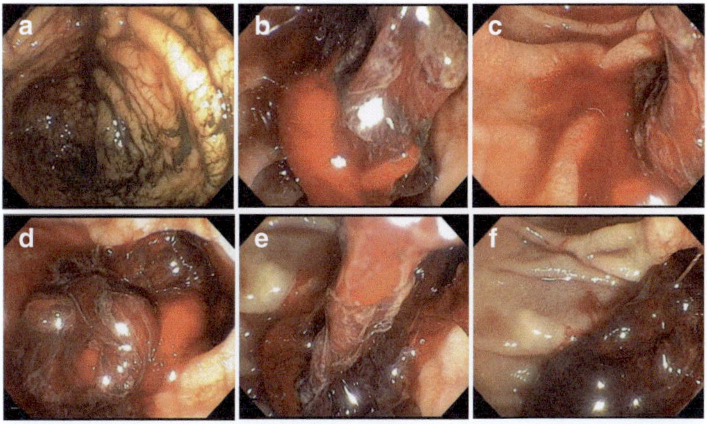

FIGURE 16.4 Case 2. (**a**) Dark-colored and fresh blood in the stomach. (**b**) Large blood clot with active bleeding at the major papilla. (**c**) Injection of epinephrine slowed the bleeding. (**d–f**) Large clot within the periampullary diverticulum removed with cold snare

seen in the stomach. Large blood clot with active bleeding was noted at the major papilla. The major papilla could not be identified initially despite suctioning and aggressive irrigation. The area was injected with 8 cc of epinephrine (1:10,000), and this slowed the bleeding. Large clots were noted at the level of the major papilla and within the periampullary diverticulum. These clots were removed with a snare. The major papilla was then identified with active bleeding at the site of sphincterotomy. The site was injected again with 2 cc of epinephrine (1:10,000). The bile duct was cannulated and cholangiogram was normal. Balloon sweep was performed and nothing was found. Given the significant bleeding, decision was made to place a fully covered self-expandable metal stent (SEMS) (Fig. 16.5). A 10 mm × 4 cm

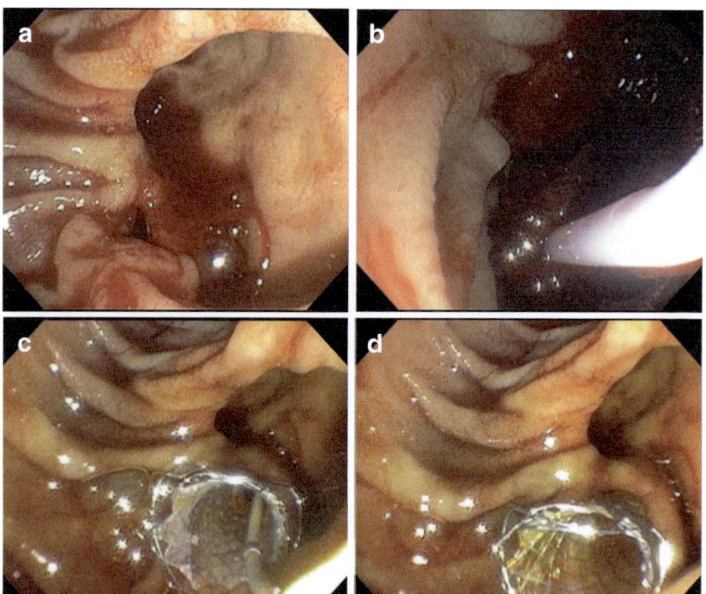

FIGURE 16.5 Case 2. (**a**) Active bleeding at site of previous sphincterotomy. (**b**) Bile duct cannulation. (**c**) Placement of transpapillary fully covered metal stent (WallFlex, 10 mm × 4 cm). (**d**) Stent in place with bile drainage and no bleeding

transpapillary covered metal stent (WallFlex) with no internal/external flaps was placed 3 cm into the common bile duct with consideration to not occlude the opening of the cystic duct. Bile flowed through the stent. The patient had no further bleeding and did well clinically.

Diagnosis/Assessment

Bleeding in the post-ERCP patient should be approached systematically using specific features to diagnose the etiology. Important questions can guide the assessment and management.

1. Does the patient have risk factors for bleeding? Antiplatelet or anticoagulant, thrombocytopenia, bleeding diathesis, cirrhosis?
2. Are there procedure-related factors that increase the risk of bleeding such as performance of sphincterotomy?

The Sandblom triad of gastrointestinal bleeding (GIB) (melena), biliary colic, and jaundice traditionally used to describe traumatic hemobilia can also be seen after bile duct manipulation (iatrogenic hemobilia) [7].

In the first case, a young female on anticoagulation underwent a biliary and pancreatic sphincterotomy for papillary stenosis and 4 days later has a significant drop in her hemoglobin. CTA was performed as the initial diagnostic test given the absence of any overt gastrointestinal bleeding (GIB). When intraluminal blood was identified, ERCP was deemed the most appropriate next step. In the second case, an elderly gentleman with gallstone pancreatitis underwent biliary sphincterotomy and stone removal via balloon sweep, with a hospital course complicated by NSTEMI for which he was started on dual antiplatelet therapy with subsequent melena. The suspicion was highest for post-sphincterotomy bleed in the setting of dual antiplatelet therapy; thus, urgent ERCP was performed.

Risk Factors for Bleeding

When evaluating a patient with post-ERCP bleeding, it is critical to define the patient profile. This includes medical comorbidities, anatomical variants, and concomitant medications. A landmark paper by Freeman et al. in *NEJM* 1996 described the rate of adverse events after endoscopic biliary sphincterotomy according to the patient, procedure, and endoscopic technique [2]. In a multivariate analysis, five risk factors were identified as significantly increasing the risk for post-endoscopic sphincterotomy (ES) bleeding. These included coagulopathy before procedure (OR 3.32, 95% CI, 1.54–7.18), initiation of anticoagulation <3 days after procedure (OR 5.11, 95% CI, 1.57–16.68), cholangitis before procedure (OR 2.59, 95% CI, 1.38–4.86), endoscopist mean case volume (OR 2.17, 95% CI 1.12–4.17), and bleeding during procedure (OR 1.74, 95% CI 1.15–2.65). Interestingly, they found that use of aspirin or nonsteroidal anti-inflammatory drugs (NSAIDs) within 3 days did not increase the risk of post-ES bleeding. They also found that ampullary tumor, extension of prior sphincterotomy, and length of incision were not associated with bleeding. Similar findings were seen in a retrospective cohort study evaluating 2715 therapeutic ERCPs with 122 hemorrhagic complications. Univariate analysis showed that aspirin/clopidogrel use (OR 1.84; 95% CI, 1.45–2.88) and anticoagulant use (OR 1.65, 95% CI 1.15–2.89) were significant risk factors for post-sphincterotomy bleeding; however in multivariate analysis they were not independent predictors [8].

The risk of post-ERCP bleeding in the setting of coagulopathy of liver disease seems to be more nuanced. A retrospective review of 129 ERCPs performed in cirrhotic patients compared to 392 in non-cirrhotic patients found that cirrhosis was a risk factor for post-ERCP gastrointestinal bleeding (GIB) (OR = 3.58; 95% CI, 1.22–10.47) as well as sphincterotomy during ERCP (OR 3.22; 95% CI, 1.05–9.94). Interestingly, multivariable analysis demonstrated that INR was not a predictor of GIB (OR 2.09; 95% CI, 0.85–5.12) suggesting possible limited value in using this laboratory test for risk stratification or preprocedure planning [9]. A recent South Korean study looked at the timing of restarting anticoagulation and its impact on post-sphincterotomy bleeding in 96 patients on warfarin bridged with heparin therapy around the time of their procedure. They found no difference in bleeding in very early (<24 h), early (24–48 h), and late resumption (>48 h); however, there was an increased risk of thromboembolic events in the late resumption group (0 vs. 0 vs. 24%) [10]. The precise role of the newer direct-acting, non-vitamin K oral anticoagulants (dabigatran, rivaroxaban, apixaban, and edoxaban) on risk of bleeding requires further investigation.

Prevention

Prevention of ERCP-related bleeding requires a thoughtful approach to the clinical scenario and various procedure-related techniques. Here we offer some practical suggestions.

The importance of having an accurate list of patient medications before and after ERCP cannot be overstated. An elective procedure provides the luxury of preprocedure planning. The endoscopist should take a detailed history on use of antiplatelet or anticoagulants and follow the ASGE guidelines on how to manage these in the periprocedural period [11]. Although a complete review is beyond the scope of this chapter, these detailed recommendations emphasize weighing the procedural risk for bleeding with the risk of cardiovascular or thromboembolic event. ERCP with biliary or pancreatic sphincterotomy poses a high-risk for bleeding, especially while on therapeutic anticoagulation, though less so while on aspirin [11]. ERCP with stent placement or papillary balloon dilation without sphincterotomy is a low-risk procedure. Patients at high risk of thromboembolic events (mechanical valves, atrial fibrillation with a history of CVA, or a CHADS-VASC of >2) can be bridged with heparin in the periprocedural period. The novel oral anticoagulants should be stopped

>2 half-lives before the procedure, which depends on the specific agent and the patient's renal function. Generally aspirin can be continued, but thienopyridine should be stopped 5–7 days prior to the procedure if possible. When sphincterotomy is anticipated, anticoagulation should be held if possible. It is prudent to avoid sphincterotomy in patients with coagulopathy and instead perform balloon dilation. Finally, correction of coagulopathy may be required after endoscopic sphincterotomy to prevent post-procedure bleeding.

Use of meticulous procedural technique is imperative. Care should be taken to achieve the preferred angle for cutting, which is usually 11 o'clock for biliary and 1 o'clock for pancreatic sphincterotomy. The desired extent of the sphincterotomy should be determined prior to cutting as the anatomy can become distorted. Use of smart electrocautery is advised. Our practice is to use ENDO CUT mode (ERBE, Germany), with settings effect 1, duration 2, and interval 3. The person performing the procedure is also a factor that can impact outcomes. Performance by an endoscopist with high case volume is associated with better technical success (OR 1.6, 95% CI, 1.2–2.1) and lower post-ERCP adverse events (OR 0.7, 95% CI 0.5–0.8) as demonstrated in a recent systematic review and meta-analysis [12].

Treatment/Management

Medical Management

In all cases of gastrointestinal bleeding, the importance of resuscitation and medical management cannot be overemphasized. First steps include adequate intravenous access, resuscitation with fluid and/or blood products, and medical stabilization. The majority of post-sphincterotomy bleeding can be managed with endoscopic therapy. Modalities include injection of epinephrine, balloon tamponade using occlusion balloon, clipping, thermal therapy (bipolar coagulation), and placement of a metal biliary stent. If the bleeding is refractory to endoscopic therapy including metal stent, then CTA and assistance from interventional radiology for embolization should be pursued. It is rare that surgery would be needed.

Endoscopic Therapies

Bleeding may occur in the seconds to minutes following sphincterotomy or hours to days later, and timing will likely dictate endoscopic therapy. Wilcox et al. described post-sphincterotomy bleeding patterns in a prospective study of 506 patients who underwent 550 procedures [13]. Bleeding within the first 5 minutes was characterized as oozing (42%), trickle (27%), pulsatile (6%), or none (24%). In a total of 79 of these cases (14%), injection of 1:10,000 diluted epinephrine (median 0.55 cc, range 0.5–4 cc total) as monotherapy achieved acute hemostasis. The use of epinephrine injection alone has also been demonstrated to achieve hemostasis in delayed post-sphincterotomy bleeding, even when compared to use in combination with thermal therapy [14].

Although there is some data for epinephrine injection alone for post-sphincterotomy bleeding, the larger body of literature describing approaches and outcomes in endoscopic hemostasis in non-variceal upper GIB is relevant. Societal guidelines emphasize that epinephrine should always be combined with a second endoscopic therapy such as cautery or clips (high-grade recommendation) [15]. This recommendation can be applied to other clinical scenarios. A few particular cautions in the post-endoscopic sphincterotomy bleed deserve mention. Caution should be applied not to place a clip over the pancreatic orifice, and thermal therapy should be avoided in close proximity as pancreatitis can occur. There is no specific guideline on how to avoid or prevent this other than careful attention to the anatomy. In case 1, since the bleeding vessel was just inferior to the pancreatic orifice, a prophylactic pancreatic duct stent was placed prior to use of hemostatic clips and thermal therapy.

Over the past decade, fully covered self-expandable metal stents (SEMS) have been used for post-sphincterotomy bleeding with good clinical outcomes [16–18]. They can be particularly effective in cases where primary endoscopic intervention fails, to obviate the need for angiography or surgery. In a case series from Japan of 11 patients with post-sphincterotomy bleeding where epinephrine injection and balloon tamponade were unsuccessful at controlling the bleeding, subsequent placement of a SEMS achieved hemostasis for all cases [19]. One patient was found to have subsequent stent dislodgment, and rebleeding occurred. Additional data comes from the CEASE study where 67 patients with post-endoscopic sphincterotomy bleeding and primary intervention failure were treated with either fully covered SEMS ($n = 23$) or nonstent therapy ($n = 44$) [20]. The stent group had higher risk of bleeding (40% vs. 9%, p value 0.008) but lower bleeding rate at 72 h (0.66 g/dL vs. 1.98 g/dL, $P < 0.001$).

There have been no head to head trials comparing clipping, cautery, or metal stents for post-sphincterotomy bleeding. As illustrated in our two cases, various approaches can be utilized. In the first case presented, injection of diluted epinephrine, placement of hemostatic clips, and bipolar thermal therapy achieved primary hemostasis. This approach utilizes the fundamental tools traditionally applied in other luminal causes of gastrointestinal bleeding. In the second case presented, injection of epinephrine and removal of clot with snare allowed for improved visualization of the bleeding source, followed by placement of SEMS with short- and long-term hemostasis.

Outcomes

Both of these cases demonstrate ERCP-related bleeding from sphincterotomy that was successfully controlled with endoscopic methods. In the first case, the patient presented initially with post-ERCP pancreatitis followed by bleeding. Of note, her anticoagulation was resumed at <3 days post procedure, timing which has been associated with increased risk of bleeding. In the second case, the patient had comorbidities (diabetes, hypertension, hyperlipidemia, elderly) that placed him at higher risk with subsequent cardiorespiratory event. It is likely that initiation of dual antiplatelet therapy did contribute to his post-sphincterotomy bleed. He also was noted to have a periampullary diverticulum. Increased risk of post-endoscopic sphincterotomy bleeding with periampullary diverticulum has been suggested [21]; however, other studies point against it (OR 0.96, 95% CI 0.53–2.06) [8] so the significance remains unclear. Important predictors of rebleeding after initial hemostasis include severity of initial bleeding and serum bilirubin level of greater than 10 mg/dL [22].

Pearls/Pitfalls

- ERCP-related bleeding adverse events are relatively uncommon, but the endoscopist needs to be skilled at prevention and management.
- Prevention involves appropriate use of anticoagulation prior to procedure, consideration for balloon dilation when appropriate, and performance by a skilled endoscopist.
- Endoscopic therapy options include epinephrine injection, hemostatic clips, thermal therapy, and placement of metal biliary stent.
- ERCP-related bleeding rarely requires angiography or surgery.
- Endoscopists performing ERCP should be aware of the ASGE/ACG established quality metrics and adverse event reporting system and monitor their performance in practice [23].

Disclosures SW is a consultant for Boston Scientific and Medtronic.

Funding This study was supported by a grant from the University of Colorado, Department of Medicine, Outstanding Early Scholars Program (SW) and the NIH Gastrointestinal Diseases Training Grant T32 DK007038 (JK).

References

1. Rustagi T, Jamidar PA. Endoscopic retrograde cholangiopancreatography-related adverse events. General overview. Gastrointest Endosc Clin N Am. 2015;25:97–106.
2. Freeman ML, et al. Complications of endoscopic biliary sphincterotomy. N Engl J Med. 1996;335:909–19.
3. Chavalitdhamrong D, Donepudi S, Pu L, Draganov PV. Uncommon and rarely reported adverse events of endoscopic retrograde cholangiopancreatography. Dig Endosc. 2014;26:15–22.
4. Chandrasekhara V, et al. Adverse events associated with ERCP. Gastrointest Endosc. 2017;85:32–47.
5. Cotton PB, et al. Endoscopic sphincterotomy complications and their management: an attempt at consensus. Gastrointest Endosc. 1991;37:383–93.
6. Cotton PB, et al. A lexicon for endoscopic adverse events: report of an ASGE workshop. Gastrointest Endosc. 2010;71:446–54.
7. Sandblom P. Hemorrhage into the biliary tract following trauma; traumatic hemobilia. Surgery. 1948;24:571–86.
8. Katsinelos P, et al. Risk factors for therapeutic ERCP-related complications: an analysis of 2,715 cases performed by a single endoscopist. Ann Gastroenterol. 2014;27:65–72.
9. Adike A, Al-qaisi M, Baffy NJ, Kosiorek H, Pannala R. International normalized ratio does not predict gastrointestinal bleeding after endoscopic retrograde cholangiopancreatography in patients with cirrhosis. N Engl J Med. 2017;10:177–81.
10. Paik WH, et al. Optimal time of resuming anticoagulant after endoscopic sphincterotomy in patients at risk for thromboembolism: a retrospective cohort study. Surg Endosc. 32(9):3902–8.
11. Acosta RD, et al. The management of antithrombotic agents for patients undergoing GI endoscopy. Gastrointest Endosc. 2016;83:3–16.
12. Keswani RN, Qumseya BJ, O'Dwyer LC, Wani S. Association between endoscopist and center endoscopic retrograde cholangiopancreatography volume with procedure success and adverse outcomes: a systematic review and meta-analysis. Clin Gastroenterol Hepatol. 2017;15:1866–1875.e3.
13. Wilcox CM, Canakis J, Mönkemüller KE, Bondora AW, Geels W. Patterns of bleeding after endoscopic sphincterotomy, the

subsequent risk of bleeding, and the role of epinephrine injection. Am J Gastroenterol. 2004;99:244–8.
14. Tsou YK, et al. Treating delayed endoscopic sphincterotomy-induced bleeding: epinephrine injection with or without thermotherapy. World J Gastroenterol. 2009;15:4823–8.
15. Hwang JH, et al. The role of endoscopy in the management of acute non-variceal upper GI bleeding. Gastrointest Endosc. 2012;75:1132–8.
16. Abdel Samie A. Fully covered self-expandable metal stents for treatment of malignant and benign biliary strictures. World J Gastrointest Endosc. 2012;4:405.
17. Shah JN, Marson F, Binmoeller KF. Temporary self-expandable metal stent placement for treatment of post-sphincterotomy bleeding. Gastrointest Endosc. 2010;72:1274–8.
18. Canena J, Liberato M, Horta D, Romão C, Coutinho A. Short-term stenting using fully covered self-expandable metal stents for treatment of refractory biliary leaks, postsphincterotomy bleeding, and perforations. Surg Endosc Other Interv Tech. 2013;27:313–24.
19. Itoi T, et al. Endoscopic hemostasis using covered metallic stent placement for uncontrolled post-endoscopic sphincterotomy bleeding. Endoscopy. 2011;43:369–72.
20. Cochrane J, Schlepp G. Comparing endoscopic intervention against fully covered self-expanding metal stent placement for post-endoscopic sphincterotomy bleed (CEASE Study). Endosc Int Open. 2016;04:E1261–4.
21. Leung JWC, Chan FKL, Sung JJY, Chung SCS. Endoscopic sphincterotomy-induced hemorrhage: a study of risk factors and the role of epinephrine injection. Gastrointest Endosc. 1995;42:550–4.
22. Lee MH, et al. Predictors of re-bleeding after endoscopic hemostasis for delayed post-endoscopic sphincterotomy bleeding. World J Gastroenterol. 2016;22:3196–201.
23. Adler DG, Lieb JG 2nd, Cohen J, et al. Quality Indicators for ERCP. Gastrointest Endosc. 2015;81(1):54–66.

Chapter 17
ERCP in Surgically Altered Anatomy

Srinivas Gaddam

Abbreviations

CT	Computer tomography
ERCP	Endoscopic retrograde cholangiopancreatography
EUS	Endoscopic ultrasound
MRCP	Magnetic resonance cholangiopancreatography
PDAC	Pancreatic ductal adenocarcinoma

Case Presentations

Case 1

An 80-year-old woman with a history of Roux-en-Y gastric bypass 20 years ago and a history of cholecystectomy 15 years ago presents with generalized weakness, chills, and altered mental status. Her white cell count is 13,000 μL, and bilirubin

S. Gaddam (✉)
Division of Digestive and Liver Diseases, Cedars-Sinai Medical Center, Los Angeles, CA, USA

D. K. Mullady (ed.), *Dilemmas in ERCP*,
https://doi.org/10.1007/978-3-030-12741-1_17

is 4.2 mg/dL. Patient is found to have Gram-negative bacteremia. Work-up for source of infection is negative. A right upper quadrant ultrasound shows a dilated common bile duct with a 5-mm hyperechoic density associated with shadowing, within the common bile duct. What is the next step?

Case 2

A 52-year-old male with a history of resectable pancreatic ductal adenocarcinoma (PDAC) in the head of the pancreas that was detected 2 years ago. Soon after, he underwent an R0 classic pancreaticoduodenectomy. Subsequently, adjuvant chemotherapy and radiation were administered. He has done well since then. He now presents with elevated liver function tests, right upper quadrant pain, and fever. Gram-negative bacteremia was noted on blood culture. A computer tomography (CT) scan of the abdomen showed dilated biliary tree. What is the most likely cause for these abnormal findings?

Case 3

A 60-year-old male with history of Roux-en-Y gastric bypass approximately 20 years ago presents with right upper quadrant pain, nausea, emesis, and elevated liver function tests. He currently takes amlodipine for primary hypertension. He is otherwise healthy. A right upper quadrant ultrasound was performed in the emergency department. This showed evidence of cholelithiasis, with gallbladder wall thickening and a small amount of pericholecystic fluid. The common bile duct was dilated to 12 mm. The distal common bile duct and pancreas were obscured by bowel gas. What is the best management option?

Case 4

A 60-year-old male with a history of partial gastrectomy now presents with jaundice, fevers, chills, nausea, and vomiting. An

MRI/MRCP was performed and showed a 2 cm stone within the common bile duct. What is the choice of endoscope in this patient with altered surgical anatomy?

Case 5

An 85-year-old female with history of hypertension, hyperlipidemia, and Roux-en-Y hepaticojejunostomy about 35 years ago presents with isolated elevation in alkaline phosphatase (440 μL). She lives alone and her ECOG performance grade is 0. An MRI/MRCP shows an isolated left intrahepatic duct stricture. What is the next step?

Introduction

ERCP was first described in 1965 mainly as a diagnostic procedure [1], and in the following years, cannulation technique was described in 60 patients with a successful cannulation occurring in 73% of patients [2]. Over the ensuing decades, the development in dedicated duodenoscopes along with new therapeutic accessories has transformed ERCP into an effective procedure for the management of pancreaticobiliary diseases. The role of ERCP has evolved mainly into a therapeutic role with the advent of newer and safer alternative imaging techniques such as magnetic resonance cholangiopancreatography (MRCP) and endoscopic ultrasound (EUS) [3, 4].

Surgical procedures on the biliary tract have decreased over the past decades [3]; however, there has been an increase volume of non-biliary gastrointestinal surgery [5, 6]. This can result in alteration of the luminal or biliopancreatic anatomy which presents unique challenges to the endoscopist. There are no specialized endoscopes to access the biliary or pancreatic ducts in this subgroup of patients. Endoscopists are therefore compelled to achieve biliopancreatic access with endoscopes that are generally used for luminal endoscopy. Technical challenges include identification and intubation of the biliopancreatic limb, reaching and visualizing the papilla or pancreaticobiliary-enteric anastomosis, limited dedicated accessories, and cannulation without the help of an endoscope equipped with an elevator [7, 8].

The aim of this article is to review the common alterations in surgical anatomy and challenges and possible solutions to accomplishing a successful ERCP in patients with either altered luminal or pancreaticobiliary anatomy. Limited data exist to support the endoscopist to make clinical decisions regarding management of these patients. The approach to patients with altered anatomy may vary widely depending on local expertise. This article reviews commonly used techniques and tools when performing an altered anatomy ERCP and provides evidence-based approach, where available.

Procedure Planning

Types of Altered Surgical Anatomy

A thorough understanding of the type of surgery and nomenclature is critical to a successful altered anatomy ERCP. Review of operative reports, when available, is helpful in estimating length of the surgically altered limbs, and this can help in the right choice of endoscope and accessories while preparing for an altered anatomy ERCP. Also, knowledge of the extent of anatomic resection, length of surgically created bowel, type of reconstruction, and type of anastomosis can help in the planning of these procedures. In addition, extensive firsthand review of gastrointestinal imaging may help provide greater insight into potential difficulties and pitfalls that may be encountered during the procedure. The radiological reports may not fully convey the extent of information needed by the endoscopist, and therefore review of the actual images is highly recommended. The images can provide insight into other potential causes of cholangitis that can sometimes be easily missed on endoscopy such as chronic afferent loop syndrome. Further, it can provide an understanding of the possible postsurgical anatomy when limited information is available from the patient and medical records. If this is a repeat ERCP, previous fluoroscopic images may be reviewed while paying special attention to the small bowel anatomy and/or the orientation of the scope when in optimal position for ERCP.

The presence of altered surgical anatomy may rarely be discovered only after an endoscope is passed into the stomach. This can occur in patients who are new to the health system, have scant outside hospital records, and/or are poor historians. In such situations, when possible, it may be prudent to reschedule a non-emergent procedure with a longer length of block time to help appropriately plan and accomplish a successful ERCP. In centers with high volume of altered anatomy procedures who have well-labeled accessories set aside for this purpose, the procedure can be successfully performed in the allotted time, especially when the altered surgical anatomy is favorable (e.g., Whipple's procedure).

Standard ERCP Techniques in Altered Surgical Anatomy

Patients with prior esophagectomy with gastric pull-through, vertical band gastroplasty, laparoscopic adjustable gastric band placement, choledochoduodenostomy, sleeve gastrectomy, Billroth I surgery, and central pancreatectomy (when evaluating the bile duct or pancreatic duct in the head of the pancreas) can undergo ERCP with a conventional duodenoscope and accessories. The duodenoscope in Billroth I and in choledochoduodenostomy can be unstable without the possibility of gaining a short "hockey stick" position. To gain stability and access, it may be necessary to advance the scope in and maintain an inward tension and/or rotation of physician's axis of the body. Despite the problems with scope stability, most therapeutic interventions can be accomplished with conventional ERCP techniques.

Nonstandard ERCP Techniques in Altered Surgical Anatomy

Billroth II reconstruction, Roux-en-Y gastrojejunostomy, Whipple's procedure, and Roux-en-Y gastric bypass are the commonest types of altered surgical anatomy encountered that require nonstandard ERCP techniques. The most important part of the preparation for the procedure is the choice of endoscope. This further determines the types of accessories and the stents that can be used.

First successful antrectomy was performed in 1881 by Theodor Billroth in a patient with gastric cancer [9]. Partial gastrectomy became the standard surgery for gastric ulcer since its first publication in 1910 [10]. Partial gastrectomy is commonly performed today for malignant and rarely for benign disease. Surgical therapy is uncommon for gastric ulcers in today's post-proton pump inhibitor era. After an antrectomy, there are three common ways to restore continuity into the small bowel: Billroth I, Billroth II, and Roux-en-Y reconstructions. Billroth I surgical reconstruction involves the primary anastomosis of the resected edges of the stomach and duodenum in an end-to-end fashion. As stated above, in patients with Billroth I surgical anatomy, ERCP can be accomplished using standard tools and techniques.

Billroth II is generally performed when Billroth I cannot be performed such as in a more extensive gastrectomy. The duodenal stump is closed, and loop of jejunum is pulled up to the gastric resection site, and this is reconstructed in an end-to-side fashion. Hence, jejunal continuity is restored in this surgical technique but not the duodenal continuity. Construction of a Roux-en-Y diverts pancreaticobiliary drainage away from the stomach. In this technique, proximal jejunal limb is transected, and an end-to-side gastrojejunostomy is performed. The biliopancreatic limb is then anastomosed to the jejunum at an optimal length of about 40 cm from gastrojejunostomy. This is generally performed to overcome the problem of biliary reflux that can be seen in patients with Billroth II. A Braun's enteroenterostomy may sometimes be performed in patients with Billroth II anatomy to decompress the afferent limb and decrease alkaline reflux into the stomach.

A Whipple's procedure is performed to resect neoplastic lesions in the head of the pancreas, for chronic pancreatitis, or for duodenal lesions/injuries. This involves pancreaticoduodenectomy with partial resection of the stomach. The jejunal limb is then mobilized, and reconstruction of an end-to-side anastomotic gastrojejunostomy is performed. The proximal limb of jejunum is anastomosed with the hepatic duct and the remaining pancreatic duct. This limb is the afferent limb or the biliopancreatic limb. Several variations of this classic Whipple's procedure have been developed. These include pylorus-preserving surgery, pancreaticogastrostomy, and minimally invasive surgery, among others. Any of these variations can be encountered during your procedure, and this mainly depends on local expertise.

Roux-en-Y gastric bypass was first described in 1994 and is currently the second most common bariatric surgery performed in the United States. A 30-mL gastric pouch is created in the proximal stomach, and this is anastomosed with a jejunal limb, known as the Roux limb. The Roux limb can measure between 75 cm and 150 cm in length and connects to a biliopancreatic limb distally to form the common channel. The common alterations in surgical anatomy and their terminology are reviewed in Fig. 17.1.

Choice of Endoscope

The choice of endoscope is based on the anticipated length of the limbs and the difficulty in traversing them. In Billroth II anatomy, the ampulla can be reached with an upper endoscope, a pediatric colonoscope, an adult colonoscope, or a conventional duodenoscope. Similarly, in a patient with Whipple's procedure anatomy, biliary and pancreatic access can be gained with any of the above scopes. Occasionally, a double-balloon enteroscope (DBE) or a single-balloon enteroscope (SBE) may be required, especially in patient with adhesions or with

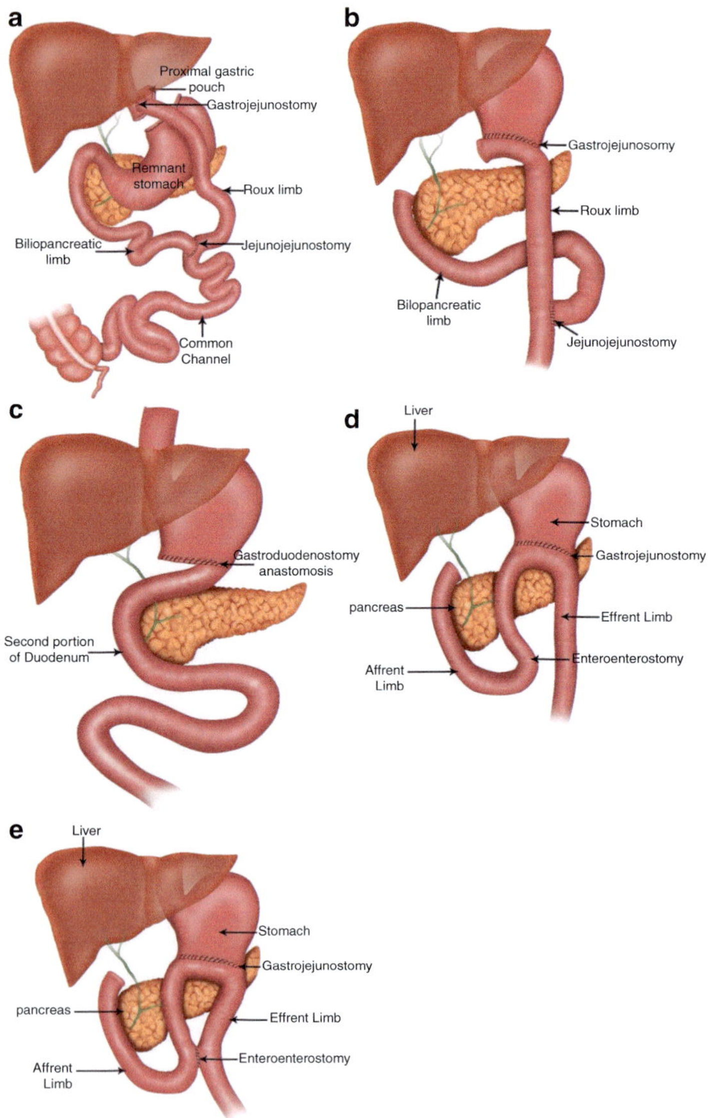

FIGURE 17.1 Types of altered surgical anatomy. (**a**) Roux-en-Y gastric bypass. (**b**) Roux-en-Y gastrojejunostomy. (**c**) Billroth I. (**d**) Billroth II. (**e**) Billroth II with Braun's enteroenterostomy

longer than usual afferent limb. The choice of scopes is also influenced by the local expertise and experience. For example, some centers routinely use a therapeutic upper endoscope for ERCP in both post Whipple's and Billroth II anatomy.

In patients with a Roux-en-Y gastrojejunostomy, access to the ampulla can be gained using a pediatric or an adult colonoscope. In case of Roux-en-Y gastric bypass, the Roux limb is generally about 100 cm, and therefore an SBE or DBE is required to access the papilla. Occasionally, a colonoscope may be adequate to reach the papilla in some patients. Table 17.1 describes the working channel diameter of each endoscope and their merits and limitations. It is ideal to start with the shortest scope with the largest caliber working channel. Please refer to Table 17.1 for details of available endoscopes and their specifications.

Support Staff

The availability of well-trained support staff is imperative for a successful procedure. This is even more important in altered anatomy ERCP. As part of planning, one should confirm that the available staff are trained in altered anatomy ERCP and are familiar with the tools.

Procedure

The skill set for an altered anatomy ERCP procedure is different from that of a conventional ERCP. While the conventional ERCP has one major rate-limiting step, i.e., cannulation, the altered anatomy ERCP has multiple major rate-limiting steps. The correct identification of the afferent limb, successful advancement of the endoscope to the papilla, cannulation without help from an elevator channel, sphincterotomy without dedicated conventional accessories, and stent placement without the conventional ability to push the stent across a tight stricture are all potential bottlenecks preventing successful completion of the procedure.

TABLE 17.1 Scopes used in altered surgical anatomy ERCP

Endoscope	Working channel length (cm)	Accessory channel diameter (mm)	Altered surgical anatomy	Biliary and pancreatic drainage	Maximum caliber of stent	Strengths	Weaknesses
Therapeutic duodenoscope	124	4.2	Esophagectomy	Native papilla	All stents	Elevator	Possible higher risk of perforation in the small bowel
			Vertical band gastroplasty	Native papilla	Standard ERCP accessories	Side-viewing endoscope	
			Laparoscopic adjustable gastric band placement	Native papilla			
			Choledochoduodenostomy	Native papilla			
			Sleeve gastrectomy	Native papilla			
			Billroth I	Native papilla			
			Billroth II	Native papilla			
			Whipple's procedure	Separate hepaticojejunostomy and pancreaticojejunostomy			
			Central pancreatectomy	Native papilla			

Therapeutic gastroscope	103	3.7	Billroth II	Native papilla	All stents (care should be taken to keep flaps down when advancing stent into the accessory channel)	Can accommodate most standard ERCP accessories	Forward-viewing endoscope
			Whipple's procedure	Separate hepaticojejunostomy and pancreaticojejunostomy		Can place 10 Fr stents	No elevator
Adult colonoscope	168	3.7	Billroth II	Native papilla	All stents (care should be taken to keep flaps down when advancing stent into the accessory channel	Can accommodate most standard ERCP accessories	Forward-viewing endoscope
			Whipple's procedure	Separate hepaticojejunostomy and pancreaticojejunostomy		Can place 10 Fr stents	No elevator

(continued)

TABLE 17.1 (continued)

Endoscope	Working channel length (cm)	Accessory channel diameter (mm)	Altered surgical anatomy	Biliary and pancreatic drainage	Maximum caliber of stent	Strengths	Weaknesses
			Roux-en-Y hepaticojejunostomy	Hepaticojejunostomy[a]		Can offer better ability to push stents	Can be difficult to advance scope
Pediatric colonoscope	168	3.2	Billroth II	Native papilla	8.5 Fr stents (care should be taken to keep flaps down when advancing stent into the accessory channel)	Easier to advance scope than adult colonoscope	Forward-viewing endoscope
			Whipple's procedure	Separate hepaticojejunostomy and pancreaticojejunostomy	Some fully covered biliary metal stents can be placed		No elevator
			Roux-en-Y hepaticojejunostomy	Hepaticojejunostomy[a]			

Single-balloon enteroscope/ double-balloon enteroscope	200 (SBE)/220 (DBE)[b]	2.8[b]	Whipple's procedure	Separate hepaticojejunostomy and pancreaticojejunostomy	7 Fr stents (care should be taken to keep flaps down when advancing stent into the accessory channel)	Scope is soft and easy to advance	Limited number of accessories
			Roux-en-Y gastric bypass	Native papilla		Ability to reach further than other scopes	Advancing stents and other accessories can be difficult
			Roux-en-Y hepaticojejunostomy	Hepaticojejunostomy[a]			Forward-viewing endoscope No elevator

[a]In patients with Roux-en-Y hepaticojejunostomy, while a new bilioenteric anastomosis is created, the pancreatic ductal orifice remains at the major papilla
[b]Newer DBE scopes with shorter length (152 cm) and wider caliber of working channel (3.2 mm) are available

Identification of the Afferent Limb

In patients with Billroth II and Whipple's anatomy, once the gastrojejunal anastomosis has been reached, it is not uncommon to easily locate one of the limbs of small bowel. This is usually the efferent limb. The afferent limb oftentimes is located on the same side as the lesser curvature of the stomach. This is generally the difficulty of the two limbs to find or intubate. Careful evaluation of the peristaltic wave can sometimes help with identification of the limbs. The peristaltic waves travel in a craniocaudal fashion inside the reconstructed afferent and efferent limb. On careful observation, subtle indications in the small bowel peristalsis can generally help identify the afferent limb. The presence of bilious material is a poor predictor of the afferent limb.

If a presumed afferent limb has been intubated, the scope is then advanced as far distally as possible. If the papilla or the bilioenteric anastomosis is not encountered, further evaluation of the possibility of a longer afferent limb can be performed by injection of contrast through the working channel under fluoroscopic guidance. Injection of contrast into the lumen can sometimes result in reflux into the stomach and increase the risk of aspiration. It is prudent to recommend general anesthesia in those patients known to have a history of failed or difficult ERCP. Upon injection of contrast, if the contrast flows to the blind limb or a cholangiogram is noted on contrast injection or there is flow of contrast into the right upper quadrant, it may indicate that the endoscope is in the afferent limb. If further advancement is not possible, change in patient position, abdominal pressure, or change to a SBE or DBE may be warranted. On the other hand, if the contrast seems to flow into the right lower quadrant, it is less likely to be the afferent limb. The endoscope is then pulled back, to the gastrojejunal anastomosis and then advanced into the other limb. It is not uncommon that endoscopists with limited experience in altered anatomy can often fall back and inadvertently readvance back into the same limb. Taking a biopsy of the mucosa at the entrance of the limb or withdrawing the scope while exchanging for a wire can help identify the two limbs and avoid this pitfall.

Identification of the afferent limb at the jejunojejunostomy can be challenging. Here again, careful examination to identify the direction of peristalsis can give a clue regarding the afferent limb. Experts generally recommend "crossing the anastomosis" as an effective strategy in differentiating the afferent limb from the common channel. The presence of bile, although often advocated, is not a reliable predictor of the afferent limb. In patients who have had revisions of RYGB or have had multiple surgeries in the past, the identification and advancement of scope may be much more challenging. When viewed on fluoroscopy, the scope may assume unusual paths, and therefore many of the above rules may not apply. Acute angulations and inability to advance the scope may be encountered. Changing to a thinner caliber scope can help with angulation issues. Often, acute angles can be the result of excessive torqueing of the scope, insufflation, or looping. When it is impossible to pass and advance the scope, withdrawal of the scope by a 30–50 cm and readvancing can help. At the same time, care should be taken to minimize air insufflation. Changes in patient position and abdominal pressure may be applied if necessary. Just as in all altered anatomy endoscopy, there is not a single solution to addressing issues with scope advancement in patients with history of multiple surgeries. However, difficulty in accomplishing ERCP in this subgroup of patients is significantly higher.

Despite following the above general principles, identification of the afferent limb can sometimes be challenging. Often, the appearance of the anastomosis, relative location of the afferent limb at the anastomosis, and the limb lengths can vary based on local surgical expertise and techniques. It is not uncommon to have difficulty in accomplishing altered anatomy ERCP in patients who present from a different health system or who have undergone surgery several decades ago.

Cannulation

Cannulation is a procedure-limiting step in ERCP. This is further complicated in altered anatomy for several reasons: approach to the papilla from a retrograde or from a caudal approach, use of forward-viewing scope without an elevator, and the use of tools designed for standard ERCP.

Native Papilla

The caudal approach of the papilla alters the endoscopic appearance of the relative locations of biliary and pancreatic orifices. From a caudal view, the biliary and pancreatic orifices are reversed by 180 degrees when compared to standard ERCP. Sometimes, rotation of the scope by 180 degrees such that the papilla is in the bottom half of the screen may be required for successful cannulation. A combination of fluoroscopic and endoscopic images can help identify the correct orientation and angulation that is required for successful cannulation. The use of clear cap can further aid in exposure of the papilla and possibly in straightening of the distal common bile duct. The tools that can be used for cannulation can vary depending upon the type of scope. SBE- and DBE-assisted ERCPs tend to have the greatest limitation in availability of ERCP accessories.

Bilioenteric or Pancreaticoenteric Anastomosis

Identification of the hepaticojejunostomy and pancreaticojejunostomy can be facilitated using a clear cap fitted at the tip of the endoscope. The hepaticojejunostomy can be identified after advancing the tip of the scope to the area of the hilum of the liver on fluoroscopic images. After adequate insufflation of the lumen, the cap maybe used effectively to move the small bowel folds aside to locate the anastomosis. Identification of the anastomosis can be challenging when patient has anastomotic stricture or small bowel luminal strictures. Luminal strictures can form because of tumor infiltration or radiation. Underwater examination of the afferent loop can sometimes help in identifying the orifice. After identification, cannulation can be achieved with a wire and extraction balloon. When hepaticojejunostomy is performed higher up in the bile duct, two anastomotic orifices can be seen within the lumen.

Therapeutics

It is often desirable to access selective intrahepatic bile ducts to evaluate and treat biliary disease in the liver. This can often be challenging despite the use of curved hydrophilic guidewires. This may be due to acute angulation of the common bile duct, lack of alignment of the scope to the common bile duct, or acute angulation of intrahepatic ducts after extended liver resection. Appropriate changes to the scope tip under endoscopic and fluoroscopic guidance can help improve alignment of the scope to the bile duct. This provides the best opportunity to obtain biliary access to the desired intrahepatic duct. Further, this can help in increasing the chances of a successful stent placement. Changes to patient body position may be attempted as the last resort (i.e., change from prone to semi-prone or supine position) if all other corrective measures have been unsuccessful. The common therapeutic maneuvers are described below.

Sphincterotomy

Sphincterotomy can be achieved with a needle-knife or a special S-shaped Billroth II sphincterotome. Freehand needle-knife sphincterotomy can be associated with higher risk of complications. Often, stents are placed into the bile duct, and an over-the-stent needle-knife sphincterotomy is performed to decrease risks. Alternatively, a small needle-knife sphincterotomy followed by sphincteroplasty can be safe and effective.

Stone Extraction

Stone extraction is a common maneuver performed in altered anatomy ERCP. The caudal approach of the forward-viewing scope to the ampulla alters the angles, and therefore the principles of stone extraction in standard ERCP cannot be applied to these patients. Stone extraction in altered anatomy requires a generous sphincteroplasty. If balloon sweeps alone are not adequate for stone removal from the common bile duct, a combination of balloon and enteroscope may need to be pulled back to facilitate stone removal. Alternatively, long baskets are available to remove stone from the bile duct. However, the use of rescue lithotripsy can be limited, especially in SBE or DBE ERCP.

Stent Placement

Stent placement can be challenging without an elevator on the enteroscope. The caliber of the working channel of the enteroscope severely limits the size of stent that can be placed. The ability to traverse a stricture is severely limited in altered anatomy ERCP. When a stent is being placed to traverse a stricture, it is imperative to perform adequate dilation to accommodate stents. As described above, corrections to the tip of the scope to correct alignment of scope to the bile duct are recommended to achieve successful stent placement. Care should be taken to keep the flaps down when advancing a stent into the working channel. This can be achieved using a positioning sleeve that is supplied with the stent.

Alternatives to Peroral ERCP

Even with experienced endoscopists, altered anatomy ERCP can be unsuccessful. Several alternative approaches to ERCP are available. These maybe performed when altered anatomy ERCP has failed or if equipment or expertise for altered anatomy ERCP is unavailable. For choledocholithiasis, patients may proceed to cholecystectomy and then undergo common bile duct exploration. If this is successful, ERCP can be avoided.

Laparoscopic-Assisted Transgastric ERCP

When the indication for ERCP is urgent, laparoscopic-assisted transgastric ERCP may be performed in the operating room where the surgeon accesses the gastric remnant with a large-bore trocar that can be used to traverse a duodenoscope. This method offers the added advantage of being able to perform endoscopic ultrasound (EUS) at the same time if needed. In addition, cholecystectomy can also be performed in the same setting, if indicated.

Newer Techniques

In patients with RYGB who have biliary disease that requires multiple ERCPs, it may be necessary to create an access to the gastric remnant either by creation of a gastrogastric fistula or by creation of a gastrocutaneous fistula. The former can be achieved by endoscopic ultrasound-guided placement of a lumen-opposing stent to create a fistula between the gastric pouch and the gastric remnant [11, 12]. The latter can be achieved by placement of a push or pull percutaneous endoscopic gastrostomy (PEG) tube placement with the help of a DBE or a surgically placed gastrostomy tube. These access points can be dilated after maturation of the tract to help with passage of a duodenoscope. These techniques are helpful for nonurgent procedures.

EUS-guided antegrade biliary access has been described. In this procedure, access to a dilated left intrahepatic bile duct is obtained under endosonographic visualization from the proximal stomach. This access point is used to further direct therapy in an antegrade fashion [13]. Another approach, endoscopic ultrasound-directed transgastric ERCP (EDGE) describes

EUS-guided placement of a PEG tube into the gastric remnant for transgastric access [14]. Further research is needed to evaluate the efficacy and safety of these newer techniques.

Percutaneous Transhepatic Cholangiography

In patients that require emergent access to the bile ducts in the setting of acute cholangitis with hemodynamic instability or when local expertise in altered surgical anatomy is not available, PTC may be performed. This is also an option when altered surgical anatomy ERCP has been unsuccessful. When the failure is primarily due to unsuccessful cannulation, EUS rendezvous or PTC rendezvous may be considered for antegrade passage of wire across the papilla to facilitate retrograde ERCP cannulation.

Outcomes

Studies in altered anatomy ERCP are highly variable in their outcomes. The outcomes' endpoint may be access to the papilla, cannulation, therapeutic success, or overall success. Further, studies in this area have been over several decades. Over the study duration, there have been changes to endoscopes and technology in ERCP accessories. This makes comparison of the study difficult. The underlying altered surgical anatomy likely determines the difficulty, success, and safety of the procedure.

Case Outcomes

Case 1

Patient was taken for an urgent altered anatomy ERCP with a DBE enteroscope fitted with cap at the tip. The afferent limb was selectively intubated by "crossing the anastomosis." Selective biliary cannulation was successfully performed with a 600-cm-long wire with a hydrophilic tip and a 320-cm-long sphincterotome. A small sphincterotomy was performed with a needle-knife, and common bile duct stone was extracted using 350-mm-long stone retrieval balloon. After multiple balloon sweeps, an occlusion cholangiogram was performed and was normal. Patient tolerated the procedure well, and her mental status improved dramatically after the procedure. Older patients with cholangitis can present with altered mental status more often than younger patients (43% vs. 23%) [15].

Case 2

Patient's CT scan images were carefully evaluated. In addition to the dilation of the bile ducts, there was evidence of dilation of small bowel loops which appeared to be in the afferent limb. Based on these findings, there was clinical suspicion for afferent loop syndrome. ERCP was performed with a therapeutic upper endoscope. At the gastrojejunal anastomosis, the afferent limb appeared to be stenosed, and abnormal mucosa, suspicious for tumor infiltration, was noted. This was biopsied. Dilation of the stenosis was performed to 10 mm, and the endoscope was advanced into the afferent limb. The entire lumen of the afferent limb which was dilated with large amounts of bilious material was noted. The hepaticojejunostomy was widely patent. Cholangiography showed mildly dilated biliary tree without obstructing stone or lesion. A fully covered 10 mm by 6 cm self-expanding metal stent with both internal and external flanges was placed across the stricture at the gastrojejunostomy. Efferent limb was widely patent. Patient tolerated the procedure well and improved clinically. The biopsies showed recurrent adenocarcinoma consistent with PDAC. He was presented at the tumor board for discussion regarding future management.

Case 3

This patient has high probability of choledocholithiasis. Local surgeons have expertise in common bile duct exploration. Patient was referred to minimally invasive surgery and underwent laparoscopic cholecystectomy and CBD stone removal by exploration. Patient recovered well after procedure and was discharged home.

Case 4

Further review of MRI showed that patient may have undergone Billroth I surgery. Previous records were unavailable for review. Based on this finding, the procedure was begun with a duodenoscope. Careful evaluation of the gastroenteric anastomosis confirmed that this was Billroth I. Using standard ERCP techniques, common bile duct stone was removed. Postoperative course was uneventful. Patient improved clinically and was discharged the following day.

Case 5

A family meeting was conducted in clinic. Patient did not wish to undergo surgical resection should that stricture be cholangiocarcinoma; however she was open to chemotherapy, if indicated. A decision was then taken to perform ERCP to obtain a tissue diagnosis.

A DBE ERCP was performed. Choledochojejunostomy was widely patent. Biliary cannulation was achieved with a 350-mm-long stone retrieval balloon and a 600-mm-long guidewire with a straight hydrophilic tip. The common bile duct appeared sigmoid in shape. The isolated left intrahepatic duct stricture was visualized on cholangiography; however, this could not be selectively accessed despite the use of a fully hydrophilic guidewire. Patient was then sent to interventional radiology, and a PTC was performed, and brushings of the stricture were obtained. The brushings were nondiagnostic.

Patient was brought in for a repeat ERCP 6 weeks later. The PTC was removed after advancing a wire through it into the jejunum under fluoroscopic guidance. The tract was dilated, and a thin caliber scope was advanced into the bile duct through the percutaneous route. Water infusion was performed without any air insufflation to minimize risk of air embolization. The stricture was endoscopically visualized, and biopsies were obtained. The biopsies showed cholangiocarcinoma, and patient was referred to oncology for discussion about treatment options.

Pearls and Pitfalls

- Successful completion of an altered anatomy ERCP requires a thorough understanding of the indication, type of altered anatomy, pre-procedure planning (Table 17.2), selection of appropriate scope and accessories, and a keen eye for safety.
- A review of cross-sectional imaging, when available, can provide insights into anatomy that might otherwise be missed on reading the reports alone.
- Familiarizing oneself with the available accessories and organizing them into one labeled cabinet is often helpful. As with standard ERCP, ensuring that there is an appropriate indication for procedure is vital.
- The use of fluoroscopy and a clear cap fitted at the tip of the scope can be invaluable in identifying the afferent limb and major papilla or hepaticojejunostomy. It can also help expose the papilla better and aid in cannulation.
- Reducing and creating a stable scope position at the papilla and evaluating the angles between the scope and bile duct can be time-consuming; however, they are imperative to a successful altered anatomy ERCP.
- When advancing the stent into the working channel, care should be taken to keep the flaps down. This can be achieved with a positioning sleeve that is generally supplied with the stent.
- Advancement of stent into the biliary tree requires a complex maneuver beyond the manual advancement of the stent through the accessory channel. This can include advancement of scope and the use of right/left or up/down control knobs to advance the scope tip closer to the biliary orifice.
- Finally, a multidisciplinary approach with involvement of surgical team in the decision-making process is recommended for optimal outcomes from ERCP in patients with altered surgical anatomy.

Table 17.2 Pre-procedure planning checklistsss for ERCP in patients with altered surgical anatomy

Ensure that the procedure is being performed for appropriate indication.
Obtain relevant history from the patient regarding type of surgery and previous failed ERCP attempts, if any.
Discuss patient in multidisciplinary meeting. Discuss with surgeon and interventional radiologist.
Obtain an informed consent. Discuss openly with the patient regarding risks, benefits, and alternatives.
Review operative reports to understand type of surgical reconstruction.
Consider other alternatives based on local expertise, e.g., surgical common bile duct exploration.
Review cross-sectional images when available.
Consider the use of clear cap affixed at the tip of the endoscope.
Based on above information, pick an appropriate endoscope with widest working channel possible.
If previous history of failed ERCP is noted, consider modification of tools and accessories. Review records to understand the cause of failed prior attempt.
Check GI lab for availability of appropriately trained support staff.
Ensure that appropriately trained staff are available in the procedure room.

Suggested Reading

Suggested reading articles are marked with an *

References

1. Rabinov KR, Simon M. Peroral cannulation of the ampulla of Vater for direct cholangiography and pancreatography. Preliminary report of a new method. Radiology. 1965;85(4):693–7.

2. Cotton PB, et al. Cannulation of papilla of vater via fiberduodenoscope. Assessment of retrograde cholangiopancreatography in 60 patients. Lancet. 1972;1(7741):53–8.
3. Huang RJ, et al. Evolution in the utilization of biliary interventions in the United States: results of a nationwide longitudinal study from 1998 to 2013. Gastrointest Endosc. 2017;86(2):319–326.e5.
4. Mazen Jamal M, et al. Trends in the utilization of endoscopic retrograde cholangiopancreatography (ERCP) in the United States. Am J Gastroenterol. 2007;102(5):966–75.
5. He J, et al. 2564 resected periampullary adenocarcinomas at a single institution: trends over three decades. HPB (Oxford). 2014;16(1):83–90.
6. Nguyen NT, et al. Trends in use of bariatric surgery, 2003–2008. J Am Coll Surg. 2011;213(2):261–6.
7. *Committee AT, et al. Devices and techniques for ERCP in the surgically altered GI tract. Gastrointest Endosc. 2016;83(6):1061–1075.
8. *Gomez V, Petersen BT. Endoscopic retrograde cholangiopancreatography in surgically altered anatomy. Gastrointest Endosc Clin N Am. 2015;25(4):631–656.
9. Pach R, Orzel-Nowak A, Scully T. Ludwik Rydygier--contributor to modern surgery. Gastric Cancer. 2008;11(4):187–91.
10. Sablinski T, Tilney NL. Ludwik Rydygier and the first gastrectomy for peptic ulcer. Surg Gynecol Obstet. 1991;172(6):493–6.
11. Kedia P, et al. EUS-directed transgastric ERCP for Roux-en-Y gastric bypass anatomy: a minimally invasive approach. Gastrointest Endosc. 2015;82(3):560–5.
12. *Ngamruengphong S, et al. Endoscopic ultrasound-guided creation of a transgastric fistula for the management of hepatobiliary disease in patients with Roux-en-Y gastric bypass. Endoscopy. 2017;49(6):549–552.
13. Binmoeller KF, Nguyen-Tang T. Endoscopic ultrasound-guided anterograde cholangiopancreatography. J Hepatobiliary Pancreat Sci. 2011;18(3):319–31.
14. Kedia P, et al. Endoscopic ultrasound-directed transgastric ERCP (EDGE) for Roux-en-Y anatomy: a novel technique. Endoscopy. 2015;47(2):159–63.
15. Sugiyama M, Atomi Y. Treatment of acute cholangitis due to choledocholithiasis in elderly and younger patients. Arch Surg. 1997;132(10):1129–33.

Chapter 18
ERCP in Pregnancy

Jaclyn Kagihara and Larissa Fujii-Lau

Case Report

A 34-year-old woman who is 24 weeks pregnant with her first child presents to the emergency room with a 2-week history of right upper quadrant abdominal pain. She initially attributed her discomfort to acid reflux as the pain was primarily postprandial, but the use of over-the-counter H2 blockers provided no symptom relief. On presentation, she noted a 3-hour episode of persistent pain, associated with nausea, non-bloody emesis, and generalized fatigue. She denied fevers and jaundice.

In the emergency room, she was found to have temperature 98.5 °F and pulse 114 beats per minute (bpm). Labs were significant for aspartate transaminase 159, alanine transaminase 210, alkaline phosphatase 280, and total bilirubin 1.2. On transabdominal ultrasound, the visualized portions of the extrahepatic bile duct were seen to be dilated to 8 mm (Fig. 18.1) with sludge seen in the gallbladder (Fig. 18.2). Her heart rate improved to 86 bpm with the administration of normal saline fluids. Both gastroenterology and general surgery were consulted.

J. Kagihara · L. Fujii-Lau (✉)
University of Hawaii, Queens Medical Center, Honolulu, HI, USA
e-mail: llau@queens.org

D. K. Mullady (ed.), *Dilemmas in ERCP*,
https://doi.org/10.1007/978-3-030-12741-1_18

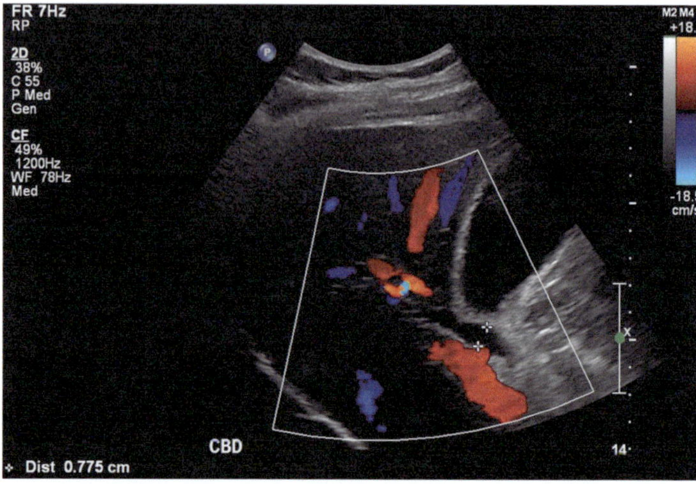

Figure 18.1 Transabdominal ultrasonography revealing a dilated common bile duct (8 mm) but no choledocholithiasis

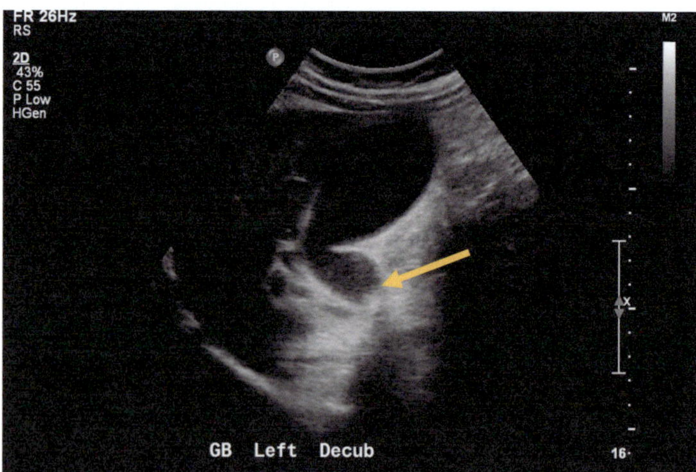

Figure 18.2 Transabdominal ultrasonography revealing shadowing sludge within the gallbladder neck (arrow)

The patient's case posed a handful of dilemmas in management:

- Is an endoscopic retrograde cholangiopancreatography (ERCP) indicated?
- Is immediate action necessary or can the patient be medically managed with therapeutic intervention delayed until after delivery?
- Should a confirmatory test be performed to determine if the patient has choledocholithiasis, if so should it be a magnetic resonance cholangiopancreatography (MRCP) or endoscopic ultrasound (EUS)?
- What risks does ERCP pose to the mother and the fetus?
- How must standard ERCP techniques be tailored in a pregnant patient?

Introduction

Pregnancy is a known risk factor for developing gallstones. During pregnancy, elevated levels of estrogen and progesterone increase bile lithogenicity and decrease gallbladder wall motility, favoring the formation of gallstones [1–3]. These physiologic alterations in pregnancy can even provoke the recurrence of biliary tract disease in patients who have already undergone cholecystectomy [4].

Pancreaticobiliary disease is estimated to complicate as many as 3.3–12.2% of pregnancies [5, 6]. In a prospective study, sludge and/or stones were found by ultrasound in 5.1% and 7.9% of pregnant women by the second trimester and third trimester, respectively, as well as in 10.2% of women by 2–4 weeks postpartum [7]. Fortunately, most pregnant women remain asymptomatic, such that the frequency of disease requiring therapeutic intervention has been reported be as few as 1 in 1200 deliveries [8]. Furthermore, in the postpartum period, sludge and stones are spontaneously cleared in 61% and 28% of women, respectively, as hormone levels return to their prepregnancy state [9]. Despite this phenomenon, significant complications of cholelithiasis including acute cholecystitis, cholangitis, and pancreatitis can still develop in up to 10% of symptomatic pregnant females and may lead to potentially life-threatening consequences for both the mother and the fetus. Surgery, once considered to be the mainstay in management for gallstone disease, is now understood to carry an increased risk of maternal and fetal compromise [10]. ERCP, therefore, has emerged as the treatment of choice, and interventional endoscopists treating pregnant patients need to be experienced and comfortable with this procedure. In this chapter we review the special considerations that should be reviewed when ERCP is considered for a pregnant patient.

Diagnosis/Assessment

Indications for ERCP

The role of ERCP in pregnancy is strictly therapeutic. The primary indications are similar to those in nonpregnant patients and are listed in Table 18.1. In rarer instances, ERCP has been performed in pregnant patients with choledochal cysts [11], parasitic infection of the biliary tree [12], and pancreatic adenocarcinoma [12].

Justifying the need for ERCP in a pregnant patient begins with the appropriate diagnosis. Transabdominal US has tradi-

TABLE 18.1 Indications for ERCP during pregnancy

Symptomatic choledocholithiasis
Cholangitis
Gallstone pancreatitis
Obstructive jaundice
Biliary or pancreatic ductal disease (i.e., leak, stricture)

tionally been the initial imaging study of choice in patients with suspected choledocholithiasis, but its use may be limited when considering the changes in body habitus and the anatomy that occur in pregnancy. The use of MRCP and EUS to confirm the presence of choledocholithiasis prior to ERCP has recently been gaining popularity. However, due to the limited studies on the use of MRI during pregnancy, the International Commission on Non-Ionizing Radiation Protection recommends avoiding this as much as possible during the first trimester of pregnancy [13]. They state that MRI should only be pursued after critical risk-benefit analysis has been undertaken for each individual patient. Data supports the use of EUS prior to ERCP, especially in cases where transabdominal US and/or MRCP are nondiagnostic and the clinical suspicion for CBD stones remains high. Several studies have emphasized the utility of EUS-guided ERCP in patients with suspected choledocholithiasis as up to 40% of ERCPs may be avoided by the lack of biliary pathology seen on initial EUS [14–16].

Ultimately, treatment should not be delayed for patients with a clear diagnosis that requires intervention. In a retrospective study, patients managed conservatively for symptomatic gallstones were more likely to develop recurrent symptoms, require emergency room or hospital visits, and undergo cesarean section operations than those treated with either ERCP and/or cholecystectomy [17]. For patients in whom an indication is not straightforward, the decision to undergo ERCP should be individualized, based on the clinical status of the mother and the fetus and expert opinions of the endoscopist, anesthesiologist, obstetrician, and surgeon.

Pregnancy Testing

Rapid pregnancy testing is commonplace and should be considered standard of care prior to ERCP in any woman of childbearing age. The importance of pregnancy screening is highlighted in a case series on the safety and efficacy of standard ERCP in pregnancy in which 3 out of 23 women did not know they were pregnant at the time of ERCP [8].

Consent

As with any intervention, a thorough informed consent process is mandatory prior to ERCP. All patients should be told of available alternatives in management, the proposed plan for ERCP, along with any potential adverse events. In addition to the immediate risks of ERCP to the patient and the fetus, the possible long-term risk of radiation exposure to the fetus should be discussed with the patient [18].

Fetal Monitoring

Prior to ERCP, an obstetrician consultation is required for assistance in the perioperative care of the patient and the fetus. Their support should also be readily available throughout the procedure in the event there is fetal or patient distress. The decision to monitor fetal heart rate should be individualized based on the recommendation of the obstetrician, which is typically guided by gestational age of the fetus and available resources. Before 24 weeks gestation, Doppler confirmation of the presence of an adequate fetal heart rate before and after the procedure is sufficient. After 24 weeks gestation, simultaneous monitoring of electronic fetal heart and uterine contraction should be performed before and after the procedure [19].

Timing

There is scarce evidence in regard to the optimal timing of ERCP in pregnancy. The second trimester of pregnancy theoretically provides the safest opportunity [19]. In the first trimester, the fetus is undergoing organogenesis and is therefore most susceptible to the teratogenic effects of ionizing radiation [20]. Studies from atomic bomb survivors suggest that the effects of radiation on the central nervous system are highest during weeks 8–15 of gestation [21]. In the third trimester, the mother's gravid uterus may present anatomic alterations that make it difficult for even the most skilled endoscopists to access the ampulla.

In a retrospective review, patients who underwent ERCP in the first trimester had the lowest percentage of term pregnancy (73.3%), highest risk of preterm delivery (20.0%), and highest-risk low-birth-weight newborns (21.4%) [22]. The authors suggested that the adverse outcome in those undergoing first-trimester ERCP was attributed more to the hepatobiliary disease itself rather than the ERCP procedure itself. Reassuringly, none of the 59 patients in this study experienced adverse events such as stillborn or fetal malformations.

Sedation and Antibiotics

Sedation is high risk in pregnancy and therefore should be administered under the guidance of an anesthesiologist. All agents should be used with great caution and vigilance and given in slow titration and at the lowest dose to avoid hemodynamic and respiratory changes in the mother and the fetus.

Physiologic changes to the respiratory system during pregnancy include a 20% increase in oxygen consumption and a 20% decrease in pulmonary function residual capacity, which can lead to a rapid decrease in partial pressure oxygen in situations with maternal apnea [23]. Furthermore, airway protection is of concern in pregnant patients, as swelling of the oropharyngeal tissues and a decreased caliber of the glottic opening can make intubation challenging. Additionally, progesterone causes relaxation of the lower esophageal sphincter, thereby increasing the risk of aspiration in an unconscious pregnant patient [24]. Noteworthy hemodynamic changes during pregnancy include a 40% increase in blood volume and cardiac output and a 20% dilutional decrease in hematocrit, rendering the fetus sensitive to maternal hypoxia and hypotension [23]. Great care, therefore, must be taken to avoid oversedation of pregnant patients [19].

The risk of drug teratogenicity in the fetus is related to the inherent toxicity of the medication, the dosage and the duration of exposure, and the period of fetal development when introduced [25]. Recommendations are based on scant data from case series and reports and from the Food and Drug Administration (FDA) drug categorization. Since 2014, the FDA no longer uses the five categories (A, B, C, D, and X) to determine the safety of over-the-counter and prescription drugs in pregnancy. Because most information about drug safety during pregnancy came from animal studies, uncontrolled studies, and postmarking surveillance, the old FDA classification system led to confusion and difficulty applying available information to clinical decisions. In 2015, the FDA enlisted a new labeling of all drugs in a consistent format called the "Pregnancy and Lactation Labeling (Drugs) Final Rule (PLLR)." The information required by the FDA has three subsections: pregnancy (8.1), lactation (8.2), and females and males of reproductive potential (8.3) [26]. A summary of the commonly used sedative drugs using the new FDA classification is provided in Table 18.2.

The indications for antibiotics are the same in pregnant and nonpregnant patients. Antibiotics are often given prophylactically during ERCP particularly if contrast is used to decrease the risk of infection of inadequately drained contrast. In general, penicillins, cephalosporins, erythromycin, and clindamycin are considered to be safe during pregnancy and lactating, while quinolones and tetracyclines should be avoided in all trimesters [19]. Metronidazole should not be used in the first trimester, and sulfonamides and nitrofurantoin should not be given to pregnant patients in their third trimester. During breastfeeding, sulfonamides, quinolones, and metronidazole should be avoided.

Treatment/Management

Positioning

The optimal position for pregnant women undergoing ERCP should minimize fetal radiation exposure (discussed further below) and avoid vascular compression. In the second and

Table 18.2 Sedative medication for ERCP during pregnancy. (From the FDA website for each medication)

Drug	Old FDA pregnancy safety category	PLLR	
		Pregnancy (8.1)	Lactation (8.2)
Meperidine (DEMEROL®)	B	Available data with meperidine are insufficient to inform a drug-associated risk for major birth defects and miscarriage Formal animal reproduction studies have not been conducted with meperidine Meperidine administration to pregnant hamsters during organogenesis reportedly caused neural tube defects (exencephaly and cranioschisis) at a dose 0.85 and 1.5× the recommended human dose, 1200 mg/day	Meperidine appears in the milk of nursing mothers receiving the drug
Fentanyl citrate	C	Available data with fentanyl are insufficient to inform a drug-associated risk for major birth defects and miscarriage Fentanyl administration to pregnant rats during organogenesis has been shown to be embryocidal at doses within the range of the recommended human dose	Fentanyl appears in the milk of nursing mothers receiving the drug Infants exposed to fentanyl through breast milk should be monitored for excess sedation and respiratory depression

(continued)

Table 18.2 (continued)

Drug	Old FDA pregnancy safety category	PLLR	
		Pregnancy (8.1)	Lactation (8.2)
Midazolam (VERSED®))	D	Available data with midazolam are insufficient to inform a drug-associated risk for major birth defects and miscarriage Midazolam administration to pregnant rabbits and rats showed no evidence of teratogenicity at doses 5 and 10× the recommended human dose, 0.35 mg/kg	Midazolam appears in the milk of nursing mothers receiving the drug
Diazepam (VALIUM®)	D	Available data with diazepam are insufficient to inform a drug-associated risk for major birth defects and miscarriage Diazepam administration to pregnant mice and hamsters during organogenesis has been shown to cause cleft palate and encephalopathy at a dose 8× the recommended human dose, 1 mg/kg/day	Diazepam appears in the mild of nursing mothers receiving the drug

Propofol (DIPRIVIAN®)	D	Available data with propofol are insufficient to inform a drug-associated risk for major birth defects and miscarriage Propofol administration to pregnant rats either prior to mating, during early gestation, or during late gestation and early lactation has been shown to cause decreased pup survival and increase maternal mortality at a dose less than the recommended human dose, 15 mg/kg/day	Propofol appears in the mild of nursing mothers receiving the drug

third trimester, patients should avoid being placed in the supine position as the gravid uterus can compress the aorta or the vena cava, resulting in maternal hypotension and inadequate placental perfusion [19]. In most studies, patients are placed in the left lateral position with a wedge or pillow placed under the patient's right hip to help maintain safe orientation.

Electrocautery

Amniotic fluid can serve as a conduit for electrical current to the fetus [27]. When sphincterotomy is used, the uterus should not lie in the path between the sphincterotome and the grounding pad. Placement of the grounding pad on the posterior thoracic wall therefore is more ideal than placement on the thigh. If available, monopolar electrocautery can be used to avoid the need for a grounding pad and decrease the risk of current passing through the gravid uterus [19].

Radiation Exposure and Risk

The consequences of radiation exposure during standard ERCP with fluoroscopy are a major and highly debated concern. Knowledge regarding the effects of radiation are largely derived from epidemiologic and observational studies from exposed human populations and animal studies. Radiation harm to the fetus can be divided into two types. Deterministic effects of radiation include malformation and disturbances in growth and development, the likelihood and severity of which are proportional to the radiation dose. Stochastic effects include disturbances in genetics and cancer, which follow a "no-threshold" model regardless of radiation dose [28].

There are three possible sources of radiation during standard ERCP [29]. The first occurs when the X-ray source emits a focused beam of radiation directly toward a subject. The second form is the major source of exposure to the endoscopists and staff, as well as the fetus, as the X-ray "scatters" throughout the room. It occurs when a source emits a focused beam of radiation that strikes an object and ricochets from its original path. The third form is often negligible and occurs when radiation escapes or "leaks" from the X-ray source.

Ionizing radiation can be quantified in a variety of ways [30]. The *absorbed dose* is the amount of energy per unit mass of tissue through which the radiation passed and is expressed in units of gray (Gy). The *effective dose* is expressed in units of sievert (Sv). It combines the amount of radiation absorbed and tries to estimate the effect of the radiation, based on radiation type and radiation-sensitivity of different organs. This measurement is used to assess long-term risk of radiation exposure, such as cancer. The *dose-area product (DAP)* or *kerma-area* product is a measure of radiation dose integrated across the entire exposed field. It is derived from the absorbed dose multiplied by the area irradiated and is expressed in units of gray per square centimeters (Gy/cm^2).

The 2017 American College of Obstetricians and Gynecologists Guidelines for Diagnostic Imaging During Pregnancy and Lactation state, "fetal risk of anomalies, growth restriction, or abortion have not been reported with radiation exposure of less than 50 mGy, a level above the range of exposure for diagnostic procedures." [20]

Several authors, therefore, have attempted to quantify radiation exposure during ERCP to both the mother and the fetus using different methodologies. Using thermoluminescent dosimeters (TLDs), Kahaleh et al. found mean estimated fetal radiation exposure to be 0.4 mGy (range 0.01–1.8 mGy) [31]. Another group used a non-anthropomorphic phantom to estimate the entrance dose and subsequently measured fetal dose exposure at 3 mGy (range 1.02–5.77 mGy) with a mean fluoroscopy time of 3.2 minutes (range 1.1–6.1 minutes) [32]. Samara et al. presented an intriguing model utilizing data obtained from 24 nonpregnant patients for estimating conceptus radiation dosage for a specific patient procedure [28]. The study was performed in two stages. The first step involved collecting data on technical and physical parameters for fluoroscopy and radiography. The second step involved the use of a Monte Carlo-N-particle code, a mathematical phantom, to calculate the normalized conceptus dose for a range of exposure techniques, patient size, and gestational age. This model allows for a more accurate estimation of fetal radiation exposure when compared with traditional methods. Their data revealed that fetal dose exposure may occasionally exceed 50 mGy (range 3.4–55.9 mGy), above the level deemed "safe" by ACOG. Despite these authors' efforts and the recommendations laid forth by ACOG, a clear-cut safe or harmful radiation dose for ERCP in pregnancy is still unknown. We recommend the lowest dose of radiation necessary to complete the procedure successfully be used.

Because standard ERCP has the potential to deliver elevated doses, dose reduction techniques are of the utmost importance to protecting the mother and the fetus. Table 18.3 contains a list of general rules for safe and effective fluoroscopy use. Patients should be strategically positioned relative to the expected trajectory of the X-ray beam. Wagner et al. proposed that a posteroanterior projection of the X-ray beam would result in 3–7× less entrance dose compared to a lateral approach, as the mother has more tissue in this direction to provide shielding [33]. A lead should be used in all cases of ERCP with fluoroscopy. The use of a radiation-attenuated drape (made of heavy metals bismuths and antimony) hung

Table 18.3 Techniques to minimize radiation exposure in standard ERCP

Use short "taps" of fluoroscopy
Use the last-image-hold or fluoroscopy loop recording feature for image analysis
Use low-dose-rate setting Avoid recorded images
Avoid use of magnification
Collimate X-ray beam to the smallest field possible
Place the patient close to the image receptor and far from the radiation source
Use lead shielding

around the image intensifier in one study reduced radiation dose exposure to the endoscopists and the staff by ~90% [29]. Room setup is important and should be arranged so that the image receptor is kept as close to the patient as possible and the X-ray beam as far from the patient as possible. Endoscopists should use pulse (not continuous) fluoroscopy at a low-dose frame rate setting. If image noise becomes a problem at the low-dose frame rate, then endoscopists should collaborate with a medical physicist or work with a vendor service representative to adjust image processing settings to optimize image quality [34]. The number of recorded spot images should be limited, keeping in mind that digital image capture requires a lower dose compared with film radiography, if images are necessary. For image analysis the last-image-hold or loop recorder feature is useful. Magnification mode should be used sparingly as the radiation dose is compounded as the field of view decreases. Routine reminder of demagnification may be useful as endoscopist may have the habit of staying in magnification mode while preoccupied with other facets of ERCP [35]. Collimating the X-ray beam to the smallest field possible accomplishes several advantages including decreasing the amount of scatter radiation striking the fetus and image receptor, improving the fluoroscopic image quality, and reducing the chance of direct exposure to the fetus [34]. The importance of ERCP in pregnant patients being performed by skilled endoscopists in properly equipped and staffed healthcare institutions cannot be reinforced enough. It has been shown that radiation exposure is significantly higher with endoscopists who perform less than 200 ERCPs per year. In a study by Liao et al., the differences in median radiation exposure to patients essentially doubled when the procedure was performed by a low-volume endoscopist [36].

Non-radiation ERCP

The goal of non-radiation ERCP is to achieve biliary cannulation without radiation exposure, thereby negating the risks of radiation to the patient and fetus. However, the lack of fluoroscopy may increase the risk of retained stones or missing biliary pathology (i.e., strictures, leak). Therefore, the benefit of the lack of fetal radiation exposure needs to be weighed against the risk of the more technically challenging ERCP. Multiple techniques have been suggested including needle-knife fistulotomy, two-stage process with biliary stenting, and bile aspiration. Further studies are needed to determine the role of each of these techniques in pregnancy.

In 1990, Binmoeller and Katon published a landmark case of NR-ERCP in a pregnant female with an impacted stone at the ampulla that caused displacement and obstruction of the papillary orifice, prohibiting standard papillotomy and biliary cannulation [37]. Using the needle-knife papillotome, a large choledochal-duodenal fistula was created allowing spontaneous passage of the stone. Several other authors have reported use of the needle-knife papillotome to facilitate biliary cannulation in patients that fail conventional methods [38, 39]. The needle-knife allows for flexibility in orientation and ease of maneuverability and can cut with little current. The authors note that the incision should be done over the calculus as this will function as a safety buffer. Safety of needle-knife was examined by Huibregtse et al. who found the rate of duodenal perforation to be less than that of standard endoscopic papillotomy with no difference in bleeding rates but a higher risk of pancreatitis with use of needle-knife [40].

Bile aspiration is another proposed technique for non-radiation ERCP. Uomo et al. first described this technique in 1994 where a catheter was inserted into the bile duct followed by aspiration of fluid [41]. The technique is based off the assumption that if bilious fluid is aspirated, then bile duct cannulation is confirmed. If clear fluid is seen, then placement in the pancreatic duct is presumed and cannulation is reattempted. Shelton et al. performed wire-guided cannulation and confirmed biliary cannulation by observing bilious fluid around the guidewire while moving the guidewire back and forth to facilitate fluid drainage [42]. The bile aspiration technique has several potential drawbacks. The method does not differentiate between cannulation of the cystic duct versus the common hepatic duct, and it may be difficult to discern whether the duct has been cannulated beyond the level of obstruction. Additionally, confirmation that the biliary duct has been swept of all biliary stones or sludge is not always clear. Shelton et al. overcame this by performing choledochoscopy to confirm ductal clearance in five patients, while transabdominal ultrasound was performed after ERCP in another case series [43].

The use of stents in the setting of pregnancy is controversial. Axelrad et al. was the first group to implement prophylactic bile duct stenting in a pregnant patient with choledocholithiasis who had recurrent pain after sphincterotomy and balloon extraction [44]. Repeat ERCP demonstrated retained gallstones prompting placement of a CBD stent to prevent recurrence. Opponents of biliary stents as temporary treatment for choledocholithiasis in pregnancy argue that stent placement requires fluoroscopy and a second procedure to remove the stent, with the added potential complication of stent occlusion and cholangitis. Proponents, on the other hand, reason that it is a safe technique with minimal adverse events. In a case series of ten pregnant patients who underwent placement of a 10 Fr biliary stent without sphincterotomy, all the patients delivered healthy babies at term with postpartum ERCP with sphincterotomy and stent extraction [45]. In two patients, the stent remained in place for 7 and 8 months throughout gestation without cholangitis. Sharma et al. performed a similar study but opted for sphincterotomy plus stenting of a 7Fr double-pigtail CBD stent [46]. In the postpartum period, patients were subjected to definitive ERCP with stent removal, cholangiogram, and stone removal. One patient presented for her second ERCP 3 years after the first and in the interim had another asymptomatic pregnancy with normal delivery. Four patients were found to have completely blocked stents with bile drainage seen around the stent. The authors recommend therefore that a sphincterotomy be performed prior to stenting as it allowed drainage of the bile even in the event of stent occlusion, decreasing the risk of complications.

Imaging tool-guided ERCP entails the use of transabdominal US, EUS, or choledochoscopy to directly visualize the biliary duct to facilitate cannulation and clearance. Transabdominal US requires the patient to be moved from the left lateral position to supine with the ERCP equipment in place [47, 48]. This is time-consuming and difficult, making it not an optimal technique for ERCP. As discussed earlier, EUS before ERCP can determine the actual necessity of intervention. It can also provide information regarding the location, size, and number of stones present to directly guide biliary intervention. Vohra et al. used EUS to confirm the presence of choledocholithiasis prior to ERCP, and the number of stones extracted at ERCP matched the number of stones seen during EUS [15]. Two patients underwent direct peroral choledochoscopy to confirm stone clearance due to fragmentation of a stone during extraction. There were no immediate procedure-related complications, and no patient required a repeat procedure. A more recent trial by Netinatsunton et al., however, seems to yield more concerns and questions regarding the efficacy and safety of EUS-guided ERCP without fluoroscopy when compared to that of standard ERCP with fluoroscopy [49]. While the cannulation success rates, adverse event rates, and total procedure times were similar in both groups, the stone clearance rate in the EUS-guided ERCP group was inferior to that in the standard ERCP group. Peroral choledochoscopy provides direct visualization of the duct and is performed by insertion of a cholangioscope through the working channel of a duodenoscope. Few reports have utilized this technique; however a promising case series by Shelton et al. used the SpyGlass Direct Visualization System (Boston Scientific, Marlborough, MA) to confirm biliary cannulation and document stone clearance without the need for fluoroscopy [42]. The main limitations of choledochoscopy are its high cost and exhaustive technical and time demands, such that it should be used selectively in pregnant patients after conventional ERCP methods have been unsuccessful.

Outcomes

Adverse Events

Complications of ERCP whether performed during pregnancy or not include pancreatitis (2–9%), post-sphincterotomy hemorrhage (0.5–5%), cholangitis (<1%), and perforation (<1%) [50, 51]. Post-ERCP pancreatitis (PEP) is an important and potentially preventable complication of ERCP. Patient-related risk factors for PEP include young age and female gender. Procedural risk factors include difficult cannulation, need for precut sphincterotomy, and passage of a guidewire deep into the pancreatic duct.

A retrospective cohort study of the National Inpatient Sample compared standard ERCP outcomes among 907 pregnant women with 2721 nonpregnant women [52]. There was no difference in rates of perforation, infection, and bleeding between both groups. However, PEP occurred in 12% of pregnant women versus 5% of nonpregnant women. Pregnancy was an independent risk factor for PEP, even when controlling for the lower rate of pancreatic duct stent placement in the pregnant women. The authors proposed several theories to explain this including more difficult cannulation due to minimizing of radiation use and physician hesitancy to give large volumes of intravenous fluid and prophylactic rectal indomethacin. Muniraj and Jamidar et al. reviewed the outcomes of 11 large studies using standard ERCP in pregnancy and found PEP and post-sphincterotomy bleeding to comprise 9.5% and 1.0% of maternal complications, respectively [53]. There were no maternal deaths. Fetal complications included preterm birth (4.0%), spontaneous abortion (0.5%), and pre-eclampsia (1%). There was one neonatal death, but no clear causal relationship to the ERCP procedure was established.

Wu et al. analyzed the outcomes of 12 large studies of NR-ERCP in pregnancy [54]. The overall morbidity rate in the series was found to be 15.6%. Significant maternal complications included incomplete stone clearance (6.7%), hemorrhage (2.2%), stent occlusion (2.2%), PEP (1.1%), and stent migration (1.1%). Fetal complications included preterm birth, intrauterine growth restriction, and spontaneous abortion at a rate of 2.6%, 2%, and 0.6%, respectively. There were no therapeutic abortions or postpartum infant deaths after ERCP, and with fetal mortality <1%, the procedure is seen to be relatively safe. Again, because the protocol for NR-ERCP eliminates ionizing exposure altogether, there is no need to consider the potential effects the fetus or child may experience.

Case Presentation Follow-up

In the presented case of the pregnant patient with complicated gallstones, an obstetrician was present to assist the patient and the fetus throughout the perioperative period. The patient was determined to be at indeterminate risk of choledocholithiasis based on ASGE guidelines and therefore underwent an EUS, which confirmed the presence of one stone within the bile duct (Fig. 18.3).[GIE 2010 71; 1] An

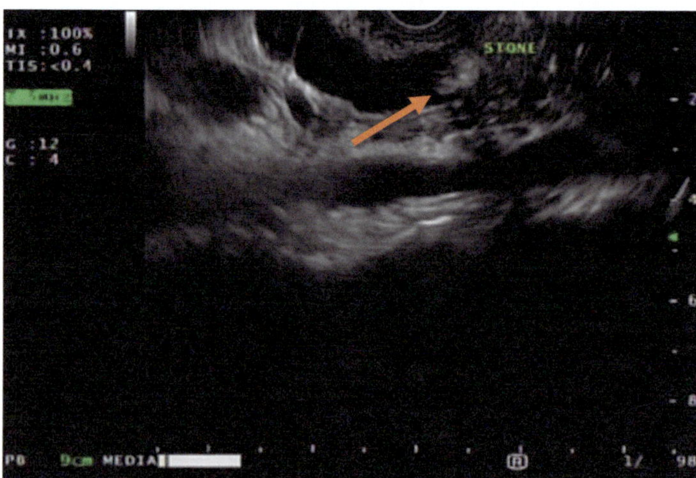

FIGURE 18.3 Endoscopic ultrasonography reveals a shadowing stone (arrow) in the distal common bile duct

immediate ERCP was performed with fluoroscopy used to only confirm biliary placement of the wire. A sphincterotomy was performed and the one stone was swept from the duct. Further balloon sweeps yielded nothing and were without resistance to suggest the presence of additional stones. The next day the patient underwent a laparoscopic cholecystectomy. She went on to have an uncomplicated pregnancy and delivered a full term baby without further biliary issues.

Conclusions

ERCP with or without the use of fluoroscopy is efficacious and safe in pregnant patients. It should be emphasized that this procedure be performed under the appropriate indications and when otherwise conservative management poses a life-threatening risk. Although the use of ERCP without fluoroscopy has the benefit of avoiding fetal exposure to radiation, the procedure becomes much more advanced and technically challenging. Therefore, each therapeutic endoscopist needs to have an arsenate of skill sets and should provide a comprehensive informed consent that includes the risks to both the patient and the fetus.

Pearls/Pitfalls

- ERCP with or without fluoroscopy is safe in all trimesters of pregnancy.
- ERCP should not be delayed in patients with a clear indication.
- EUS is theoretically preferred over MRCP for confirmation of bile duct pathology in the first trimester.
- Perioperative fetal monitoring and an obstetrician consultation should be considered in all patients.
- There is no known threshold for "safe" or "harmful" radiation to the fetus, so radiation reduction strategies should be employed in all patients.

- Non-radiation ERCP can be utilized in pregnant patients but makes the procedure more technically challenging.
- Therapeutic endoscopists with low ERCP volumes should consider transferring pregnant patients to a tertiary center with higher volumes.

Suggested Reading

The highly significant articles are marked in * in the reference section.

References

1. Everson GT. Pregnancy and gallstones. Hepatology. 1993;17(1):159–61.
2. Everson GT, McKinley C, Kern F Jr. Mechanisms of gallstone formation in women. Effects of exogenous estrogen (Premarin) and dietary cholesterol on hepatic lipid metabolism. J Clin Invest. 1991;87(1):237–46.
3. Marzio L. Factors affecting gallbladder motility: drugs. Dig Liver Dis. 2003;35(Suppl 3):S17–9.
4. Bani Hani MN, Bani-Hani KE, Rashdan A, AlWaqfi NR, Heis HA, Al-Manasra AR. Safety of endoscopic retrograde cholangiopancreatography during pregnancy. ANZ J Surg. 2009;79(1–2):23–6.
5. Basso L, McCollum PT, Darling MR, Tocchi A, Tanner WA. A study of cholelithiasis during pregnancy and its relationship with age, parity, menarche, breast-feeding, dysmenorrhea, oral contraception and a maternal history of cholelithiasis. Surg Gynecol Obstet. 1992;175(1):41–6.
6. Valdivieso V, Covarrubias C, Siegel F, Cruz F. Pregnancy and cholelithiasis: pathogenesis and natural course of gallstones diagnosed in early puerperium. Hepatology. 1993;17(1):1–4.
7. Ko CW, Beresford SA, Schulte SJ, Matsumoto AM, Lee SP. Incidence, natural history, and risk factors for biliary sludge and stones during pregnancy. Hepatology. 2005;41(2):359–65.

8. Jamidar PA, Beck GJ, Hoffman BJ, Lehman GA, Hawes RH, Agrawal RM, et al. Endoscopic retrograde cholangiopancreatography in pregnancy. Am J Gastroenterol. 1995;90(8):1263–7.
9. Maringhini A, Ciambra M, Baccelliere P, Raimondo M, Orlando A, Tine F, et al. Biliary sludge and gallstones in pregnancy: incidence, risk factors, and natural history. Ann Intern Med. 1993;119(2):116–20.
10. Brodsky JB, Cohen EN, Brown BW Jr, Wu ML, Whitcher C. Surgery during pregnancy and fetal outcome. Am J Obstet Gynecol. 1980;138(8):1165–7.
11. Hewitt PM, Krige JE, Bornman PC, Terblanche J. Choledochal cyst in pregnancy: a therapeutic dilemma. J Am Coll Surg. 1995;181(3):237–40.
12. Shah OJ, Robanni I, Khan F, Zargar SA, Javid G. Management of biliary ascariasis in pregnancy. World J Surg. 2005;29(10):1294–8.
13. NRP B. Protection of pregnant patients during diagnostic medical exposures to ionising radiation. Doc NRPB. 2009:3–16.
14. Shah JN, Bhat YM, Hamerski CM, Kane SD, Binmoeller KF. Feasibility of nonradiation EUS-based ERCP in patients with uncomplicated choledocholithiasis (with video). Gastrointest Endosc. 2016;84(5):764–9.
15. Vohra S, Holt EW, Bhat YM, Kane S, Shah JN, Binmoeller KF. Successful single-session endosonography-based endoscopic retrograde cholangiopancreatography without fluoroscopy in pregnant patients with suspected choledocholithiasis: a case series. J Hepatobiliary Pancreat Sci. 2014;21(2):93–7.
16. Zaheer A, Anwar MM, Donohoe C, O'Keeffe S, Mushtaq H, Kelleher B, et al. The diagnostic accuracy of endoscopic ultrasound in suspected biliary obstruction and its impact on endoscopic retrograde cholangiopancreatography burden in real clinical practice: a consecutive analysis. Eur J Gastroenterol Hepatol. 2013;25(7):850–7.
17. Othman MO, Stone E, Hashimi M, Parasher G. Conservative management of cholelithiasis and its complications in pregnancy is associated with recurrent symptoms and more emergency department visits. Gastrointest Endosc. 2012;76(3):564–9.
18. Friedel D, Stavropoulos S, Iqbal S, Cappell MS. Gastrointestinal endoscopy in the pregnant woman. World J Gastrointest Endosc. 2014;6(5):156–67.
19. *Shergill AK, Ben-Menachem T, Chandrasekhara V, Chathadi K, Decker GA, Evans JA, et al. Guidelines for endoscopy in pregnant and lactating women. Gastrointest Endosc. 2012;76(1):18–24.

20. *Committee Opinion No. 723: guidelines for diagnostic imaging during pregnancy and lactation. Obstet Gynecol. 2017;130(4):e210–e6.
21. Hall EJ. Scientific view of low-level radiation risks. Radiographics. 1991;11(3):509–18.
22. Tang SJ, Mayo MJ, Rodriguez-Frias E, Armstrong L, Tang L, Sreenarasimhaiah J, et al. Safety and utility of ERCP during pregnancy. Gastrointest Endosc. 2009;69(3 Pt 1):453–61.
23. Cheek TG, Baird E. Anesthesia for nonobstetric surgery: maternal and fetal considerations. Clin Obstet Gynecol. 2009;52(4):535–45.
24. Baron TH, Richter JE. Gastroesophageal reflux disease in pregnancy. Gastroenterol Clin N Am. 1992;21(4):777–91.
25. Cragan JD, Friedman JM, Holmes LB, Uhl K, Green NS, Riley L. Ensuring the safe and effective use of medications during pregnancy: planning and prevention through preconception care. Matern Child Health J. 2006;10(5 Suppl):S129–35.
26. Adminisration USFaD. PLR requirements for prescribing information. Available from: https://www.fda.gov/Drugs/GuidanceComplianceRegulatoryInformation/LawsActsandRules/ucm084159.htm.
27. Einarson A, Bailey B, Inocencion G, Ormond K, Koren G. Accidental electric shock in pregnancy: a prospective cohort study. Am J Obstet Gynecol. 1997;176(3):678–81.
28. Samara ET, Stratakis J, Enele Melono JM, Mouzas IA, Perisinakis K, Damilakis J. Therapeutic ERCP and pregnancy: is the radiation risk for the conceptus trivial? Gastrointest Endosc. 2009;69(4):824–31.
29. Muniraj T, Aslanian HR, Laine L, Farrell J, Ciarleglio MM, Deng Y, et al. A double-blind, randomized, sham-controlled trial of the effect of a radiation-attenuating drape on radiation exposure to endoscopy staff during ERCP. Am J Gastroenterol. 2015;110(5):690–6.
30. Rehani MM, Ciraj-Bjelac O, Vano E, Miller DL, Walsh S, Giordano BD, et al. ICRP Publication 117. Radiological protection in fluoroscopically guided procedures performed outside the imaging department. Ann ICRP. 2010;40(6):1–102.
31. Kahaleh M, Hartwell GD, Arseneau KO, Pajewski TN, Mullick T, Isin G, et al. Safety and efficacy of ERCP in pregnancy. Gastrointest Endosc. 2004;60(2):287–92.

32. Tham TC, Vandervoort J, Wong RC, Montes H, Roston AD, Slivka A, et al. Safety of ERCP during pregnancy. Am J Gastroenterol. 2003;98(2):308–11.
33. Wagner L, Lester R, Sladana L. Exposure of the pregnant patient to diagnostic radiations. 2nd ed. Madison; 1997.
34. Baron TH, Schueler BA. Pregnancy and radiation exposure during therapeutic ERCP: time to put the baby to bed? Gastrointest Endosc. 2009;69(4):832–4.
35. Binmoeller KF, Nett A. ERCP: time to take the lead off? Gastrointest Endosc. 2017;86(6):1066–9.
36. Liao C, Thosani N, Kothari S, Friedland S, Chen A, Banerjee S. Radiation exposure to patients during ERCP is significantly higher with low-volume endoscopists. Gastrointest Endosc. 2015;81(2):391–8.e1.
37. Binmoeller KF, Katon RM. Needle knife papillotomy for an impacted common bile duct stone during pregnancy. Gastrointest Endosc. 1990;36(6):607–9.
38. Marshall JB, Stassen WN. Multiquadrant precut papillotomy for extraction of large impacted common bile duct stone. Gastrointest Endosc. 1985;31(5):336–8.
39. Schapira L, Khawaja FI. Endoscopic fistulo-sphincterotomy: an alternative method of sphincterotomy using a new sphincterotome. Endoscopy. 1982;14(2):58–60.
40. Huibregtse K, Katon RM, Tytgat GN. Precut papillotomy via fine-needle knife papillotome: a safe and effective technique. Gastrointest Endosc. 1986;32(6):403–5.
41. Uomo G, Manes G, Picciotto FP, Rabitti PG. Endoscopic treatment of acute biliary pancreatitis in pregnancy. J Clin Gastroenterol. 1994;18(3):250–2.
42. Shelton J, Linder JD, Rivera-Alsina ME, Tarnasky PR. Commitment, confirmation, and clearance: new techniques for nonradiation ERCP during pregnancy (with videos). Gastrointest Endosc. 2008;67(2):364–8.
43. Llach J, Bordas JM, Gines A, Mondelo F, Teres J. Endoscopic sphincterotomy in pregnancy. Endoscopy. 1997;29(1):52–3.
44. Axelrad AM, Fleischer DE, Strack LL, Benjamin SB, al-Kawas FH. Performance of ERCP for symptomatic choledocholithiasis during pregnancy: techniques to increase safety and improve patient management. Am J Gastroenterol. 1994;89(1):109–12.

45. Farca A, Aguilar ME, Rodriguez G, de la Mora G, Arango L. Biliary stents as temporary treatment for choledocholithiasis in pregnant patients. Gastrointest Endosc. 1997;46(1):99–101.
46. Sharma SS, Maharshi S. Two stage endoscopic approach for management of choledocholithiasis during pregnancy. J Gastrointestin Liver Dis. 2008;17(2):183–5.
47. Freistuhler M, Braess A, Petrides AS. Ultrasound-controlled endoscopic papillotomy in pregnancy in severe biliary pancreatitis. Z Gastroenterol. 1999;37(1):27–30.
48. Parada AA, Goncalves MO, Tafner E, Arago JM, Borges SL, Branco PR, et al. Endoscopic papillotomy under ultrasonographic control. Int Surg. 1991;76(2):75–6.
49. Netinatsunton N, Sottisuporn J, Attasaranya S, Witeerungrot T, Siripun A, Pattarapuntakul T, et al. Prospective randomized trial of EUS-assisted ERCP without fluoroscopy versus ERCP in common bile duct stones. Gastrointest Endosc. 2017;86(6):1059–65.
50. Freeman ML. Adverse outcomes of ERCP. Gastrointest Endosc. 2002;56(6 Suppl):S273–82.
51. Freeman ML, Guda NM. Prevention of post-ERCP pancreatitis: a comprehensive review. Gastrointest Endosc. 2004;59(7):845–64.
52. Inamdar S, Berzin TM, Sejpal DV, Pleskow DK, Chuttani R, Sawhney MS, et al. Pregnancy is a risk factor for pancreatitis after endoscopic retrograde cholangiopancreatography in a national cohort study. Clin Gastroenterol Hepatol. 2016;14(1):107–14.
53. Muniraj T, Jamidar PA. ERCP in Pregnancy: ERCP: Elsevier; 2013. p. 282–7.
54. *Wu W, Faigel DO, Sun G, Yang Y. Non-radiation endoscopic retrograde cholangiopancreatography in the management of choledocholithiasis during pregnancy. Dig Endosc. 2014;26(6):691–700.

Chapter 19
ERCP in Pediatric Populations

Mayssan Muftah, Christopher Fritzen, and Field F. Willingham

Case Presentations

Case 1

A 9-year-old male without significant past medical history presented to the emergency department with persistent and worsening epigastric abdominal pain. He reported decreased appetite and non-bloody, non-bilious emesis approximately 24 hours after falling off his bike onto the handle bars. The review of systems was notable for abdominal pain radiating to his back. The physical exam revealed epigastric tenderness, guarding, and bruising to his right mid-abdomen. Laboratory testing revealed

---

M. Muftah
Department of Medicine, Emory University School of Medicine, Atlanta, GA, USA

C. Fritzen
Gastroenterology, Hepatology and Nutrition, Children's Healthcare of Atlanta, Emory University School of Medicine, Atlanta, GA, USA

F. F. Willingham (✉)
Department of Gastroenterology, Children's Healthcare of Atlanta, Emory University School of Medicine, Atlanta, GA, USA

Division of Digestive Diseases, Emory University School of Medicine, Atlanta, GA, USA
e-mail: field.willingham@emory.edu

D. K. Mullady (ed.), *Dilemmas in ERCP*,
https://doi.org/10.1007/978-3-030-12741-1_19

an elevated lipase (9173 U/L) and amylase (197 U/L). Computed tomography (CT) scanning of the abdomen and pelvis with contrast revealed an abnormal hypo-density throughout the body of the pancreas consistent with a pancreatic body laceration and contusion with peri-pancreatic fluid. He was admitted to the pediatric surgical service and was initially managed conservatively with bowel rest. His lipase and amylase were initially down-trending, and his abdominal pain improved while NPO. However, upon advance to a low-fat diet, he developed acute, sharp, epigastric abdominal pain, nausea, and non-bloody, non-bilious vomiting with recurrent elevation in the serum lipase (9085 U/L) and amylase (345 U/L). Right upper quadrant ultrasound revealed a more defined peripancreatic fluid collection. Bowel rest was resumed, total parenteral nutrition (TPN) was initiated, and he was referred for ERCP.

Case 2

A 14-year-old female with a past medical history of chronic pancreatitis, nonalcoholic fatty liver disease (NAFLD), obesity, elevated liver enzymes, vomiting, functional abdominal pain, and laparoscopic cholecystectomy presented to the emergency department with worsening abdominal pain for 2 days. She had been previously managed with ERCP with a nasopancreatic drain 4 years prior for acute pancreatitis. Her lipase was elevated (4210 U/L) at presentation. She was referred for evaluation for ERCP.

Introduction

Endoscopic retrograde cholangiopancreatography (ERCP) is an advanced endoscopic procedure that allows for diagnostic evaluation and management of pancreaticobiliary disorders. Relative to adults, there is less data on ERCP in pediatric populations. Table 19.1 includes all studies on pediatric ERCP between the years of 2004 and 2017. Notably, there has been an increase in the number of pediatric ERCPs performed and an overall rise in therapeutic procedures

TABLE 19.1 Indications for pediatric endoscopic retrograde cholangiopancreatography

Biliary
Choledocolithiasis
Biliary stricture, usually secondary to primary sclerosing cholangitis or following liver transplantation
Intra- or extrahepatic ductal dilation
Management of other etiologies of biliary obstruction
Biliary leaks following blunt abdominal trauma, cholecystectomy, or liver transplantation
Neonatal cholestasis
Preoperative evaluation of choledochal cyst and pancreaticobiliary maljunction
Evaluation of the biliary tract when less invasive diagnostic modalities are equivocal or suspected to have a false negative
Pancreatic
Gallstone pancreatitis
Chronic pancreatitis
Acute or recurrent pancreatitis of unclear etiology
Pancreatic pseudocyst drainage
Pancreatic leaks following blunt abdominal trauma
Pancreas divisum
Annular pancreas
Evaluation of the pancreas when less invasive diagnostic modalities are equivocal or suspected to have a false negative

(69% increase between 2000 and 2009) with a decline in diagnostic procedures (43% decrease) felt to be due to more widespread use of MRI and endoscopic ultrasonography [1]. There has also been an increased incidence in pancreatitis and biliary disease in pediatric populations [1]. While the need for ERCP in pediatric populations is increasingly recognized, there are no guidelines for ERCP in children, and the translation of adult practices to the pediatric population has been based largely on the clinical experience of providers. The overall technical and clinical success rates appear to parallel those seen in adults without an increase in the adverse event rate [2, 3]. This chapter aims at discussing the indications, success rates, procedural considerations, and complications associated with ERCP in pediatric populations.

Indications

ERCP is performed for pancreaticobiliary indications. In children, it is more commonly utilized in early adolescents, with a mean age range of 7–13.9 years old [2, 4–14], without a gender predominance [3]. In adults, the American Society of Gastrointestinal Endoscopy (ASGE) has clear guidelines regarding use of ERCP for diagnostic and therapeutic purposes. Although there is considerable overlap between children and adults, the distribution of indications is different in pediatrics, and while malignant indications are common in adults, they are rare in pediatric cohorts.

Table 19.2 lists indications for ERCP in children. Similar to adults, the most common indications are biliary obstruction and pancreatitis, reported at rates of 11.3–63.9% and 4–60.9%, respectively [4–6, 8, 10, 11, 14, 16, 17]. Children ages 0–6 have an equal distribution of biliary and pancreatic indications, those ages 7–12 have a predominance of pancreatic indications, and those 13 and older have a predominance of biliary indications [7]. This discussion will focus on indications unique to pediatric populations.

Traumatic Injuries

Pancreatic injury following blunt abdominal trauma is estimated at about 0.6%. In children, the most common mechanism is from motor vehicle accidents (55.8%). Other common

TABLE 19.2 Consensus classification of post-ERCP pancreatitis [15]

Requires the presence of all three of the following:

- Clinical pancreatitis
- Amylase >3 times the upper limit of normal more than 24 hours following ERCP
- Admission to the hospital following procedure or extension of hospital stay by 2–3 days in those with planned admission

Can be categorized further as mild, moderate, or severe based off duration of hospital stay, associated complications, or need for intervention

Mild	*Moderate*	*Severe*
Hospital stay lasting up to 3 days	Hospital stay lasting 4–10 days	Requires *one* of the following: • Hospital stay lasting more than 10 days • Development of hemorrhagic pancreatitis, phlegmon, pseudocyst, or infection • Need for percutaneous drainage of surgery

etiologies include bicycle accidents (19.7%), strikes to the abdomen (14.1%), and falls (8.8%) [18]. Injury to the pancreas occurs when the pancreas is compressed by anterior blunt force against the vertebral bodies posteriorly resulting in pancreatic contusion, laceration, or transection [19]. The patient presentation may include abdominal pain, fever, leukocytosis, and elevation in the serum amylase and lipase. The diagnosis may be evaluated with abdominal imaging. Ultrasound is often favored in children and may demonstrate abdominal free fluid; however it is often unable to image the pancreas due to overlying bowel gas. Contrast-enhanced CT may demonstrate the pancreatic injury and the presence of peripancreatic fluid collections and/or walled off necrosis. MRI with magnetic resonance cholangiopancreatography (MRCP) may be more involved, especially for young children due to the need for breath holding and length of time required to obtain imaging. For these reasons, sometimes general anesthesia is required to obtain MRI/MRCP in children. However, it is the best noninvasive modality for imaging the pancreatic and biliary ductal anatomy and can help discriminate between solid and liquid peripancreatic collections. ERCP is primarily indicated for therapeutic indications and is the most sensitive test for ductal anatomy and leaks.

Although rare, traumatic injuries are associated with high morbidity (26.5%) and mortality (5.3%) [18]. Pancreatic head injuries are more morbid than tail injuries due to associated damage to the inferior vena cava, portal vein, and superior mesenteric vein. Those with ductal injury have an increased risk of death within 48 hours, as leakage of pancreatic contents can lead to rapid decompensation and multiorgan failure. They also have a risk of major complications, including fistulas and abscess formation [19].

In the setting of ductal injury, the management has been traditionally operative. A recent review reported the use of ERCP for these injuries in 2.8% of patients [18]. Newer research for pancreatic duct disruption and pancreatic transection suggests a role for ERCP in the management of these conditions and may enable children with traumatic injuries to avoid major abdominal surgery and the postoperative complications of pancreatectomy.

Biliary tract injuries are rare but can occur in children following blunt abdominal trauma via motor vehicle accidents, bicycle accidents, or strikes to the abdomen. These can range from minor injuries to complete ductal transections and are estimated to occur at a rate of 0.09% [19, 20]. Patients may have a delayed presentation and can present with fever, abdominal pain, hyperbilirubinemia, or the presence of a biloma. A hepatobiliary iminodiacetic acid (HIDA) scan may confirm a biliary leak. ERCP is often the best approach to biliary leaks. Biliary sphincterotomy and stent placement can provide for physiologic flow of bile and allow for healing of the biliary injury. Bilomas may in some cases require percutaneous drainage. Stenting across duct transections and strictures has reduced the number of children requiring laparotomy and hepaticojejunostomy [20].

Multiple studies highlight the use of ERCP in managing blunt abdominal injuries. A retrospective review evaluated nine patients that underwent ERCP following blunt abdominal trauma. Seven had pancreatic injuries and two had hepatic duct injuries. Four patients were successfully treated with stents (44.4%), one was stented but required distal pancreatectomy for persistent leak, and four were managed with laparotomy following diagnostic evaluation [21]. An additional retrospective review of 22 pediatric trauma centers found that ERCP altered management or improved outcomes in 50% of patients with blunt pancreatic injury [22]. Another retrospective review evaluated 11 patients with traumatic bile leaks. All patients were diagnosed with a HIDA scan and were successfully treated with combinations of percutaneous drainage and ERCP with stenting and/or sphincterotomy [23]. A retrospective review evaluated patients with biliary tract injuries following blunt abdominal trauma. Five patients were identified, and 60% were successfully treated with ERCP and stenting. The remaining patients required laparotomy [20]. Lastly, a retrospective study demonstrated successful treatment of posttraumatic and postoperative biliary leaks with ERCP and stenting in 85.7% of patients [24].

Neonatal Cholestasis and Biliary Atresia

Neonatal cholestasis, defined as a direct hyperbilirubinemia >1 mg/dL, occurs in about 1 in 2,500 full-term infants [25, 26]. It can have intra- or extrahepatic causes and warrants further investigation. Biliary atresia is the most common extrahepatic disorder, occurring at a rate of 1 in 12,000 live births in the United States [26]. There is a female predominance and increased incidence among non-white infants [27]. Biliary atresia typically presents 2–6 weeks following birth with jaundice and acholic stools, consistent with an extrahepatic ductal obstruction disrupting the flow of bile [25]. Initial evaluation may involve ultrasound and hepatobiliary scintigraphy. MRCP, while sensitive (99%), has poor specificity (36%) and may not be able to confirm the diagnosis. The gold standard for the diagnosis is intraoperative cholangiogram and biopsy [26]. ERCP is emerging as a less invasive diagnostic tool with higher specificity (estimated at 73–94%) than MRCP [26, 28, 29] and may spare a laparotomy and biopsy in up to 12–20% of neonates [12, 29]. Multiple studies have demonstrated that ERCP can be safe in infants with a low risk of complication [12, 28, 30]. Management of biliary atresia may necessitate liver transplantation, although a Kasai portoenterostomy may be an alternative, particularly as a bridge to transplant [31].

Choledochal Cysts and Pancreaticobiliary Maljunction

Choledochal cysts are rare congenital cystic dilations of the biliary tract. They are more common in Asians and have a female predominance. They may present in 1 in 13,000 individuals in Japan and 1 in 100,000–150,000 individuals in Western countries. Choledochal cysts may be associated with an anomalous pancreaticobiliary junction (APBJ), a congenital malformation in which the pancreatic and bile ducts join outside the duodenal wall, in approximately 30–70% of cases [32]. It can also be associated with concurrent biliary atresia [32].

Approximately 80% of patients are diagnosed within the first decade of life. Patients usually present with abdominal pain, jaundice, or a right upper quadrant mass. They may experience complications such as pancreatitis and cholangitis. Patients may be initially identified due to common bile duct dilatation concerning for choledocholithiasis or other ductal obstruction. ERCP is the gold standard for diagnosis and is also indicated in type 3 choledochal cysts (choledochoceles) in which a biliary sphincterotomy may be therapeutic. MRCP is often performed in lieu of ERCP and has a high sensitivity (70–100%) and specificity (90–100%) for the diagnosis. However, MRI does not have a therapeutic role and can miss small choledochoceles and more subtle abnormalities [32]. ERCP may also provide for better preoperative planning, particularly in cases where cross-sectional imaging is equivocal for the diagnosis. A retrospective review found that preoperative ERCP was successful in 99% of 92 patients with choledochal cysts. ERCP clearly identified pancreaticobiliary maljunction (PBM) in 79% of patients and delineated the pancreatic duct in 94% of patients [30]. PBM is another condition that may benefit from preoperative evaluation with ERCP [33]. This condition, particularly the non-cystic sub-type, does not typically cause symptoms in patients. However, diagnosis and excision are important due to the risk of malignant transformation to cholangiocarcinoma or gallbladder cancer [34]. For many choledochal cysts, the management involves surgical excision, particularly in those with high risk for malignant transformation. Some patients may require liver transplantation, and choledochoceles may be managed with ERCP alone [32].

Pancreas Divisum

Pancreas divisum is the most common anatomical variant of the pancreas in the general population, occurring at a rate of 5–10% [35]. It is a congenital abnormality in which a short duct of Wirsung drains the minor, ventral portion of the pancreas through the major papilla and the duct of Santorini drains the major, dorsal portion of the pancreas through the minor papilla. It occurs when the dorsal and ventral pancreatic buds fail to fuse during the seventh week of embryonic development [36]. Most patients remain asymptomatic; however, approximately 5% can present with chronic or recurrent pancreaticobiliary-type pain, idiopathic recurrent acute pancreatitis, and/or chronic pancreatitis due to inability to drain pancreatic secretions [36]. The diagnosis may be confirmed by MRCP; however, MRI has a sensitivity of 60–73.3% compared to ERCP [37–39]. When indicated, ERCP is the gold standard for establishing the diagnosis of a ductal abnormality. Endoscopic ultrasound may also be used with a reported sensitivity of 50–86.7% [37, 40].

Management is either endoscopic or surgical with a goal of improving pancreatic drainage through the minor papilla. The most common endoscopic therapy involves a papillotomy at the minor papilla with pancreatic duct stent placement. Other therapies include balloon dilation of the minor papilla, stone extraction, and botulinum toxin injection at the minor papilla [36]. Endoscopic therapy has a reported clinical success rate of 62.3–69.4%. It is associated with a higher risk of re-intervention; however it is much less invasive than surgical interventions which may involve a sphincteroplasty, pancreatic head resection, or Whipple procedure [35, 41]. More recently, the role of divisum in pancreatitis has been called into question, and large prospective studies in adults are being developed to define the role for interventions directed at minor papilla therapy. Overall, the clinical decision making should weigh the risks, benefits, and patient characteristics.

Complications Post Liver Transplant

Following liver transplantation, patients may develop biliary complications at a rate of 12–50%, most common of which are biliary strictures and biliary leaks occurring at the anastomotic site. These are more common in those who have a duct to duct anastomosis [42, 43]. Patients can present with abdominal pain or abnormal liver enzymes, and the work-up may involve evaluation and treatment with ERCP. ERCP has proven to be safe in the management of biliary complications following transplant in children [44, 45]. Biliary strictures can be treated via ERCP with sphincterotomy, balloon dilation, and stenting. A retrospective review evaluated children with liver transplant undergoing ERCP for abdominal pain, elevated liver enzymes, and known biliary strictures. Seventy-seven percent of these patients underwent therapeutic interventions. The overall complication rate was 2.9%, similar to that in adults and in children who have not had liver transplantation [44].

Procedural Considerations

The ASGE addresses specific procedural considerations when performing endoscopy in children [46]. General anesthesia is typically employed when performing ERCP in children; however, some studies suggest that monitored anesthesia care with propofol was equivalent to general anesthesia in regard to safety and technical success [5]. Children may be at greater risk of hypoventilation in the prone or supine position and airway obstruction due to higher airway compliance. Airway hyperreactivity can be exacerbated by recent upper respiratory infection. General anesthesia is generally favored, and at present we use general anesthesia for all patients undergoing ERCP. Contraindications to ERCP are relative and similar to those seen in adults and include neutropenia, coagulopathy, and unstable cardiopulmonary disease [46].

In regard to equipment, most pediatric procedures can be performed using an adult duodenoscope. The pediatric duodenoscope is limiting due to a diminutive 2 mm working channel [46], which severely limits the passage of devices and/or stents through the working channel as well as the ability to suction. The adult duodenoscope is recommended in any child over 2 years of age [5, 8, 46]. For children between 1 and 2 years of age, it may still be reasonable to use the adult duodenoscope if the child is larger and weighs more than 10 kg. In children less than 1 year of age, a pediatric duodenoscope may be required [46].

Pediatric ERCP has been compared to ASGE grade-matched adult controls on procedural parameters and clinical outcomes. In this study, all procedures were done for therapeutic indications with adult duodenoscopes by adult gastroenterologists. No difference was found between the two groups in regard to technical success, clinical success, or complication rates. There was also no difference in procedural duration, length of hospital stay, or the number of procedures performed on each patient. There was an increased use of general anesthesia in pediatric patients, and post-procedural admission rates were higher. Overall outcomes were equivalent between the two groups [6].

There is debate on whether adult or pediatric gastroenterologists should be performing ERCP in children. To date, most procedures are performed by high-volume adult-trained endoscopists. Previously, ERCP was exclusively performed by adult-trained endoscopists due to the technical skill and procedural proficiency needed to ensure adequate success rates and reduce the risk of adverse events [47, 48]. A pragmatic consideration is that there are no clear pathways for therapeutic pediatric advanced endoscopy fellowship training. In rare cases, pediatric gastroenterologists may pursue advanced endoscopic training in adult-based fellowships. In terms of competency, the ASGE recommends at least 200 ERCPs at a minimum [49]; however, a 2015 meta-analysis suggested that this may not be sufficient [50]. A meta-analysis evaluating rates of adverse events in pediatric ERCPs attempted to assess for differences related to the type of endoscopist performing the procedure; however, the data that currently exists is too heterogeneous to draw meaningful conclusions [3]. A 2010 retrospective review found that high-volume centers have lower rates of post-ERCP pancreatitis, despite performing ERCP on higher-risk patients, compared to low-volume centers [48]. Another retrospective review suggests an ongoing case volume of at least 50 cases a year is associated with higher success rates and lower complication rates [51].

Outcomes and Complications

The overall complication rate in children undergoing ERCP is reported at 6% [3]. This parallels that seen in the adult population [46, 52]. The most common complication is post-ERCP pancreatitis, estimated to occur at a rate of 2.8–9.2%, in line with reported rates in adults at 3–10% [52]. Other complications include bleeding, estimated at a rate of 0.8%, and infection, estimated at 0.6% [3].

Post-ERCP Pancreatitis

A consensus definition of post-ERCP pancreatitis (PEP) has been frequently used since 1991 (Table 19.3) [15]. This definition is used to report rates of PEP in most studies. There are concerns that this definition overestimates the rates of PEP because many patients have abdominal pain prior to the procedure and many patients have expected hyperamylasemia following instrumentation of the pancreatic duct [52]. There are limited data on procedural and patient characteristics associated with an increased risk of PEP in children including pancreatic duct injection, pancreatic sphincterotomy, pancreatic duct stricture dilation, and prophylactic pancreatic stenting [16, 53, 56]. In adults, prophylactic pancreatic duct stenting has been repeatedly shown to reduce the risk of PEP [52]. However, a retrospective multivariate analysis evaluating 432 pediatric ERCPs showed that pancreatic sphincterotomy and pancreatic duct injection were associated with an increased risk of PEP in children. There was no identifiable association between PEP risk and age, female gender, or prior episodes of PEP as has been found in adult cohorts. Chronic pancreatitis was found to be a protective factor [56].

Given that PEP is the most common adverse event following ERCP, many studies have been performed to evaluate prophylactic interventions to reduce the risk of PEP. In a large blinded sham-controlled trial, rectal indomethacin has been shown to be protective against PEP in adults – reducing the overall incidence and severity of PEP [52]. A single dose of 100 mg rectal indomethacin is used at the time of the procedure. There have been limited data on the use of rectal indomethacin in the pediatric population. One trial examined the rates of PEP in children who received a dose of rectal indomethacin compared to those that did not. In this study, the rate of PEP was not different between the groups. There was no increase in bleeding or renal injury in the group receiving indomethacin. The study was not powered to examine an impact on the PEP rate; however, the authors recommend the use of indomethacin for prophylaxis in pediatric

TABLE 19.3 Studies on pediatric ERCP (2004–2017)

Year[a]	Focus of study	Number of procedures	Age[b]	Technical success rate[c] (%)	Complication rate[d] (%)
2004 [2]	Compared technical success and complication rates between ERCP in pediatric and matched adult cohorts	163	9.3 years	97.5	3.4
2005 [14]	Diagnostic and therapeutic yields of ERCP in children	48	10 years	97	6
2005 [13]	Indications, findings, therapies, safety, and success rates	329	12.3 years	97.9	9.7
2009 [12]	Indications, findings, therapies, safety, and success rates	99	7 years	71	4
2009 [29]	Diagnostic accuracy of ERCP in neonates with cholestasis compared to intraoperative cholangiogram	140	60 days	93	3.6
2009 [53]	Post-ERCP pancreatitis (excluded patients with chronic pancreatitis)	276	11 years		2.5
2010 [11]	Indications, findings, therapies, safety, and success rates	245	8 years	98.4	18.4
2010 [28]	Diagnostic efficacy of ERCP in evaluating neonates with cholestasis	104	7 weeks	91.3	1.0
2011 [10]	Indications, therapies, safety, and success rates	231	11.4 years		4.76
2012 [54]	Evaluation of neonatal cholestasis	27	55 days		0

Table 19.3 (continued)

Year[a]	Focus of study	Number of procedures	Age[b]	Technical success rate[c] (%)	Complication rate[d] (%)
2013 [7]	Compared indications, findings, therapies, and safety of ERCP between age groups in the pediatric population	289	11.5 years	90.7	5.9
2013 [17]	Indications, safety, success rates	429	14.9 years	95.2	7.7
2013 [55]	Safety and success rates of pediatric ERCP by pediatric gastroenterologists for choledocholithiasis	154	15.2 years	98	5
2013 [9]	Efficacy and safety of pediatric ERCP performed by adult gastroenterologists	70	12 years	97.1	7.1
2014 [23]	Traumatic bile leaks	11	11 years	100	18
2014 [1]	Pediatric ERCP trends in the United States	22,153	18 years (median)		
2014 [30]	ERCP in small children with pancreaticobiliary disorders, including choledochal cyst and biliary atresia	235	2 years	96	9.4
2015 [21]	Role in blunt abdominal trauma	9	7.8 years		55.6
2015 [56]	Factors associated with post-ERCP pancreatitis	432	12.7 years (median)		10.9
2015 [57]	Pancreaticobiliary maljunction	63			
2015 [45]	Post-transplant biliary complications	17	12 years	94	29.4
2015 [4]	Indications, therapies, and safety	75	13.9 years (median)	94.7	9.7

(continued)

Table 19.3 (continued)

Year[a]	Focus of study	Number of procedures	Age[b]	Technical success rate[c] (%)	Complication rate[d] (%)
2015 [16]	Indications, type of sedation, therapies, and safety	425	13.6 years	95	16.6
2016 [8]	Outcomes of pediatric ERCP by adult gastroenterologists using adult duodenoscopes	65	13 years	93.8	12.3
2016 [5]	Clinical outcomes of therapeutic ERCP	144	13.3 years	93.1	4.9
2016 [6]	Compared outcomes of ERCP in children compared to ASGE grade-matched adult controls	107	12.8 years	91	4.7
2016 [58]	Blunt pancreatic trauma	25	8.5 years		
2016 [3]	Systematic review of complication rates	3566			6
2017 [59]	Biliary complications following liver transplantation	25	10.7 years (at time of transplant)		
2017 [60]	Outcomes of sphincterotomy	198	8.7 years	98.9	14.1 (early); 6.1 (long-term)
2017 [61]	Efficacy and safety of rectal indomethacin for post-ERCP pancreatitis	119	13 years	95.8	4.2
2017 [62]	Demographics, indications, therapies, safety, and success rates	215	14 years	97	10

TABLE 19.3 (continued)

Year[a]	Focus of study	Number of procedures	Age[b]	Technical success rate[c] (%)	Complication rate[d] (%)
2017 [63]	Therapeutic ERCP for recurrent acute pancreatitis or chronic pancreatitis	117	11.9 years		
2017 [24]	Bile duct injuries	46	10 years	85.7	4.3
2017 [64]	MRCP vs. ERCP in evaluating chronic pancreatitis	48	12.1 years	85.4	
2017 [22]	Pediatric pancreatic trauma	28	11 years	86	16
2017 [65]	Indications, safety, and success rates	54	7.6 years	90.7	9.3

[a]Studies listed in chronological order
[b]Listed as mean age unless otherwise stated
[c]Technical success rate was typically defined as successful cannulation of the bile duct; however definitions were either omitted or varied between studies
[d]Complications were defined differently between studies, particularly that there was no consistency on whether hyperamylasemia alone was considered a complication

patients undergoing ERCP [61]. There have been many studies in adults investigating the utility of prophylactic pancreatic stenting [66], intravenous hydration [67], and cannulation techniques [68, 69] in preventing PEP. However, there are no prospective studies evaluating the efficacy of these interventions in children.

Outcome of Cases

Case 1

Due to the persistent inability to tolerate oral intake, an MRCP was performed which confirmed the formation of a peripancreatic fluid collection at the site of the laceration, measuring 2.9 × 2.6 × 3.4 cm, which was in communication with the pancreatic duct (PD). He was then transported to a quaternary children's hospital for ERCP. Pancreatogram revealed a PD stricture in the region of the neck and a PD leak with extravasation of contrast (Fig. 19.1b). A sphincterotomy was performed, and stent was placed bridging the stricture and the region of the ductal disruption. He returned to the floor with near complete resolution of his symptoms. A regular diet was advanced the following day, and he was discharged home in stable health that evening.

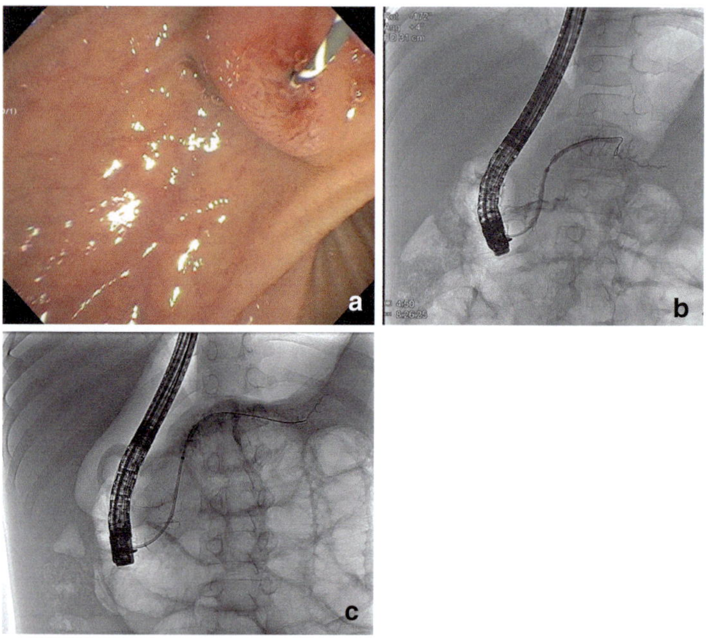

FIGURE 19.1 (**a**) Endoscopic image of the duodenoscope in the second portion of the duodenum. A wire has been inserted into the pancreatic duct to traverse the ductal disruption. (**b**) Fluoroscopic image showing the duodenoscope in the second portion of the duodenum. A wire has been advanced across the ductal disruption to the tail of the pancreas. In the central portion and overlying the spine, there is contrast extravasation confirming a transection and pancreatic duct leak. (**c**) The final fluoroscopic image on follow-up ERCP. The stent has been removed and a wire has been passed to the tail of the pancreas. The pancreatic duct leak and injury have resolved

Following discharge, he continued to thrive. He returned for repeat outpatient ERCP approximately 1 month later which showed minimal dilatation of the main PD (3 mm), improved PD stricture in the body region, and improved leak in the body/tail region. The stent was upsized again bridging the leak, and he was discharged home. A repeat right upper quadrant abdominal ultrasound was repeated 3 weeks later which showed complete resolution. His final ERCP was performed the next day, confirming resolution of the stricture and leak, and no new stents were placed at that time (Fig. 19.1c).

Case 2

Prior to proceeding with ERCP, an MRCP was performed which revealed an accessory pancreatic duct with a peripancreatic fluid collection near the head (Fig. 19.2a). There were edema and inflammatory changes surrounding the pancreas compatible with pancreatitis. The common bile duct (CBD) was dilated to 10 mm with no obstructing stones. Based on these findings, she was admitted to the pediatric gastroenterology service and underwent ERCP. The ERCP was remarkable for pancreatic duct (PD) dilation to 5 mm, with a prominent duct of Santorini and a santorinicele at the insertion. There was a frank pancreatic duct leak with free contrast extravasation at the insertion of the duct of Santorini in the region of the santorinicele (Fig. 19.2b). There was biliary ductal dilatation to 12 mm with no contrast extravasation on the cholangiography. A pancreatic duct stent was placed into the ventral PD via the major papilla, and a biliary stent was placed into the CBD; however, she remained symptomatic. The minor papilla was not patent. ERCP was repeated, and a thin stent was placed via the major papilla in an antegrade manner back into the duct of Santorini and to the region of the leak in the santorinicele, and a new stent was placed via the major papilla to the tail (Fig. 19.2c, d). She returned to the floor, and her symptoms improved almost immediately. She was discharged home in stable health. She has returned to school and remains asymptomatic tolerating a regular diet. Repeat ERCP with stent exchange has demonstrated a slowly resolving leak.

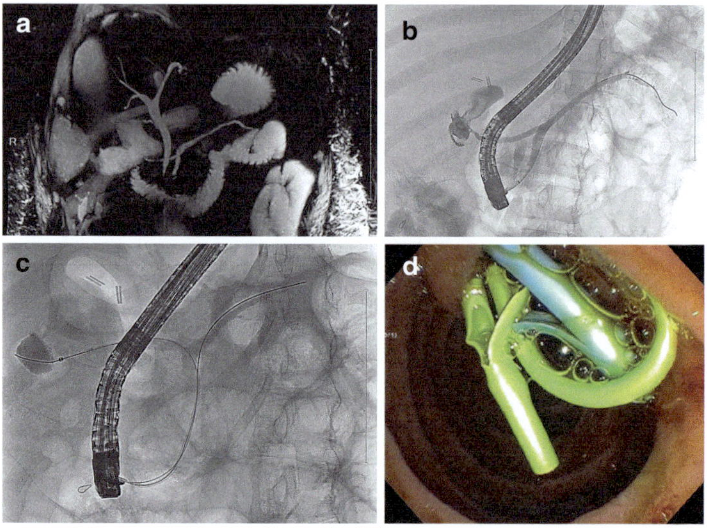

FIGURE 19.2 (**a**) MRCP revealing the pancreatic and biliary ductal anatomy. The duct of Wirsung terminates at the major papilla with the bile duct. There is a prominent duct of Santorini. There is a fluid collection and pancreatic duct leak at the insertion of the duct of Santorini on the duodenum. (**b**) Fluoroscopic image showing the duodenoscope in position. A wire and catheter have been passed to the tail of the pancreas. There is a prominent duct of Santorini and a frank pancreatic duct leak with free contrast extravasation at the insertion of the duct of Santorini on the duodenum. (**c**) Fluoroscopic image showing the duodenoscope in position. Two wires have been passed. One wire inserts at the major papilla and passed back in a partially antegrade manner into the duct of Santorini, while the second passes in a completely retrograde manner in the ventral duct to the tail of the pancreas. Stents were placed over both wires, resulting in resolution of symptoms, tolerance of an oral diet, and discharge home. (**d**) Final endoscopic image showing both pancreatic duct stents and a biliary stent in position

Conclusions

The numbers of ERCPs performed in children have been increasing, and the procedure has shown to be safe and efficacious for a growing number of indications in pediatric populations. ERCP may be critically indicated in children and may result in dramatic benefit with certain clinical presentations. There is a major role for pancreatic injuries, some pancreatitis presentations, biliary strictures, and obstructions such as stones. As the procedure becomes more widely adopted, larger prospective studies may further refine the roles the procedure plays in younger cohorts of patients.

Pearls and Pitfalls

- ERCP can be performed safely in children, with similar success and complication rates as in adult populations.
- Indications such as traumatic pancreaticobiliary leaks and congenital abnormalities may be more frequent in pediatric cohorts.
- An adult duodenoscope is typically used in children over the age of 2 years.
- The most common complication is post-ERCP pancreatitis, for which rectal indomethacin can be used safely for prophylaxis.

Grant Support

This manuscript was supported in part by a development grant from the Department of Medicine at Emory University School of Medicine.

Disclosures

The authors report no conflicts of interest with the work contained in this manuscript.

References

1. Pant C, Sferra TJ, Barth BA, Deshpande A, Minocha A, Qureshi WA, et al. Trends in endoscopic retrograde cholangiopancreatography in children within the United States, 2000–2009. J Pediatr Gastroenterol Nutr. 2014;59(1):57–60.

2. Varadarajulu S, Wilcox CM, Hawes RH, Cotton PB. Technical outcomes and complications of ERCP in children. Gastrointest Endosc. 2004;60(3):367–71.
3. Usatin D, Fernandes M, Allen IE, Perito ER, Ostroff J, Heyman MB. Complications of endoscopic retrograde cholangiopancreatography in pediatric patients; a systematic literature review and meta-analysis. J Pediatr. 2016;179:160–5 e3.
4. Kieling CO, Hallal C, Spessato CO, Ribeiro LM, Breyer H, Goldani HA, et al. Changing pattern of indications of endoscopic retrograde cholangiopancreatography in children and adolescents: a twelve-year experience. World J Pediatr. 2015;11(2):154–9.
5. Mekaroonkamol P, Nieto J, Chawla S, Freeman AJ, Alnoah Z, Keilin S, et al. Sa2065 A multicenter evaluation of therapeutic endoscopic retrograde cholangiopancreatography in pediatric populations. Gastrointest Endos. 2016;83(5):AB303–AB4.
6. Mekaroonkamol P, Nieto J, Chawla S, Freeman AJ, Alnoah Z, Keilin S, et al. Sa2067 Safety and efficacy of endoscopic retrograde cholangiopancreatography in pediatric patients: A 7-year experience. Gastrointest Endos. 2016;83(5):AB304–AB5.
7. Limketkai BN, Chandrasekhara V, Kalloo AN, Okolo PI. Comparison of performance and safety of endoscopic retrograde cholangiopancreatography across pediatric age groups. Dig Dis Sci. 2013;58(9):2653–60.
8. Yildirim AE, Altun R, Ocal S, Kormaz M, Ozcay F, Selcuk H. The safety and efficacy of ERCP in the pediatric population with standard scopes: does size really matter? Springerplus. 2016;5:128.
9. Halvorson L, Halsey K, Darwin P, Goldberg E. The safety and efficacy of therapeutic ERCP in the pediatric population performed by adult gastroenterologists. Dig Dis Sci. 2013;58(12):3611–9.
10. Otto AK, Neal MD, Slivka AN, Kane TD. An appraisal of endoscopic retrograde cholangiopancreatography (ERCP) for pancreaticobiliary disease in children: our institutional experience in 231 cases. Surg Endosc. 2011;25(8):2536–40.
11. Jang JY, Yoon CH, Kim KM. Endoscopic retrograde cholangiopancreatography in pancreatic and biliary tract disease in Korean children. World J Gastroenterol. 2010;16(4):490–5.
12. Vegting IL, Tabbers MM, Taminiau JA, Aronson DC, Benninga MA, Rauws EA. Is endoscopic retrograde cholangiopancreatography valuable and safe in children of all ages? J Pediatr Gastroenterol Nutr. 2009;48(1):66–71.
13. Cheng CL, Fogel EL, Sherman S, McHenry L, Watkins JL, Croffie JM, et al. Diagnostic and therapeutic endoscopic retrograde

cholangiopancreatography in children: a large series report. J Pediatr Gastroenterol Nutr. 2005;41(4):445–53.
14. Rocca R, Castellino F, Daperno M, Masoero G, Sostegni R, Ercole E, et al. Therapeutic ERCP in paediatric patients. Dig Liver Dis. 2005;37(5):357–62.
15. Cotton PB, Lehman G, Vennes J, Geenen JE, Russell RC, Meyers WC, et al. Endoscopic sphincterotomy complications and their management: an attempt at consensus. Gastrointest Endosc. 1991;37(3):383–93.
16. Giefer MJ, Kozarek RA. Technical outcomes and complications of pediatric ERCP. Surg Endosc. 2015;29(12):3543–50.
17. Enestvedt BK, Tofani C, Lee DY, Abraham M, Shah P, Chandrasekhara V, et al. Endoscopic retrograde cholangiopancreatography in the pediatric population is safe and efficacious. J Pediatr Gastroenterol Nutr. 2013;57(5):649–54.
18. Englum BR, Gulack BC, Rice HE, Scarborough JE, Adibe OO. Management of blunt pancreatic trauma in children: review of the National Trauma Data Bank. J Pediatr Surg. 2016;51(9):1526–31.
19. Gupta A, Stuhlfaut JW, Fleming KW, Lucey BC, Soto JA. Blunt trauma of the pancreas and biliary tract: a multimodality imaging approach to diagnosis. Radiographics. 2004;24(5):1381–95.
20. Soukup ES, Russell KW, Metzger R, Scaife ER, Barnhart DC, Rollins MD. Treatment and outcome of traumatic biliary injuries in children. J Pediatr Surg. 2014;49(2):345–8.
21. Garvey EM, Haakinson DJ, McOmber M, Notrica DM. Role of ERCP in pediatric blunt abdominal trauma: a case series at a level one pediatric trauma center. J Pediatr Surg. 2015;50(2):335–8.
22. Rosenfeld EH, Vogel AM, Klinkner DB, Escobar M, Gaines B, Russell R, et al. The utility of ERCP in pediatric pancreatic trauma. J Pediatr Surg. 2017;S0022-3468(17):30660–7.
23. Kulaylat AN, Stokes AL, Engbrecht BW, McIntyre JS, Rzucidlo SE, Cilley RE. Traumatic bile leaks from blunt liver injury in children: a multidisciplinary and minimally invasive approach to management. J Pediatr Surg. 2014;49(3):424–7.
24. Keil R, Drabek J, Lochmannova J, Stovicek J, Rygl M, Snajdauf J, et al. Endoscopic treatment of bile duct post-traumatic and post-operative lesions in children. Scand J Gastroenterol. 2017;52(8):870–5.
25. Fischler B, Lamireau T. Cholestasis in the newborn and infant. Clin Res Hepatol Gastroenterol. 2014;38(3):263–7.

26. Fawaz R, Baumann U, Ekong U, Fischler B, Hadzic N, Mack CL, et al. Guideline for the evaluation of cholestatic jaundice in infants: joint recommendations of the North American society for pediatric gastroenterology, hepatology, and nutrition and the European society for pediatric gastroenterology, Hepatology, and Nutrition. J Pediatr Gastroenterol Nutr. 2017;64(1):154–68.
27. Asai A, Miethke A, Bezerra JA. Pathogenesis of biliary atresia: defining biology to understand clinical phenotypes. Nat Rev Gastroenterol Hepatol. 2015;12(6):342–52.
28. Keil R, Snajdauf J, Rygl M, Pycha K, Kotalova R, Drabek J, et al. Diagnostic efficacy of ERCP in cholestatic infants and neonates–a retrospective study on a large series. Endoscopy. 2010;42(2):121–6.
29. Petersen C, Meier PN, Schneider A, Turowski C, Pfister ED, Manns MP, et al. Endoscopic retrograde cholangiopancreatography prior to explorative laparotomy avoids unnecessary surgery in patients suspected for biliary atresia. J Hepatol. 2009;51(6):1055–60.
30. Saito T, Terui K, Mitsunaga T, Nakata M, Kuriyama Y, Higashimoto Y, et al. Role of pediatric endoscopic retrograde cholangiopancreatography in an era stressing less-invasive imaging modalities. J Pediatr Gastroenterol Nutr. 2014;59(2):204–9.
31. Gallo A, Esquivel CO. Current options for management of biliary atresia. Pediatr Transplant. 2013;17(2):95–8.
32. Soares KC, Arnaoutakis DJ, Kamel I, Rastegar N, Anders R, Maithel S, et al. Choledochal cysts: presentation, clinical differentiation, and management. J Am Coll Surg. 2014;219(6):1167–80.
33. Kamisawa T, Ando H, Hamada Y, Fujii H, Koshinaga T, Urushihara N, et al. Diagnostic criteria for pancreaticobiliary maljunction 2013. J Hepatobiliary Pancreat Sci. 2014;21(3):159–61.
34. Kamisawa T, Kuruma S, Tabata T, Chiba K, Iwasaki S, Koizumi S, et al. Pancreaticobiliary maljunction and biliary cancer. J Gastroenterol. 2015;50(3):273–9.
35. Hafezi M, Mayschak B, Probst P, Buchler MW, Hackert T, Mehrabi A. A systematic review and quantitative analysis of different therapies for pancreas divisum. Am J Surg. 2017;214(3):525–37.
36. Rustagi T, Golioto M. Diagnosis and therapy of pancreas divisum by ERCP: a single center experience. J Dig Dis. 2013;14(2):93–9.
37. Kushnir VM, Wani SB, Fowler K, Menias C, Varma R, Narra V, et al. Sensitivity of endoscopic ultrasound, multidetector com-

puted tomography, and magnetic resonance cholangiopancreatography in the diagnosis of pancreas divisum: a tertiary center experience. Pancreas. 2013;42(3):436–41.

38. Mosler P, Akisik F, Sandrasegaran K, Fogel E, Watkins J, Alazmi W, et al. Accuracy of magnetic resonance cholangiopancreatography in the diagnosis of pancreas divisum. Dig Dis Sci. 2012;57(1):170–4.
39. Carnes ML, Romagnuolo J, Cotton PB. Miss rate of pancreas divisum by magnetic resonance cholangiopancreatography in clinical practice. Pancreas. 2008;37(2):151–3.
40. Rana SS, Bhasin DK, Sharma V, Rao C, Singh K. Role of endoscopic ultrasound in the diagnosis of pancreas divisum. Endoscopic ultrasound. 2013;2(1):7–10.
41. Liao Z, Gao R, Wang W, Ye Z, Lai XW, Wang XT, et al. A systematic review on endoscopic detection rate, endotherapy, and surgery for pancreas divisum. Endoscopy. 2009;41(5):439–44.
42. Laurence JM, Sapisochin G, DeAngelis M, Seal JB, Miserachs MM, Marquez M, et al. Biliary complications in pediatric liver transplantation: incidence and management over a decade. Liver Transpl. 2015;21(8):1082–90.
43. Karakayali F, Kirnap M, Akdur A, Tutar N, Boyvat F, Moray G, et al. Biliary complications after pediatric liver transplantation. Transplant Proc. 2013;45(10):3524–7.
44. Otto AK, Neal MD, Mazariegos GV, Slivka A, Kane TD. Endoscopic retrograde cholangiopancreatography is safe and effective for the diagnosis and treatment of pancreaticobiliary disease following abdominal organ transplant in children. Pediatr Transplant. 2012;16(8):829–34.
45. Dechene A, Kodde C, Kathemann S, Treckmann J, Lainka E, Paul A, et al. Endoscopic treatment of pediatric post-transplant biliary complications is safe and effective. Dig Endosc. 2015;27(4):505–11.
46. Lightdale JR, Acosta R, Shergill AK, Chandrasekhara V, Chathadi K, Early D, et al. Modifications in endoscopic practice for pediatric patients. Gastrointest Endosc. 2014;79(5):699–710.
47. Troendle DM, Barth BA. Pediatric Considerations in Endoscopic Retrograde Cholangiopancreatography. Gastrointest Endosc Clin N Am. 2016;26(1):119–36.
48. Testoni PA, Mariani A, Giussani A, Vailati C, Masci E, Macarri G, et al. Risk factors for post-ERCP pancreatitis in high- and low-volume centers and among expert and non-expert

operators: a prospective multicenter study. Am J Gastroenterol. 2010;105(8):1753–61.
49. Committee ASoP, Faulx AL, Lightdale JR, Acosta RD, Agrawal D, Bruining DH, et al. Guidelines for privileging, credentialing, and proctoring to perform GI endoscopy. Gastrointest Endosc. 2017;85(2):273–81.
50. Shahidi N, Ou G, Telford J, Enns R. When trainees reach competency in performing ERCP: a systematic review. Gastrointest Endosc. 2015;81(6):1337–42.
51. Kapral C, Duller C, Wewalka F, Kerstan E, Vogel W, Schreiber F. Case volume and outcome of endoscopic retrograde cholangiopancreatography: results of a nationwide Austrian benchmarking project. Endoscopy. 2008;40(8):625–30.
52. Committee ASoP, Chandrasekhara V, Khashab MA, Muthusamy VR, Acosta RD, Agrawal D, et al. Adverse events associated with ERCP. Gastrointest Endosc. 2017;85(1):32–47.
53. Iqbal CW, Baron TH, Moir CR, Ishitani MB. Post-ERCP pancreatitis in pediatric patients. J Pediatr Gastroenterol Nutr. 2009;49(4):430–4.
54. Shteyer E, Wengrower D, Benuri-Silbiger I, Gozal D, Wilschanski M, Goldin E. Endoscopic retrograde cholangiopancreatography in neonatal cholestasis. J Pediatr Gastroenterol Nutr. 2012;55(2):142–5.
55. Troendle DM, Barth BA. ERCP can be safely and effectively performed by a pediatric gastroenterologist for choledocholithiasis in a pediatric facility. J Pediatr Gastroenterol Nutr. 2013;57(5):655–8.
56. Troendle DM, Abraham O, Huang R, Barth BA. Factors associated with post-ERCP pancreatitis and the effect of pancreatic duct stenting in a pediatric population. Gastrointest Endosc. 2015;81(6):1408–16.
57. Hiramatsu T, Itoh A, Kawashima H, Ohno E, Itoh Y, Sugimoto H, et al. Usefulness and safety of endoscopic retrograde cholangiopancreatography in children with pancreaticobiliary maljunction. J Pediatr Surg. 2015;50(3):377–81.
58. Keil R, Drabek J, Lochmannova J, Stovicek J, Rygl M, Snajdauf J, et al. What is the role of endoscopic retrograde cholangiopancreatography in assessing traumatic rupture of the pancreatic in children? Scand J Gastroenterol. 2016;51(2):218–24.

59. Karthik SV, Quak SH, Aw MM. Endoscopic retrograde cholangio-pancreatography in the management of biliary complications after paediatric liver transplantation – a retrospective study. Transpl Int. 2018;31(3):313–7.
60. Cho JM, Jeong IS, Kim HJ, Oh SH, Kim KM. Early adverse events and long-term outcomes of endoscopic sphincterotomy in a pediatric population: a single-center experience. Endoscopy. 2017;49(5):438–46.
61. Mekaroonkamol P, Shah R, Nieto J, Chawla S, Freeman AJ, Sauer CG, et al. Sa2079 Efficacy and safety of rectal indomethacin for prevention of post endoscopic retrograde cholangiopancreatography pancreatitis in a pediatric population. Gastrointest Endosc. 2017;85(5):AB287–AB8.
62. Rosen JD, Lane RS, Martinez JM, Perez EA, Tashiro J, Wagenaar AE, et al. Success and safety of endoscopic retrograde cholangiopancreatography in children. J Pediatr Surg. 2017;52(7):1148–51.
63. Troendle DM, Fishman DS, Barth BA, Giefer MJ, Lin TK, Liu QY, et al. Therapeutic endoscopic retrograde cholangiopancreatography in pediatric patients with acute recurrent and chronic pancreatitis: data from the INSPPIRE (International study group of pediatric pancreatitis: in search for a cure) study. Pancreas. 2017;46(6):764–9.
64. Kolodziejczyk E, Jurkiewicz E, Pertkiewicz J, Wejnarska K, Dadalski M, Kierkus J, et al. MRCP versus ERCP in the evaluation of chronic pancreatitis in children: which is the better choice? Pancreas. 2016;45(8):1115–9.
65. Felux J, Sturm E, Busch A, Zerabruck E, Graepler F, Stüker D, et al. ERCP in infants, children and adolescents is feasible and safe: results from a tertiary care center. United European Gastroenterol J. 2017;5(7):1024–9.
66. Vadala di Prampero SF, Faleschini G, Panic N, Bulajic M. Endoscopic and pharmacological treatment for prophylaxis against postendoscopic retrograde cholangiopancreatography pancreatitis: a meta-analysis and systematic review. Eur J Gastroenterol Hepatol. 2016;28(12):1415–24.
67. Zhang ZF, Duan ZJ, Wang LX, Zhao G, Deng WG. Aggressive hydration with lactated ringer solution in prevention of postendoscopic retrograde cholangiopancreatography pancreatitis:

a meta-analysis of randomized controlled trials. J Clin Gastroenterol. 2017;51(3):e17–26.
68. Tse F, Yuan Y, Bukhari M, Leontiadis GI, Moayyedi P, Barkun A. Pancreatic duct guidewire placement for biliary cannulation for the prevention of post-endoscopic retrograde cholangiopancreatography (ERCP) pancreatitis. Cochrane Database Syst Rev. 2016;(5):Cd010571.
69. Tse F, Yuan Y, Moayyedi P, Leontiadis GI, Barkun AN. Double-guidewire technique in difficult biliary cannulation for the prevention of post-ERCP pancreatitis: a systematic review and meta-analysis. Endoscopy. 2017;49(1):15–26.

Index

D. K. Mullady (ed.), *Dilemmas in ERCP*,
https://doi.org/10.1007/978-3-030-12741-1

C

N

O

P